GOING LONG

TRAINING FOR TRIATHLON'S ULTIMATE CHALLENGE

2ND EDITION

Joe Friel

Gordon Byrn

VELO press

BOULDER, COLORADO

VeloPress®, a division of Competitor Group, Inc.
1830 55th Street
Boulder, Colorado 80301-2700 USA
303/440-0601; Fax: 303/444-6788; E-mail: velopress@competitorgroup.com

To purchase additional copies of this book or other VeloPress books, call 800/234-8356 or visit us on the Web at velopress.com.

Distributed in the United States and Canada by Publishers Group West

Cover photo by Delly Carr
Cover design by Andrew Brozyna
Interior design and composition by Erin Johnson Design
Illustrations by Todd Telander

Library of Congress Cataloging-in-Publication Data

Friel, Joe.
  Going long : training for triathlon's ultimate challenge / Joe Friel and Gordon Byrn. — 2nd ed.
    p. cm.
  Includes index.
  ISBN 978-1-934030-06-6 (pbk. : alk. paper)
  1. Ironman triathlons. 2. Triathlon—Training. I. Byrn, Gordon. II. Title.
  GV1060.73.F735 2008
  796.42'57—dc22
                    2008041521

Printed in the United States of America

09 10 11 / 10 9 8 7 6 5 4 3 2

CONTENTS

Foreword by Scott Molina v
Foreword by Ryan Bolton vii
Prefaces ix
Acknowledgments xi

■ PART I: Getting Started
Chapter 1   The Iron Journey 3
Chapter 2   Approaches to Training 13
Chapter 3   Understanding Fitness 23
Chapter 4   Equipment 33

■ PART II: Ironman Training
Chapter 5   Training Overview 57
Chapter 6   Training for the Swim 95
Chapter 7   Training for the Bike 123
Chapter 8   Training for the Run 161

■ PART III: Beyond the Basics
Chapter 9   Strength Training 187
Chapter 10   Nutrition: The Fourth Discipline 211
Chapter 11   Training the Mind 237
Chapter 12   Case Studies 251

■ PART IV: Finishing Strong
Chapter 13   Recovery and Wellness 279
Chapter 14   Peaking for Your Ironman 301
Chapter 15   Racing Long 313

Epilogues 331
Appendix A: Defining Your Training Zones by Sport 333
Appendix B: Testing and Warm-up Protocols 343
Appendix C: Swimming Glossary 349
Appendix D: Brick Workouts 351
References and Recommended Reading 355
Index 365
About the Authors 372

FOREWORD BY SCOTT MOLINA

I've considered myself a good "student" of this sport for over twenty years. For me, the first step to achieving excellence in triathlon has always been to seek out the best sources of information in order to make informed decisions about my training. I remember poring over all the old issues of *Runner's World, Track and Field News, VeloNews,* and *Swimming World* magazines in the library for months and months instead of studying for my exams in college.

There have been more than a few books written on the various aspects of triathlon since then, many of them very good. Most of the physiological principles of training we've learned from other sports have certainly stood the test of time. But triathlon is still a relatively new sport, and there is still a lot of progress to be made. This is one of the things that keeps me interested in the sport, along with the physical challenge of trying to get ready for events.

I respect Gordo and his opinions because he takes a similar, if not a more extreme, approach to his triathlon education. He's humble enough to recognize that his knowledge base, like his training base, can always be increased. To say he's consumed by the journey of finding out how to do this sport better would be an understatement. He lives triathlon 24/7, and this book is the end result of that affliction to date.

I met Gordo in 2000 when a mutual friend introduced us on a training ride. Over the last few years, I've watched his development as a coach and an athlete. Although there is a broad range of strategies that can be employed to achieve athletic success, this book will provide you with a safe and effective strategy for approaching the challenges of Ironman-distance racing.

Whether you are training for your first or your fortieth Ironman-distance race, I would encourage you to remember the following key points that I have learned from my years of racing.

"It ain't brain surgery." My longtime confidant Kenny Souza used to say this to me regularly over the years to remind me to try not to overanalyze things. Don't stray to anything too exotic. You can think a lot, but there still has to be some regular, basic training done to improve your body.

"Little and often fills the purse." Training principles follow the basic laws of physics and human behavior. A regular dose of exercise every day isn't a new paradigm, but it will get you there as surely as saving a bit in the bank every month.

"Train hard; eternal youth doesn't come cheap." Take a good look around at the average guy today. It's not a pretty sight, is it? This sport is demanding, and if you want to achieve, it's going to take discipline and work.

In this book Gordo gives you a reference to come back to time and time again to keep you on track. He's done the research and put himself through every technique to put together a very concise guide to save you hundreds of hours poring over hundreds of magazines and years of frustrating experiences. I'm sure reading this book will be a very valuable investment of your time.

—Scott Molina,
The TERMINATOR

FOREWORD BY RYAN BOLTON

In 1997, when I started racing triathlons professionally, I hired Joe Friel to coach me. My primary goal at that point was to make the Olympic team in 2000. My long-term goal was to succeed in Ironman-distance racing. Since then, I earned a spot on the U.S. Olympic team and competed in Sydney, switched my focus to long-course racing in 2001, and had immediate success under Joe's coaching. Having the wealth of information, training guidelines, and feedback from Joe has been pivotal to my success.

Going Long contains comprehensive data and instruction about long-course training, racing, and schedules that Joe has made available to me in the past few years. It is presented in a manner that is easy to understand and apply to one's particular training and racing goals. It will educate, motivate, and inspire any athlete to perform at his or her fullest potential. Using periodization and the latest innovations based on extensive research, *Going Long* will help one tailor one's training to one's specific physiology, goals, and time schedule.

Given the duration and intensity of long-course races, it is helpful to adhere to a regimented schedule. In my training with Joe, I have used periodization, which takes the athlete through several stages of training. It starts with preparation, which Joe refers to as "training to train." This is followed by the Base training period, during which the athlete focuses on longer workouts with lower intensity. Then the athlete moves on to the Build period, in which volume is decreased but intensity is increased. Next, in the Peak period, volume drops even more and race intensity is further emphasized. The culmination of these periods leads to the race period, which is when the athlete is in prime condition to race and the focus is on maintaining sharpness. The last, and not the least important, is the Transition period, when the athlete rests and recovers.

Ironman training is extremely time consuming. The typical Ironman athlete is faced with balancing not only long hours of swimming, biking, and running but also family, friends, work, and other interests. To add to it all, nutrition and rest are essential elements that cannot be forgotten. The principles that Joe has applied to my training are presented in *Going Long* to assist the athlete by providing a training timeline that allows him or her to effectively incorporate all essential elements of his or her lifestyle. This allows the athlete to maintain the very necessary balance between triathlon and life beyond triathlon.

Joe Friel is among the most respected coaches in the sport of triathlon. He has years of experience with racing and coaching in addition to an analytical and well-rounded approach that is influenced by his commitment to stay abreast of the latest research in the field. It is with his expertise and passion that *Going Long* is able to provide the reader with the finest long-course training resource available.

Work hard and keep it fun.

—Ryan Bolton,
Professional Triathlete,
Christchurch, New Zealand

PREFACE BY JOE FRIEL

In 2000 Gordon Byrn flew in from Hong Kong and spent a weekend with me in Colorado. I was highly impressed not only with how well he understood the training principles I had described in *The Triathlete's Training Bible* but also with his enthusiasm for learning. He wanted to know everything there was to know about training for triathlon. I had never met anyone with such a thirst for knowledge. Unfortunately, I was not quite able to fully satisfy his thirst, as I was then, and still am, only up to about 1 percent of all that must be known about the sport. Gordo is soon to pass me, I'm sure.

After running into him at races and sharing several e-mail conversations over the next few months, I realized that Gordo was not a fluke and that he was destined to be one of the most knowledgeable coaches in the sport. In self-defense, I decided to ask him to join Ultrafit Associates, my personal coaching business. With his passion for people, solid head for business, love of all things triathlon, and gentle nature, he was immediately accepted by our coaches.

It soon became clear that Gordo and I thought alike on almost every matter. One day I suggested we write a book together on training for triathlon. As usual, he was already one step ahead of me and had put together a rough outline in his head while out for a long ride. And so the project began.

What you are about to read here is information-dense. I don't expect you'll be able to grasp it all with just one reading, although I'd suggest you give it a try. Once you have gotten through it the first time, this book will best serve as a reference as you buy equipment, set up a training program, confront your mental demons, peak for a race, make dietary choices, or consider any of the thousands of factors that go into successful long-distance triathlon racing. I'd suggest marking it up to personalize and better internalize the information. As you run into questions, contact us through our Web site at www.TrainingPeaks.com. We look forward to hearing from you and promise to help however we can.

PREFACE BY GORDON BYRN

When I bought my copy of *The Triathlete's Training Bible* in 1998, I knew very little about our sport, had never completed a triathlon, and couldn't swim more than a hundred meters without stopping. Through the application of Joe's principles, I was able to dramatically increase my performance in a relatively short period of time. I have been fortunate to study not only with Joe but also under other leading coaches of our sport (Scott Molina, John Hellemans, Dave Scott, and Mark Allen). In writing this second edition of *Going Long,* I have included all the techniques that I have learned to date.

This book is a summary of what we believe are the most effective training methods for long-course racing. Although there is a lot of detail inside, we encourage you to seek to understand the philosophy that underlies each chapter of the book. Take the essence of each section and apply it to your own personal needs. Expose yourself to as many different coaches, athletes, sports scientists, and mentors as you can. Learn what you can from each of them, and then choose the path that you think is best.

To achieve your absolute best as an athlete requires fanatical devotion. This degree of focus can liberate, or imprison, your life. Pause annually to make sure that your participation in our sport remains healthy in spirit, mind, and body.

There will be times when you need to make ethical choices. Choose wisely.

ACKNOWLEDGMENTS

This book project turned out to be a great match between Gordo and me. Gordo wrote most of what you are about to read. My input was largely a matter of ensuring that we didn't stray too far from the principles I have been learning over the past thirty years. It was a match made in writers' heaven; I would not have thought it possible for two people to agree so often on so many matters over the course of six months. We seldom disagreed, and never on substantive issues. When we did find differences, Gordo typically bowed to my greater experience and let me have my way. Thanks, Gordo.

—Joe Friel

I'd like to acknowledge my coauthor, Joe Friel. In 2000 Joe took a chance by hiring an athlete with little coaching experience (me). By believing that I would make a good coach, he set in motion a chain of events that greatly improved my life. With the passing years, my understanding of triathlon deepens and my respect for Joe grows.

When I think back over my triathlon career, I recall many people who have had a positive impact on my life. Specifically, I would like to acknowledge Scott Molina, John Hellemans, John Newsom, and Clas Björling. If I achieved my potential over the past ten years, then it is due directly to the patience, and example, of these four men. There is no easy way.

Ultradistance triathlon is an extreme event that attracts extreme people. Thinking about the crazy characters that I have met over the years brings a smile to my face. Ian, Luke, Claire, David, Jonas, Martin, Steve, John, Chris, Sam, Ben, Barry, Billy, Dennis, Justin, Chuckie, Christian, Will, Brandon, Bobby, Roly, Tim, Eric, Doug, Albert, Mark, Kevin, Dan, Ron, Kristine, Tom, Brent, Stephen, and many more. Thanks.

—Gordon Byrn

Getting Started

PART I

CHAPTER 1

THE IRON JOURNEY

The spirit of Ironman® is much more than a race, more than a simple time goal. It is about the process of preparing yourself for one of the greatest endurance challenges you will ever face. Race day is but one aspect of your overall journey.

> " *Life is achievement. . . . Give yourself an aim, something you want to do, then go after it, breaking through everything, with nothing in mind but your aim, all will, all concentration, and get it.*
>
> —AYN RAND

"CAN I DO IT?"

Nearly every athlete will ask this question at some point over the course of a successful triathlon career. The truth is, anyone can do the distance if they want it badly enough, and every Ironman race includes a large number of first-timers. There is no bigger challenge in triathlon than the Ironman distance, and ultimately the decision is yours and yours alone. The right answer lies inside you. You will do the training, you will make the necessary commitments, and you will miss out on certain other aspects of your life. For many, the trade-off is worth it.

An athlete is never "ready" for an Ironman-distance race. The event is far too big for that. However, we firmly believe that anyone (and we mean anyone) can complete the distance so long as they have one ingredient: will. The will to train and, most important of all, the will to finish. You have to be doing this for yourself. You have to want to finish, badly. There will be many moments in your training when you will want to quit, but by not quitting you will learn a lot about yourself. You will get stronger; you will change. There aren't many things in life that give us the opportunity to test our inner strength. The Ironman distance is one of those things.

In all honesty, these events are tough. That is what makes them so rewarding. You have to believe in yourself and trust that your preparations will get you to the finish line. It is a true test of mental and physical strength. Your mind and body will beg you to slow down, so your spirit must push to overcome that resistance.

Many athletes wait before committing to a race until they have the confidence that they can complete the full distance the way they want. Others arrive at the start line with little background and have a positive experience—regardless of their finishing time—and some who finish at the front of the pack don't have a positive experience. Everyone should remember that there is no rush to take on the Ironman distance. The races will be there when you are ready. There are no right or wrong answers, and you should go with what feels right to you. If you don't think you are ready, wait until you have greater confidence in your abilities.

We all race the full distance for ourselves. Preparing for the race is such a large undertaking that it is tough to do it for any other reason. If you are racing for yourself, only you can evaluate your result. It's like this for everything in life. If you do your best in preparation and execution, you should be satisfied with whatever result you get.

So how do you know you are ready to go long? You don't. You commit, train, and pray.

TRAITS FOR SUCCESS

Go to any triathlon and watch the top athletes prepare. You may notice a common air among them. Successful athletes have certain personality traits that give them an edge over the rest of the field. The following are seven such traits.

Confidence. Talented athletes know they have what it takes physically to succeed. The most successful ones never brag about this, at least not out loud. However, their self-assurance is obvious to anyone who watches the way they behave and carry themselves. There is no doubt that they are cocky, but they don't talk about how good they are. They know that if they tried to dominate their peer group, their fellow athletes' support would not be there when needed. Unabashedly cocky athletes usually wind up competing against everyone, including their teammates. Few are truly good enough to achieve all of their goals entirely alone.

There are two types of confidence: respect for yourself as a person and respect for your athletic abilities. The successful athlete scores high in both areas. But confidence in either area can be easily lost, usually through our own initiative, because inside each of us is a small voice that likes to criticize. It often points out our shortcomings and limiters. Success comes in large part from merely learning to control that voice while providing constant positive feedback. You would be hard-pressed to find an athlete who would not benefit from increased self-confidence. Always act as if you are confident. It's amazing what that does for self-perception.

Focus. During times when an important outcome is on the line, such as a race or a hard workout, successful athletes have the ability to concentrate their mental and physical energy on the task at hand. Their mental wanderings from the immediacy of what they are doing are brief. During easy workouts they may take a mental siesta, but they don't daydream during the important sessions and tend to concentrate on the present, not the future or the past. They repeatedly scan their energy reserves and movement patterns to make sure all is going well. Lacking this ability to focus, less successful athletes speed up and slow down repeatedly and later on can't understand why they were unable to maintain pace. Less successful athletes also dwell on the outcome of the race or workout and what others are doing rather than on their immediate situation. To improve, they must learn to do only what is required at the present moment and let the results take care of themselves.

Self-sufficiency. Successful athletes also take full responsibility for their actions during a race. They take calculated risks to try to win rather than trying not to lose. They are decisive and intuitively know that it's better to fully commit to a bad decision than to be uncommitted to the right decision. With the right mental state, it is sometimes possible to pull off what others may see as nearly impossible, but weak commitment is a sure loser.

Adaptability. Successful athletes have the ability in the heat of competition to analyze the situation, problem-solve, and adapt to a new set of circumstances. In time-oriented triathlon, there is a constant barrage of changing circumstances—wind, heat, humidity, fatigue, equipment, and competitors. Mother Nature can force midevent course changes, sometimes without any warning to competitors out on the course. Many athletes freak out and stop. Others adapt, keep their cool, and race on. How adaptable are you?

Emotional stability. Some athletes cannot maintain an even keel emotionally. In the course of a workout or race, they experience fear, anger, frustration, disappointment, excitement, elation, and anticipation. All of this takes its toll on energy levels and focus and can often lead to lackluster race performances despite physical ability.

Mental clarity. This point differs from focus, by which we mean the ability to concentrate on a task. By mental clarity, we mean knowing why we are doing a task and maintaining perspective and a sense of balance regarding the overall goal or project.

In their daily activities, the most successful athletes are concerned about the well-being of those closest to them, including their competitors, who are often close friends and training partners. However, in the heat of competition they really don't care about the feelings and emotions of their challengers, and they expect others to feel the same way about them. When the going gets hard, mentally tough athletes hang in there. This doesn't mean they never DNF (did not finish). There are circumstances when it is fully acceptable to decide this just isn't your day. However, this decision should never be made because the competition was greater than expected.

Being appropriately psyched. There is an optimal level of arousal necessary for every sport and for different situations within a given sport. For example, going into an Ironman-distance race with a high level of arousal is a sure way to blow up. Successful athletes know how much mental psyching is necessary and respond accordingly.

No athlete is perfect in all of these areas. Each of us has one or more that need work, and some have more to work on than others. Just as with your physical limiters, you need to determine where your mental limiters lie and initiate strategies to improve them. These strategies are discussed in greater detail in Chapter 11.

ESSENTIAL ATTRIBUTES OF A COACH

So you have signed up for an Ironman-distance race. You are excited and a little scared. You think you know that you have what it takes to finish, but you want to get the most out of the limited time you have to train. You have significant commitments in your nontriathlon life and would like to minimize the disruption for your family and coworkers. You need some advice to get you through your Iron journey and are thinking that a coach could be the way to go.

Having been on both sides of the athlete-coach relationship, we want to share some ideas on how to get the most out of your coach. Following are some key things to remember when considering a potential coaching relationship.

Trust. You will be trusting your entire season to another person. You should check the coach's credentials, experience, and background. Ask for references and speak to current clients. Review sample workout plans and discuss the coach's approach to building the season.

Goals. Communicate your key goals for the season. The best results are achieved by having a limited number of quantitative as well as qualitative goals. Set the goals early in the season and tailor the year toward achieving them.

Personality and style. There are a lot of coaches out there and just as many training philosophies. Different strategies work for different folks. You should make sure your coach's training style matches your needs. Particular things to watch for are the approaches to intensity, volume, and recovery. This is where the variation can be greatest and will have the most significant impact on your performance (both positively and negatively).

The plan. Many coaches offer different levels of service and price points. Make sure you choose the plan that best fits your needs. If you are looking for frequent interaction, then make sure your coach will be happy with the level of assistance you require. Make your expectations known in advance and see what the coach recommends.

Share of mind. If you are paying for individual coaching, make sure you will get an adequate share of mind (that is, the coach's time and attention). Find out how many athletes are currently being coached by that person. Discuss your coach's other commitments. Be sure you are confident that your plan will get the focus it deserves. Once again, make your expectations clear in advance. In our opinion, if your interaction is limited, then you are not being coached.

Communication. You are buying your coach's advice, experience, and support. Ask a lot of questions. Understand what lies behind the yearly, monthly, and weekly planning. You will become a better athlete if you understand the reasons behind each session. It is also your job to make sure your coach understands how you are doing. Take advantage of every opportunity to update the coach regarding your progress. You need to be totally honest. If you were so tired you couldn't get out of bed, then make sure that message gets across. Be open and clear about what is happening. This is even more important in an online relationship because of the lack of visual feedback (tough to hide fatigue at the track but easy on the keyboard). Don't BS your coach! This honesty is essential when you are tired, injured, or not coping. Know when to back off—that is, know when to rest, know when you have done enough training, and know when you may be trying too hard.

One plan. Once you have committed, paid your cash, built the season up ... do the program. This sounds easy, but in fact, many people second-guess their coach and adjust the plan that has been created for them. There should be a reason behind every workout. If you have doubts, ask questions until you are satisfied. You are paying for expert advice, so use it.

Belief. Coaches should have the ability to create and enhance athletes' belief in their ability to achieve their goals. The power of belief is one of the strongest forces in life. The best coaches, friends, and training partners share a belief in the ability of the athlete. People who do not serve this power of belief are best avoided. In our opinion, creating and enhancing the power of belief is the central role of the coach.

Structure. Because of their experience, coaches should have the ability to provide athletes with a structured environment that will enable them to move safely and consistently toward their goals. Structure gives athletes a feeling of control and confidence, thereby strengthening the power of belief and increasing the chances of success.

Clarity. There are two aspects of clarity: (1) Coaches should be able to explain goals, sessions, technique, and strategies in a clear manner that the athlete can understand; and (2) coaches should strive not to become personally invested in an athlete's results so they can offer the athlete the benefit of an objective opinion.

Knowledge. Coaches should be constantly seeking new training techniques and expanding their knowledge about all aspects of training, nutrition, and recovery. The goal of every coach should be to become a mind-body master. Likewise, athletes who want to perform at the highest levels should make it a priority to understand the purpose of each session and to become mind-body masters in their own right.

Openness. Coaches should be open to (and with) their athletes. Athletes should know that they will not be judged by their coaches. Openness builds trust between coach and athlete, increasing the effectiveness of the relationship.

Responsibility. Coaches must take full responsibility for the programs they create. Likewise, athletes must take full responsibility for executing the coach's program to the best of their ability. When doubts arise, the coach and athlete should review the program together and agree on the overall strategy. This builds trust and strengthens the power of belief.

WHAT DOES IT TAKE?

In coaching hundreds of athletes through successful race experiences, we have seen a wide range of effective training strategies. In our opinion the single most important attribute for ultraendurance success is a deep enjoyment of endurance training. A consistent, long-term approach is required to achieve athletic success. Moreover, the skills learned along your "Iron journey" can be integrated into your larger life for a deeper level of success.

■ *Time Commitment*

Most highly motivated athletes research the level of training required to achieve a predetermined race goal and try to cram their training regimen into an already overscheduled life.

In our experience, the most effective way for athletes (of all levels) to plan is to consider the amount of time currently available within their daily activities. Ensure that your weekly training schedule fits comfortably, and harmoniously, within the realities of your life. If you fall into the trap of overextending yourself, you will suffer from exhaustion and the emotional ups and downs that come with it. You will enjoy far more success from consistently achieving a moderate plan.

To adequately prepare for an Ironman race, you will need to build up your endurance to the point that you can complete the following key workouts: one long swim of 75–100 minutes (min.); one long ride of 4–5 hours (always run for 15–30 min. after you finish your long bike); and one long run of 90–135 min. (during the week but not immediately after the long ride). These key workouts are done over the course of first a month, then a fortnight, then a week, and finally a weekend.

Always remember that you are training for an extremely long day that will be completed very close to your maximum endurance limits and very far from your maximum speed limits. It is far more important by any measure to develop your aerobic stamina than your speed. Focus on achieving a deep level of aerobic fitness—"fast" follows "fit."

■ *Training*

The most important aspects of long-distance training are surprisingly elementary. It's often difficult, however, to convince athletes at all ability levels of the significance of these simple lessons. Those who accept and follow them always reach a higher level of success than those who don't.

Set a few clear and simple goals for the year. More than three usually causes confusion. One is often enough to keep you on track. A good goal provides direction for training, but it needs to be posted someplace where you'll see it every day. The cover of your training log is a good place. Don't get lost in just working out and racing.

Have a plan for achieving your goals. Goals without plans are wishes. A plan is like a road map—it points you in the right direction but may be changed along the way, as some "roads" are found to be better than others. Make notes on a calendar when a few measurable benchmarks of steady progress are needed to reach the goal.

Rest when you are tired. It's amazing how few self-coached athletes understand the significance of rest for improving performance. It must be the high work ethic so necessary for success in sport that causes them to disregard or trivialize feelings of fatigue. When athletes take rest seriously, both the quality of their workouts and their overall fitness improve. This leads to the next simple lesson.

Make the hard days hard and the easy days easy. Most highly focused athletes wind up doing just the opposite: They make their easy days too hard, and because of that, the hard days are too easy. All workouts gravitate toward the middle. When you regularly include days off from training and extremely light workouts, the workouts meant to push the fitness envelope do just that.

As you get started on your Iron journey, these training principles will offer you good direction. When you are well into the everyday ritual of training, this more specific list of reminders will prove helpful:

- There is no easy way. The achievement of meaningful goals requires sustained, consistent effort over an extended period.
- Intensity is not a substitute for volume. There's nothing "fast" about Ironman-distance racing. The highest-intensity sessions are the least specific in your program. Inappropriate intensity is responsible for most nutritional, recovery, and biomechanical breakdowns.
- When faced with a decision between Base and Build, choose Base.
- Recovery is essential. Schedule recovery within your week, month, and year. Most athletes spend the majority of their competitive seasons exhausted. Many ultra-endurance athletes are at their best in the late spring because Mother Nature forces them to rest.
- Running fitness is meaningless if you are too tired to use it. Marathon performance for this event is built on superior cycling fitness.
- Pace your year. Your best training performance should be four to six weeks prior to your most important competition.
- All the fitness in the world is useless if you are sick or injured on race day. The closer you get to your event, the greater caution you must apply.

As you probably already know from your triathlon experience, the weekends are an invaluable time for training, especially if you are keeping up with a challenging job. That said, you should avoid the "death" weekends that many people recommend. For better recovery, plan your long run for midweek and your longest training day for the weekend. For example, you might opt to ride long on Sunday, swim long on Friday, and run long on Wednesday.

Be wary of triathletes who bait you with talk of their megaweeks. Train safely and within your own limits. Fatigue is part of the process, but you should only feel tired for twelve to thirty-six hours after your key training days. If you are tired longer than this, back off. If you are stiff and it doesn't go away, back off.

It bears repeating: Smart training is the key to Ironman-distance success.

APPROACHES TO TRAINING

Nothing is more important than consistency, moderation, and recovery when you are training for an Ironman-distance event. Whether you are a novice or a seasoned pro, long-term success in the sport of triathlon requires that you make these three rules your mantra. Keep in mind that your optimal training program is the one that you will be able to comfortably repeat across many seasons. In terms of exploring your ultimate potential, you are playing a five- to ten-year game. It is human nature to overestimate what we can achieve in a season and underestimate what we can achieve in a decade. The top athletes in your division have likely been students of the sport for most of their adult lives.

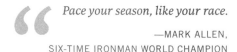

Pace your season, like your race.

—MARK ALLEN,
SIX-TIME IRONMAN WORLD CHAMPION

Most training breakdowns are due to illness, injury, burnout, and overtraining. Extended or frequent training breaks caused by such problems inevitably result in a loss of fitness. Too many athletes do that one extra workout or push hard into that one last interval. Pushing the body past endurance, strength, and speed limits rapidly increases the chances of a breakdown. The intelligent athlete trains within the body's limits and infrequently stretches them just a little. Long-term consistency, moderation, and recovery are the only way to achieve your potential.

When a workout becomes very hard, your speed decreases noticeably, or your technique changes, it is time to call it a day. Athletes with a strong work ethic find calling a halt hard to do. This is where a coach is beneficial because his or her objective, unemotional guidance will help to avoid breakdowns. The self-coached athlete will often be unsure whether or not to continue training. When unsure, always remember: If in doubt, leave it out.

Although challenging workouts are important, they are beneficial only to the extent that they guide your overall fitness toward a peak and do not result in extended recovery periods. For this reason, most athletes schedule such workouts infrequently and, normally, only in the weeks immediately preceding a major race. Moderation in training leads to consistency in training, and consistency in training leads to continual improvement.

Recovery is the aspect of training that is most neglected by highly motivated athletes. Few fully appreciate the physiological benefits that accrue during rest, especially during sleep. While asleep, the body releases growth hormone to repair damage from the day's training stresses and to shore up any physiological systems weakened by training. Without adequate sleep, fitness is lost regardless of how intense or long the workouts were. A well-rested athlete looks forward to workouts, enjoys them, feels sharp and in control, and grows stronger after training. Most working athletes find that an extra hour of sleep is the most beneficial change they can make to improve performance.

Every triathlete will make training decisions based on these three principles—consistency, moderation, and recovery—but of course not every triathlete will train the same way. Your experience in the sport and, more importantly, your experience with the Ironman distance will change your focus. Regardless of where you fall on the experience spectrum, here are some guidelines to help you realize whatever your goal may be. Remember, it never hurts to review the basics. We have used some specific examples and applications to better illustrate these points, most of which will be more thoroughly explained later in the book.

TRAINING TO FINISH: GETTING THE BASICS

For many athletes who are contemplating their first attempt at the Ironman distance, the goal is just to finish the race. Period. If they can also skip the medical tent and manage a smile, great. They are looking for advice on how to make their journey as satisfying (and pain-free) as possible. If this profile sounds familiar, then you will find this section helpful.

Before attempting an Ironman-distance race, it is recommended that you have two to five years of experience in triathlon or other endurance sports. The purpose of this period is to build a solid base of technical skills, strength, and endurance. However, many athletes are able to complete the distance, although not usually comfortably, on a lesser base.

At a minimum, you should be able to finish a half-Ironman-distance race in under 8 hours, swim 3,000 meters (m), ride 5 hours, and run 2 hours without requiring extended recovery time. (Please note that these are separate workouts!)

You don't have to kill yourself in training. You know the race is grueling, so you think you will get tough by signing up for two marathons; a half-dozen century rides; and a 3-mile, rough-water swim. Not recommended!

Successful endurance training is exactly like turning a Styrofoam cup inside out. So long as you take it slowly, you'll be able to do it. Try to rush things and—*rip!*—you'll tear the cup. You are the cup.

Build technique and endurance in your first year. If you are making the jump from Olympic- or half-Ironman-distance racing, your greatest limiter is aerobic stamina. Laying out a sketch of the year is essential. The core of your week is your longest endurance workout in each sport. Plan to build your swim up to 4,000 m, your ride up to 5 hours, and your run up to 2.5 hours. Build up very slowly: three weeks forward, one week back, repeat. Never add more than 5–10 percent in terms of duration to any week or any long workout—with your running, you would be wise to build less than 10 percent per month. You have a lot of time, even if you are racing early in the season.

Every athlete has his or her own idea of appropriate workout distances and durations; however, it is best to be a little conservative about the long stuff. This approach will enable you to recover quickly, maintain consistency, and avoid injury. The two most likely times for injury are during high-intensity training and when you run long after a long ride (short runs are routine after the long ride, but the long ride and long run should not take place consecutively). Avoid these kinds of sessions.

A classic "Iron weekend" is a 6-hour ride on Saturday followed by a 3-hour run on Sunday. These sessions are typically billed as "confidence builders." However, experience shows that such sessions are counterproductive. Lying on a couch with the ceiling gently spinning on a Sunday night can leave your confidence more shattered than built. Separate your key sessions by several days for best results.

In your second season of racing long, you should continue to focus on technique and endurance. At this stage, most athletes will also benefit from increasing (or adding) an appropriate strength training program. Each year you should plan on returning to, and improving, the foundations of your sport (skills, endurance, and strength).

Focus on your key sessions, and make your key sessions focused. With your key sessions laid out, the rest of the week is easy to plan. Add other workouts so you get three sessions of each sport, including the key workouts. You have one goal each week: to hit your key sessions fresh and injury-free. Everything else is maintenance. If you are whipped, take a rest day. If you are a little tired, use the session for skill and technique work. If you feel good, do some endurance work, but be sure to finish wanting more. Do what it takes to begin your key sessions feeling fresh.

This approach leads nicely to volume. It seems counterintuitive, but you will achieve the most by aiming for less than you think you can handle. Focus on completing your training week and use key session performance to benchmark your progress. Your training volume is a result, not a goal, of training. A word on your key sessions: If you are following these guidelines, make sure your long workouts are high-quality. Avoid long breaks, and make sure the key sessions are true endurance workouts that build your stamina. Know your intensity zones, and stay within them. Endurance training always feels "easy" at the start, but after a few hours, you will be working no matter what the effort. Place your "best" performances at the end of your longest workouts—always finish strong.

Sleep is more valuable than training. Do you drag yourself out of bed at all hours because your schedule says you have to ride X minutes at Y heart rate? By far the best thing you can do if you are exhausted is sleep. Better to miss a short workout on Thursday than a whole weekend because of an unexpected illness. Persistent fatigue is a clear sign that your program needs to be moderated.

Of course, going to bed an extra hour early every night is a better option than missing training. Weekend naps are also great for the working athlete. Keep them under an hour and preferably before 2 p.m. for best results.

Forget about anaerobic endurance and high-intensity sessions. Extended steady-state aerobic training is the most specific, and important, training for the ultraendurance athlete. A track session can toast you for twelve to thirty-six hours. Get tired the right way, by generating fatigue in the way that is most specific to long-course success.

Schedule weekly, monthly, and annual recovery. Make sure you drop the volume way down every three to four weeks. Many excellent athletes give a blank stare when asked about their recovery strategy. Your recovery strategy is the most important, and overlooked, part of your plan. Appropriate nutrition, sleep, and hydration will help you get the most from your training.

You should end each training cycle feeling fresh and ready to get back to training. If you don't feel ready to go, then your training load is too high. Try to stay active during your recovery periods. Maintain workout frequency, but drop the volume and intensity.

Train with humility and control. Know your session goals before you start, and do everything you can to stick to your goals. Group training workouts are the most risky situations for highly motivated athletes. The pace slowly creeps up, and before you know it . . . hammer time! For that reason, choose your training partners with care. Over the years, we have found that small-group training is the best way to go. With the right group, there is someone to keep the pace in check and someone to maintain workout momentum. We will cover the subject of humility in more detail in Chapter 11.

Be wary of goal inflation. Remember your goals when you decided to start this journey, and keep the training fun. There is no point in putting all this time into the sport unless you are having a heck of a good time. When it all becomes a bit much (and it will), back off and reassess. The right answers will come to you.

When you signed up, you might have been thinking it would be nice just to finish. By the time the race comes around, you might start thinking that a time of 10:15 and a Kona slot are a very real possibility. Where did that idea come from? Until you are experienced at the distance and confident of your mental skills, keep your time goals to yourself. At 7 a.m. on race day, you'll have plenty of pressure. There is no need to make things tougher on yourself.

TRAINING FOR A PERSONAL BEST: FINDING ROOM FOR IMPROVEMENT

What are the key components of achieving a personal best? In reviewing countless races with the athletes whom we coach, we have found certain recurring themes. Again, other parts of this book will cover the specifics of how to address these points. You may find that they contain the formula to take you to the next level.

Better mental focus. The ability to focus is probably the single greatest limiter for most athletes. It is very difficult to stay oriented on a task for the eight to seventeen hours of an Ironman-distance race. You can, and should, use shorter-duration races and your key workouts to strengthen the ability to focus. When athletes are able to focus, they are able to execute their race strategy and keep their "process" on target.

In any long race, this process tends to give out before an athlete's "performance" gives out. As athletes, each of us has a personal breaking point—the point in a training session, in a race, or in life at which we "crack," slow, quit, or break down. The art of training is to lean against our breaking points from time to time, thereby pushing our boundaries further out. When we push too hard, we get injured, become depressed, and/or break down in some other way. All are signs that we have gone too far. Elites (in life and sport) have the ability to push themselves, but, more importantly, they know when to back off. Racing well is demanding. If you want to race well, then you must practice the ability to maintain mental strength when your body and mind start to doubt.

Train your mind slowly over time. Many people get down on themselves for not being able to maintain a fighting spirit for a whole race. The truth is, most people can't. That is why many "slow" athletes can be relatively competitive at the Ironman distance: They have trained their minds never to quit. All it takes is practice. Rest assured that when you are hurting, everyone else is feeling the same.

Smarter nutrition. Nutrition is every bit as important as swimming, biking, and running for the long-course triathlete. If you want to race at your very best, then you have to fuel your body appropriately. The nutritional tips contained in this book will benefit your recovery, strength, body composition, and race performance.

Stronger cycling. Cycling muscular endurance is the heart of Ironman-distance racing. The bike leg is the longest element of the race, so one reason is obvious. However, the benefits of superior bike fitness are not truly realized until the marathon.

These strategies for reaching your personal best are discussed further in Chapter 3. Ultimately, success is not about being "fast." It is about being able to swim smart, ride strong, and run tough. The training philosophy outlined in this book will help you do exactly that.

TRAINING TO QUALIFY

Many triathletes have the desire to race the Hawaii Ironman® or to qualify to represent their country at a World Championship event. With the increasing number of athletes in our sport and increasing knowledge about effective training and racing techniques, qualification will continue to become more challenging. You can increase your odds of qualification at any event with the following tips.

Identify your limiters and strengths. What are your limiters? Does your race pacing strategy result in your fastest overall time? Very few people are able to optimally pace a long-distance triathlon. What about your strengths? Once you have done a personal analysis, it's time for the tough part: You need to build a program that specifically addresses your limiters while doing the minimum to maintain your strengths. If you come from a single-sport background, you may be thinking, "But if I don't run, bike, or swim five times a week, then I will lose my edge." Rest assured that you will maintain your sport-specific strengths and become a better triathlete if you work on your limiters.

Build strength and endurance during winter. For most athletes, weight training in the winter is essential. Your strength program should follow the formula in this book (see Chapter 9 for the program). As a direct result of getting stronger in the weight room, you can expect several breakthroughs in the pool and on the bike. Female, veteran, cycling-limited, and novice athletes have the most to gain from strength training.

With all that lifting, you are likely to slow down a bit in the pool and on the bike (running won't be affected as much). This slowdown can be a mental challenge, but the program will pay off if you stick with it. If you are going into many of your sport-specific sessions a little tired, then focus on skills and endurance. Gradually bump up your long swim workouts to 4,000–5,000 m, and also do several 3- to 4-hour small-chainring rides. Riding extended periods of time in the small chainring sounds easy, but do not doubt how tough it is. Two hours of spinning at 100 rpm or more is feasible, but by the 3-hour mark you will be dying to use the big ring.

What about running? Keep your weekly long run between 90 and 120 min., and focus on run frequency. Running often is the safest way to build mileage and increase your durability. If you are cycling indoors, bricks (various combinations of swimming, riding, and running) and duathlon-type workouts will help break up the monotony of indoor riding. Mix it up, do many different types of bricks, and vary your cadence, position, effort, and order of the sports.

Racing. A duathlon or running race once a month will maintain your threshold performance. Avoid racing when you are in a period of high-intensity strength training.

Key race selection. If you can, choose three qualifying races (but no more than two Ironman-distance races), and have specific reasons for choosing each of them. Why three? You don't want to put all your eggs in one basket. You never know when you will hit one of those special days, or when you will hit one of those very painful days. You are likely to hit either one at any season.

Mental skills. We discuss this topic in detail in Chapter 11. We all have our mental weak spots. Experience shows that improved race performance comes from working on these areas. The best part is that your body can recover while your mind strengthens.

Consistency and commitment. Adopt a no-excuses policy with regard to workouts. Train in challenging conditions, and if your training buddies cancel on you, head out anyhow and be thankful for the opportunity to get stronger. Always remember that you need to "back it up" the next day. Pace your season so that your best training occurs three to five weeks before your A-priority race.

Recovery. Take a complete rest day once per week, or take plenty of active rest days by shortening the workout and/or lowering the intensity when you are feeling tired. Make a commitment to get an extra hour of sleep every night and a nap on Saturday and Sunday. The extra sleep will make a huge difference to both your state of mind and the quality of your training.

Muscular endurance. If you are weak on the bike, use the tips in Chapter 7 to improve your cycling. Athletes will find that increased cycling fitness has a great impact on their overall race performance. If you can get off the bike relatively fresh, then your race will be far easier. Most often, weak run splits result from poor swim/bike pacing and an overall lack of stamina rather than a specific run limiter.

Seek advice. Take every opportunity to get additional information. Books, newsgroups, Web sites, e-mail lists, online coaching, race expos, professional athletes, videos—try them all. Not everything makes sense, but it is all useful information and forms a background against which you can tailor your program to your specific needs. There are a lot of experienced people out there who love to talk training.

Race smart. The final point is a little obvious but worth making. The longer the distance, the more important it is to show patience in the race. Many people (pros included) try to succeed by hammering the swim and the first half of the bike. This strategy nearly always results in underperformance. You are likely to set all your personal bests by focusing on superior execution of your race strategy. The race will become difficult on its own. There is no need to rush the process.

ENJOYMENT: THE FINAL INGREDIENT

A question that all athletes have from time to time is "How fast can I get?" or "How good can I be?"

If you are an age-group athlete, your potential is limited first and foremost by your commitment and desire to do what is needed. Basically, this means doing your very best to intelligently implement the tools that are contained in this book and other sources of knowledge. The path to athletic success can be difficult, and movement toward our goals can be slow, even nonexistent, at times. However, we each have the ability to achieve success beyond our wildest dreams.

This means a dedication to fundamentals—nutrition, skills, endurance, and flexibility. The lifestyle of a committed athlete is not for everyone. There must be a deep joy associated with this path and an understanding that hard work is what leads to a payoff. The notion of "hard work" is nearly always misunderstood in this context. The underlying philosophy of this book is that successful athletes are those who equate "hard work" with "focused play."

We can all become excellent athletes—but whether we become the best athlete (or person) that we can be is determined by whether it is fun for us to do what it takes.

3

UNDERSTANDING FITNESS

*E*very triathlete wants to know how to achieve better fitness. If you are training for an Ironman race, you already have a solid level of fitness. It can be increasingly difficult to realize improvements in performance because they will probably seem

 It takes a long time to get good.

—SCOTT MOLINA,
IRONMAN WORLD CHAMPION

modest in comparison to your first year or two in the sport. But you can always become a better, smarter triathlete. It begins with knowing which components of fitness you can control.

THE COMPONENTS OF FITNESS

How can we measure physical fitness? Science measures fitness by three of its most basic components—aerobic capacity, functional threshold, and economy. The top endurance athletes have excellent values for all three physiological traits, which we'll explore in more detail in Chapter 5.

■ *Aerobic Capacity*

Aerobic capacity is a measure of the amount of oxygen the body can consume during all-out endurance exercise. It is also referred to as VO_2max—the volume of oxygen the body uses during maximal aerobic exercise. VO_2max can be measured in the lab during a "graded" test in which the athlete increases the intensity of exercise every few minutes until exhaustion while wearing a device that analyzes oxygen and carbon dioxide levels. Lab tests aren't practical for everyone, so we've included a test that will estimate your VO_2max in Appendix B. VO_2max is expressed in terms of milliliters of oxygen used per kilogram of body weight per minute (ml/kg/min.).

World-class male athletes usually produce numbers in the 70–80 ml/kg/min. range. For comparison, normally active male college students typically test in the range of 40–50 ml/kg/min. On average, women's aerobic capacities are about 10 percent lower than men's.

Absolute aerobic capacity is largely determined by genetics and is limited by such physiological factors as heart size, heart rate, heart-stroke volume, blood hemoglobin content, aerobic enzyme concentrations, mitochondrial density, and muscle-fiber type. It can, however, be enhanced by training to a certain extent. A well-trained athlete typically requires six to eight weeks of high-intensity training to achieve peak values.

As we get older, our aerobic capacity usually declines by as much as 1 percent per year after age 25 in sedentary people. For those who train seriously, especially by regularly including high-intensity workouts, the loss is far smaller and may not occur at all until the late 30s.

Aerobic capacity is not a good predictor of endurance performance. If all athletes in a race category were tested for aerobic capacity, the race results would most likely not reflect their VO_2max test values because the athletes with the highest VO_2max values would not necessarily finish high in the category rankings. However, the highest percentage of VO_2max that one can maintain for an extended period of time is a good predictor of racing capacity. This sustainable percentage of aerobic capacity is a reflection of functional threshold.

■ *Functional Threshold*

Functional threshold (FT), also sometimes called anaerobic threshold or lactate threshold, is the level of exercise intensity above which lactate begins to rapidly accumulate in the blood as metabolism quickly shifts from dependence on the combustion of fat and oxygen in the production of energy to dependence on glycogen—the stored form of carbohydrate. The body is always creating lactate even when sleeping and resting. At such times, it may be in the range of about 1 millimole of lactate per liter of blood (mmol/L). As you start to exercise, more carbohydrate is used, so the lactate concentration of the blood rises.

FT typically occurs around 4 mmol/L. This is approximately the level at which an Olympic-distance triathlon or a 40K time trial is typically done. An Ironman-distance race would be done at a substantially lower level. For comparison, an all-out, 800 m run may put a runner at 20 mmol/L. Appendix B includes testing to pinpoint your FT.

Knowing only lactate concentrations in the blood tells you absolutely nothing about readiness to race. Lactate levels in the blood must be compared with some measure of performance to have meaning. Usually this measure is pace (swimming and running) or power (cycling). Over the course of several weeks, if lactate concentrations go down for any given pace or power, or if pace or power rises for any given lactate level, then fitness is typically improving. Compared with aerobic capacity, FT is highly receptive to enhancement by training.

■ *Economy*

Economy is a measure of the energy exerted as compared to the work produced. This is the single most important difference between an elite athlete and a recreational sports enthusiast. Elite athletes use less oxygen to hold a given steady submaximal velocity. Thus, the elite athletes are using less energy to produce the same power or pace.

Studies reveal that an endurance athlete's economy improves if he or she has a high percentage of slow-twitch muscle fibers (largely determined by genetics), low body mass (weight-height relationship), and low psychological stress; uses properly fitting, light, and aerodynamic equipment that limits body frontal area exposed to the wind at higher velocities; and eliminates useless and energy-wasting movements.

Fatigue negatively affects economy as muscles that are not normally called on are recruited to carry the load. That's why it's critical to go into important races well rested. Near the end of a race, when economy deteriorates due to fatigue, you may sense that your swimming, pedaling, and running skills are getting sloppy. This deterioration will waste precious energy. The longer the race, the more critical economy becomes in determining the outcome.

Like FT, economy can be materially improved by training. Not only does it improve by increasing all aspects of endurance but it also rises as you refine sport-specific skills. This is why drill work is critical in the base training phases as well as a component of the year-round training regimen.

In an ultraendurance event, metabolic efficiency can become a factor in exercise performance. As exercise intensity increases toward maximal output, the body's ability to generate fuel from fat oxidation is diminished. Given that glycogen stores and the rate of carbohydrate metabolism are limited, fat oxidation can be a limiting factor for certain athletes. Most elite ultraendurance athletes are able to access a greater percentage of their fuel from fat (for a given subthreshold intensity) and maintain this capacity at higher intensities than age-group athletes.

Modern metabolic testing methods are available to calculate the energy required, and fuel mix used, for a given exercise intensity. By analyzing the athlete's "exhaust" (expired air), the tests can determine the amount of fuel consumed. This is valuable information for deciding what type of training will most benefit your performance.

THE TRAINING TRIAD

■ *Endurance*

Ironman-distance racing is an endurance event. It doesn't matter how good any other aspect of fitness is—if endurance is poor, race fitness will also be poor. Endurance is the ability to finish the longest of races, to persevere regardless of pace, to merely continue for a long time.

Endurance training also benefits the metabolic efficiency required to fuel your race. If you come from a short-course background or have a history of primarily high-intensity training, then your ultraendurance performance could receive a big boost from focusing on endurance.

■ *Force*

This element, which could also be called strength, is the ability to apply force to the pedal, to the ground, and to the water. Successful Ironman-distance racing does not require significant maximal force but does require excellent muscular endurance (the product of force and endurance), particularly on the bike. Many athletes who ride a lot of hills find that their flat time trialing will suffer, specifically the ability to push a solid gear in the flats—an essential skill for success in long-course racing.

A general recommendation is that force workouts should be different from high-end aerobic training. When seeking to build force, it is worth keeping the heart rate (and cadence) down.

KEEPING HEART RATE AND CADENCE "DOWN" can mean different things for different people. A novice long-distance triathlete would stay down in, or below, heart rate Zone 3, whereas an elite athlete would stay down at, or below, threshold.

With cycling, be very cautious about riding hills at cadences under 50–60 rpm. When training on hills at a low cadence, an athlete should aim for a moderate heart rate and not seek to drive it sky-high. Of course, this goal takes a certain level of cycling endurance. Most new cyclists will find their heart rates very high on any hill—for them, seated, gentle rollers can be a good way to safely increase cycling power.

■ *Speed Skills*

The ability to make the movements of the sport efficiently at race pace or faster is very important. For triathletes, this means technique drills in the water to minimize drag, speed drills such as isolated leg drills or spin-up drills on the bike, and strides and step counting on the run. These and other skills are explained in Chapters 5–8. Remember that "race pace" for an ultraendurance event is most often at, or below, Zone 2.

How much can you improve your speed skills? Back in the 1970s, top American miler Steve Scott decided to go after the world record for the mile. That summer he improved his economy by 7 percent. A 7 percent improvement in economy (just another way of saying speed skills) is as good as a 7 percent improvement in VO$_2$max or FT. How much work would you have to do to accomplish these latter fitness elements? A lot.

Working on speed skills year-round, but with a great emphasis in the Base period, could pay huge dividends for your racing in the spring. Because of the tendency to focus on endurance, this is the most neglected ability—yet it is also the one that holds the greatest potential for improvement among athletes at all levels.

> **SPEED SKILLS ARE NOT THE SAME AS WHAT IS COMMONLY KNOWN AS "SPEED WORK."** Speed skills involve a focus on economy of movement. However, the approach that most athletes take to speed work is similar to their approach to anaerobic endurance. Anaerobic power (critical for sprinters) and anaerobic endurance (common for short endurance events) are not limiters for a long-course athlete. Because the highest-intensity sessions are difficult, painful, and generate high levels of fatigue, many athletes believe they are the most beneficial. In fact, they are highly risky and counterproductive for most long-course athletes and all novice athletes.

ADVANCED TRAINING ABILITIES

The training triad (endurance, force, and speed skills) is the base on which you can build advanced training abilities: muscular endurance, anaerobic endurance, and power. Each advanced training ability is a combination of two elements of the triad. For the experienced long-course athlete, muscular endurance is the most critical component of fitness.

■ *Muscular Endurance*

Muscular endurance is where force meets endurance. This ability allows the athlete to apply a fairly large force for a fairly long time and is essential for cycling. Here are some examples of muscular endurance workouts for cycling:

- Ride relatively long hills, taking 15–40 min. to climb at a heart rate of 10–15 beats per minute (bpm) below your FT.
- Ride a flat route in the big ring with efforts of the same duration.
- Ride a rolling route with the same effort level.

All of these workouts are similar to what endurance athletes encounter in a race—they need to maintain a steadily high pace for a long period of time. Muscular endurance is so crucial to race fitness and takes so long to fully realize that athletes should begin working on its most basic aspects in Base 2 (see Chapter 5 for explanation of different Base periods). In Base 3, the muscular endurance work starts, but efforts are shorter—for example, rolling hill rides are done mainly in heart rate Zones 1 and 2 while staying seated on the hills to build force.

■ *Anaerobic Endurance*

Anaerobic endurance is the ability to generate superthreshold power and pace. Heart rates and power outputs are high—heart rate Zone 5b and CP6 power zone—and therefore the effort cannot be maintained for very long. High lactate levels are generated at these paces, and these workouts are painful. They are not critical for Ironman-distance success in the same way that endurance and muscular endurance workouts are.

■ *Power*

Power is the ability to apply maximum force quickly and economically. It is the combination of force and speed-skills abilities. This is the stuff that made sprinters like Mario Cipollini (cycling) and Carl Lewis (running) the great athletes they were. Like anaerobic endurance workouts, workouts focusing on power are not critical for Ironman-distance training.

LIMITERS

Most athletes train the way they *want* to train. Athletes who are able to consistently improve season after season tend to train the way they *need* to train. It can be difficult for an athlete to focus on the areas that are holding him or her back because most of us developed our strengths in our favorite training areas. The smarter athlete is constantly addressing his or her limiters.

It is important to understand your present fitness needs in order to make wise training decisions. You must be totally honest with yourself in assessing your strengths and limiters.

Using a scale of 1 to 5, with 1 being the "worst" and 5 being the "best," rate your swim, bike, and run proficiencies. A score of 5 means that you are among the best, 3 indicates average for your category, and 1 places you at the bottom of the category.

First, you must determine what is holding you back. Second, you need to rate your endurance, force, and speed skills, using the same scale, for each sport. When doing this, you must first identify the elements of fitness that are necessary for success in your goal event. For example, if the bike course has lots of hills and your cycling force is not very good, then bike force is a race-specific limiter for you. You may have found that your strength lies in shorter events, but you struggle just to finish an Ironman-distance race. This problem would indicate that endurance is a limiter, so your training plan should focus on endurance first before moving on to muscular endurance.

Also consider a focused strength training program. Athletes who are new to cycling as well as female and veteran athletes have much to gain from a properly constructed strength program. Bike strength responds well to weights, followed by muscular endurance bike work. Seated hills and big-gear cycling are also a good way to build bike strength. Although cycling helps running, running does not appear to help cycling as much. In order to ride well, you need to ride quite a bit.

What follows are some final tips that can help you refine your limiters to better reflect your goals and experience. Please note that these are generalizations that will need to be interpreted in the context of your personal athletic history.

- If you are a novice, you should assume that your key limiters are overall force, endurance, and speed skills.
- If you are looking to improve your swim time, you should assume that your sole limiter is speed skills until you are able to swim 1,000 m in 19 min. or less.
- If you are looking to improve your bike times, you should establish your endurance, then focus on muscular endurance.
- If you are looking to improve your run times, you should remember that long-course running requires very little threshold speed (see the results sheet for any Ironman-distance race). What is required is the ability to swim and bike a long way at a solid aerobic pace without accumulating substantial fatigue. Overall endurance, race pace selection, and bike muscular endurance are the key factors for being able to run well in an Ironman-distance race.
- Whenever you are unsure whether your limiter is endurance or muscular endurance, it is best to focus on endurance. Likewise, when deciding whether additional base training or build training is required, it is best to choose additional base training.

IF THE SWIM IS YOUR LIMITER, THE ABILITIES THAT YOU LACK are more than likely endurance and speed skills. Thus, you will need to focus on stroke mechanics, balance, and endurance. If you want to improve swim-specific strength, rubber stretch cords are useful and available at swim supply and general sporting goods stores. It is essential to maintain excellent form at all times in the water. Working hard with poor form will very quickly lead you to a plateau, whereas working smart with excellent form is what leads to serious breakthroughs.

- Until your sport-specific performance is in the top quarter of your age group, you should continue to focus primarily on speed skills, overall body force, and endurance.
- Until your sport-specific performance is in the top 10 percent of your age group, there is little reason to perform aerobic endurance–type workouts.

When we make progress with our limiters, we realize greatly improved performance right away. It's just like the old saying: "A chain is only as strong as its weakest link." Once you determine your weakest link (greatest limiter), your performance will improve. If you continue to work only on your strengths, your chain (race performance) will never become stronger. Patience and focused training will sort out any limiter over time.

CRITICAL SUCCESS FACTORS

Highly motivated, intelligent endurance athletes are committed to doing what it takes to attain their goals. The role of a good coach (or book) is to guide and often temper your enthusiasm to the areas where you will get the most return for your efforts. This role is even more important for the self-coached athlete because quite often these areas are the most difficult and challenging. For Ironman-distance racing, the critical success factors are focus, nutrition, strong riding, and mental strength. Of course, endurance precedes all of these factors.

■ *Focus*

The ability to successfully execute a high-quality race requires an athlete to apply a "soft" focus for the majority of the day. Sitting on the start line, often with up to 2,000 fellow athletes, is a very challenging situation. Early in the day, superior performance results from focusing on holding oneself back. As the day progresses, this focus should shift to process management and maintaining an even effort. This level of racing includes eating, drinking, going to the bathroom, racing smart, controlling effort, and staying mentally strong. Typically, it is an athlete's process rather than his or her body that gives out during a race. Forgetting to eat, forgetting to drink, and riding faster than goal effort are examples of factors that can be controlled by an athlete. You can, and should, practice your ability to focus during training. It is a critical success factor for a solid race. Athletes who have trouble focusing should start with shorter, easier workouts and progress toward harder, longer races.

◼ *Nutrition*

Many athletes underestimate the role that nutrition plays in all aspects of physical performance. The path to elite nutrition is tough. However, if you want to race to your potential, then your body needs high-quality fuel. Remember the "Key Three" (covered in detail in Chapter 10):

1. Eliminate as many processed foods as possible.
2. Get the majority of your nutrition from lean protein, fresh veggies, and whole fruits.
3. Use starches and refined sugar in moderation, and only during and after training.

◼ *Strong Riding*

Cycling is the critical leg in Ironman-distance racing. You must do the necessary preparation to be able to push a strong gear in the flats. But first build your strength and endurance. The ability to ride 112 miles and then run a marathon requires a great deal of endurance. The better your cycling endurance, the more comfortable your ride will be and the more energy you will have for the run. Greater cycling endurance also helps to delay the onset and effects of fatigue.

Once you have established your endurance, you need to practice the ability to ride at a good pace for a long time in the flats. These are probably the most difficult sessions in which to maintain an even pace. They are also the best sessions for learning how to focus. These sessions can be done with other people, but you need to keep the momentum going for the duration of the ride. No talking, no long rests—these are not social sessions. These are Ironman-distance-specific training sessions. If you want to race well, these sessions are what it takes. There isn't a much harder session to do perfectly than a four- to six-hour steady ride in the flats because that is a very long time to concentrate.

◼ *Mental Strength*

If you maximize your mental strength you will find that you can use your training to develop patience, humility, and fortitude. Mental strength can often prevail over training and talent because it teaches you to "lean" against your breaking point. If you can learn your boundaries and slowly push against them, your mind can overcome the doubts that surface in training and racing. How do you do this? Well, you race more. After all, racing is a skill that must be practiced. We all benefit from enhancing our ability to push harder.

These pushing skills are not needed at the start of a race. Anyone can push at the start, and the smart athlete is the one who is able to show patience. The end of a race is when the smart athlete spends his or her mental strength, knowing that the most time is gained then. The hard fact is that if you slow at the end of the race, it is either your process (nutrition, hydration, and/ or pacing) or your mental strength that has let you down. You should not feel like you are "racing" before the middle of the marathon.

EMPHASIZE ENDURANCE

Emphasize endurance above all else in your first five to ten years of training. Elite and experienced athletes must rebuild and maintain this ability each season. Time in the saddle; long, steady-state riding; and consistency are key to building cycling endurance.

An athlete who has excellent swim endurance will be able to swim the Ironman distance (2.4 miles) comfortably without accumulating any material fatigue. So the goal is to build endurance while improving economy and relaxation. Only then does it make sense to shift a portion of training toward muscular endurance.

Running endurance plays a major role in distance-racing success. However, owing to how hard running is on the body and its greater potential for injury, it is not recommended that you run long more than once per week, or for more than two and a half hours. Frequency and improved running economy are the keys to improving running, and your run will also enjoy endurance benefits from cycling volume. Build your run volume by consistent run frequency and remember that exceptional durability dominates threshold speed.

Overall, Ironman-distance racing is not about being fast. It is about being able to swim smart, ride strong, and run tough. Many athletes believe that they need to run hard and run a lot to perform well. Run training is important, but it is not the key to success. As coaches, we fully believe the keys to endurance racing success are outlined in this chapter.

When evaluating your own fitness, remember that the most important aspect of a successful Ironman-distance race is superior endurance combined with a realistic pacing strategy. You can do very well by keeping your program simple and focusing on endurance, fundamental skills, and excellent nutrition.

CHAPTER 4

EQUIPMENT

*B*ikes, wheels, aerobars, wetsuits, heart rate monitors, trainers, power meters, computers. . . . If you follow the various discussions in our sport, you will see that endless time is devoted to analyzing the right training protocol, the right frame material, the right

> *It's not about the bike.*
>
> —LANCE ARMSTRONG,
> SEVEN-TIME TOUR DE FRANCE WINNER

wheel set, and so on. However, when you talk with elite performers and their coaches, you will discover that what it takes to succeed is a lot of consistent work over a very long time.

The role of the intelligent athlete is to channel this work into the most effective training schedule. Although some gear is necessary, there is no need to run out and spend your life savings on every gizmo on the market.

If you are a novice, the most important gear to begin with is a properly fitted wetsuit, a properly sized bike, good-quality running shoes, and a heart rate monitor. This chapter considers additional equipment that can help you improve your technique and build muscular endurance in training. These drills and strategies will be explained in more detail in Part II.

SWIMMING EQUIPMENT

■ *Choosing a Wetsuit*

There are many brands and styles of wetsuits to choose from. It is important that you base your choice on fit and comfort. All of the established manufacturers make good-quality products, so if your selected suit fits well, then you are unlikely to have problems.

First, you will need to decide between a sleeveless and a full-sleeved wetsuit. A good-fitting full suit is generally accepted as the faster choice. However, if you are more comfortable in a sleeveless suit, you are unlikely to be giving away much time. The sleeveless suit, or Long John, lets you maintain a better feel for the water. If you have a high stroke count or you consider yourself to be less strong in the swim, you may find a sleeveless wetsuit more comfortable.

Many athletes shy away from a tight fit when it comes to selecting a wetsuit; this can be a costly mistake. Ideally, your wetsuit should feel snug and almost uncomfortably tight when you are not in the water—it should be tight around the waist and legs, and there should be no leaks around the neck (and arms for a sleeveless suit). Once you are in the water and swimming, your suit will expand slightly and feel comfortable. If your wetsuit is not snug, you will experience drag and chafing during the swim.

In addition to ensuring that your suit fits correctly, it is important to take the time to put it on correctly. Even a correctly sized wetsuit can cause you to feel as if you are moving more slowly in the water if you aren't careful in how you wear it. Begin by working the neoprene slowly up your legs. Using socks helps to slide the suit over your feet, and rubbing a lubricant such as Body Glide or PAM on your shins (and forearms for a full suit) will make the pulling-on process a little easier and aid in a speedy removal after the swim. The wetsuit should pull up snugly against your crotch to allow the top to fit properly.

If you are wearing a full wetsuit, work it up your arms the same way that you worked it up the legs: slowly. There should be no air pocket between the suit and your armpit when your suit is on correctly. Any excess rubber will collect above your shoulder. For maximum range of motion, it is critical that you wear a full suit correctly.

■ *Other Equipment for Swimming*

There are many tools that you can use in your swim training to improve your stroke technique or build muscular endurance. Many triathletes make the mistake of incorporating swimming equipment into their training to compensate for specific limiters, such as balance and stroke technique. It is important that you consider how each tool is best used and revert to the drills in Chapter 6 to address specific limiters. You can risk injury if swimming tools are not used correctly in training.

Aside from short fins for balance and kicking drills, athletes are strongly encouraged to focus nearly all of their efforts on nongear swimming with a freestyle focus. Of the items listed in Table 4.1, the most useful swim equipment is a band/pull-buoy combination. Experienced

TABLE 4.1 SWIM EQUIPMENT

GEAR	PROS	CONS	USEFUL FOR	RISKY FOR
Band	Increased resistance	Reduces body rotation Legs drop	Building strength—typically in combination with pull-buoy Band-only swimming useful only for the strongest swimmers	Athletes with shoulder problems
Paddles	Increased feel for catch phase Increased feel for hand entry	Very easy to overload shoulders if stroke mechanics are not excellent	Building strength Learning proper catch phase Increasing hand speed through the water Building increased force Improving feel for water	Athletes with shoulder problems Athletes with poor stroke mechanics
Pull-buoy	Lifts hips Enables easier focus on front end of stroke	Removal of aid can result in poor body position	Building strength in combination with band Working on front-end stroke mechanics	Athletes with balance as a swim limiter

continued >

	TABLE 4.1 CONTINUED			
GEAR	**PROS**	**CONS**	**USEFUL FOR**	**RISKY FOR**
Fins	Enable faster speed through the water	Removal of aid can result in poor body position	Working on front-end stroke mechanics	Athletes with balance as a swim limiter
	Lift hips and enable better body position for a variety of drills		Recovery swimming	
			Long-axis drills	
			Fly-kick drills	
			Balance drills if a weak kicker (best with short fins)	
			Improving ankle flexibility	
Kickboard	Makes kick sets more comfortable	"Belly" flutter kick not swim-specific; most long-axis kicking occurs on the side	Variety of longer kick sets	

SOURCES
Laughlin, Terry. *Total Immersion*. New York: Fireside, 2004.
Maglischo, Ernest W. *Swimming Even Faster*. Mountain View, CA: Mayfield Publishing Company, 1993.
U.S.A. Swimming. *Progressions for Athlete and Coach Development*. Hong Kong: U.S.A. Swimming, 1999.

swimmers can use the band/pull-buoy in conjunction with three-stroke breathing to assist with swim-specific strength, stroke timing, and pull pattern. Remember that your most important swim sessions are distance freestyle workouts done with relaxed form and structured so that you are strong at the end.

CYCLING EQUIPMENT

■ *Choosing a Bike*

To some, the choices may seem daunting—makes, geometries, wheel sizes, wheel sets, frame materials, aerobars, saddles. Keep in mind that it takes most athletes a few frames to figure out what works for them.

Bike fit, which we will explore later in this chapter, is highly personal and you can have success with all geometries and frame materials. For racing and training long, always choose comfort over aero. If you are comfortable, you will stay more aero and run better off the bike. Comfort is really all that matters for your first few Ironman-distance races. By the time you are ready to get more serious, you will have logged many miles and know what style works best for you. So what choices are there?

Material

Many talk of frame materials such as titanium, carbon fiber, aluminum, and steel. It is generally accepted that carbon-fiber frames offer a more comfortable ride, titanium frames are the lightest, steel is the most responsive, and aluminum gives the harshest ride.

Although some materials have better vibration-dampening properties than others, it is worth remembering that if any material is used incorrectly, then the bike can have a harsh ride. That said, there is only one real consideration in choosing which frame to ride: fit. A properly fitting aluminum frame will be far more comfortable than a poorly fitting carbon-fiber frame.

Geometry

Now that you've chosen your frame material, your next decision is triathlon or road geometry. Once again—other than the obvious need for a safe bike for long-distance training and racing, comfort is your number-one goal. Road bikes are often the most comfortable, with a 73-degree seat-tube geometry. This arrangement is often referred to as a "relaxed" position, placing the rider a

---

EVEN IF YOUR GOAL IS SIMPLY TO FINISH an Ironman-distance race, you will be spending a lot of time in the saddle. Your first priority is to get a bike that fits. Some of the most common and expensive errors made by new triathletes start with their first bike purchase. Here are three things to remember:

Spend less than your budget. If you like the sport, you will want to upgrade and/or purchase race wheels and other accessories. You can drop a lot of money on your bike, and it is best to learn more about your needs before spending freely.

When purchasing a bike, consider only comfort, safety, and value. Don't get caught up in the debates on frame materials or the latest paint job. A mass-market bike from a reliable manufacturer is the safest bet for your first season.

Aerobars are the only cycling accessory you really need. Race wheels and other "go-faster" products can wait until you are more experienced. If you are not constrained by budget, then feel free to have a little fun with the toys. However, remember that strength training, a smart training program, and a set of aerobars are worth more than all the other aero devices combined.

You need only two triathletes to start a debate on frame materials, frame manufacturers, wheel sizes, shifting configurations, and any other part of the bike. If you notice the diversity of equipment and positions used in our sport, then you will quickly conclude that there are no right answers.

N   NOVICE

little farther back, and is the best climbing position. A bike with triathlon- or time trial–specific geometry is more "steep," at about 78 degrees. These bikes tend to be most comfortable (and efficient) when the rider is down on the aerobars.

It would be easier if we could all afford two bikes—one triathlon-specific and one with a road frame. Since that is not possible for most of us, consider your key races, overall comfort, and training terrain when selecting the geometry most appropriate for you.

Wheel Size

Once you have determined an appropriate frame and geometry, the best wheel size will be a function of fit. Never make a frame decision based on wheel size alone; the right wheel size for your height will normally be clear once you have decided on your other purchase variables.

Shifters

Your next option is shifters. The most versatile selection would be a moderate-geometry bike with drop handlebars and Shimano Total Integration (STI) shifting, which combines the shifters with the brake levers. On the other end of the spectrum, bullhorns and bar-end shifters are appropriate for race-specific and time trial–specific bikes.

Bullhorns and bar-end shifters are slightly faster for most riders on a flat course. However, keep in mind that bar-end shifters or bullhorns take a fair amount of skill to operate. Most novice athletes with bar-ends do not shift enough, which typically means they are pushing too high a gear. With the front chainrings, they frequently shift too late, a mistake that often results in dropped chains.

Over short hills, the efficient shifting and better power often more than make up for the slight aero disadvantage of an STI setup. Generally, the steeper setups that are appropriate for bullhorns make climbing more difficult. For this reason, most athletes will find that a more traditional road setup with clip-on aerobars is more powerful and comfortable in the hills. If you live in a hilly area, ride frequently with groups of roadies, or do a significant amount of nonaerobar riding, then you should consider STI shifting.

This final decision is a personal one, and no matter what you decide, there will be plenty of athletes who agree or disagree with your selection.

Pedals and Shoes

Pedal choices range from a small, light platform to a wider, heavier platform. Be aware that some athletes can develop foot or knee problems from certain brands of pedals. Unfortunately, the only way to find out is trial and error.

When purchasing cycling shoes, think comfort and ease of getting them on and off. Some shoes are vented, which is nice for riding and racing in hot locations. Cycling shoes should fit comfortably snugly, not tightly. When shopping for your shoes, it is best to shop at the end of the day or shortly after a long ride. Your feet swell naturally throughout the day, just as they do while riding. If your shoes fit very snugly at 9 a.m. in the bike shop, chances are they will be too snug 3 hours into your 5-hour ride.

Aerobars

There are several choices for aerobars on the market. The most durable ones are generally clip-on because they are easy to put on and take off and allow you the option of adjusting the elbow pads inward or outward. Many of the integrated aerobar setups can be unstable (due to the weight over the front wheel) and uncomfortable (due to the brakes being down and away from the rider). Most riders find that a flat, round base bar offers the most comfortable and versatile solution. As we turn our focus to bike fit, we will explore the use of aerobars in more detail.

Race Wheels

The next big debate is whether or not to use race wheels and disc wheels. Conventional wisdom is that a good set of race wheels will speed you up by 1–1.5 mph. The largest speed differential comes from swapping 32-spoked training wheels for a set of aerowheels. However, the greatest benefits of aerowheels arise only at speeds in excess of about 17 mph. There is limited benefit to using aerowheels if you don't have the muscular endurance to take advantage of their properties. For most triathletes, a power meter offers more performance gains than race wheels. Of course, you need to be willing to accept and interpret your power numbers.

An athlete needs to be quite a fast Ironman-distance rider to see a noticeable difference between a disc and a deep aerowheel. Still, if you are a strong rider, then a disc will, on average, be superior to any other wheel choice.

A set of deep-rim, or trispoke, aerowheels is an excellent all-purpose race wheel set. The only exception would be when riding in heavy or gusty crosswinds, as the front wheel can be difficult to control. Make sure that your skills and confidence match your wheel selection. It takes very little stress to lose the entire benefit of a flash set of wheels!

Helmet

Now that your bike is built, you may think you're ready to go. Not so fast! Above all else is safety. Never leave home without your helmet. Always choose an ANSI/CSI-approved helmet with plenty of vents for cooling, especially when racing in heat or humidity. Elite athletes may do well with a more aerodynamic, ventless helmet because they don't spend as much time on the bike and tend to be very lean. If you have difficulties in the heat, then choose a well-vented helmet for your races.

When shopping for a helmet, choose one that fits snugly but not too tightly, as your head can swell slightly in heat or when your core temperature is elevated. Look for one with finely adjustable sizing.

■ Bike Position

In setting up your position, remember that nothing matters as much as achieving one that is comfortable. Many triathletes start with a bike position that is too aggressive for their experience, flexibility, and body structure. "Aggressive" refers to the position of the shoulders relative to the hip joint. The lower the shoulders are relative to the hips, the more aggressive the position.

Even experienced athletes need to be very cautious with aggressive cycling positions, which require excellent flexibility. Many short-course athletes find their positions to be too extreme when they begin long-distance training and racing. All triathletes should remember that the rider accounts for almost all of the air resistance on the bike. Although aerowheels and frames can save time, the largest gains are made by making your body comfortable, powerful, and aerodynamic. This is the easiest form of speed available, and it's free! We will talk more about bike fit and how to achieve a safe, effective position later in this chapter.

There are four important starting points to any good long-distance bike position. In order of importance, they are:

1. *Safety:* The athlete is stable and able to control the bike easily.

2. *Comfort:* The athlete is comfortable and able to maintain the aero position for the duration of the ride. The transition from biking to running is smooth. A very aggressive position is useless if you can't hold it for the entire ride or have trouble running.

3. *Power:* The position enables the athlete to optimize power generation.

4. *Aerodynamics:* The position has superior aerodynamic properties.

For all athletes, there is a trade-off between power and aerodynamics. When you need to make a choice between these two, you are usually best served by choosing power. It takes a lot of aero to overcome any material loss in power.

Troubleshooting Your Lower Back Pain

Back pain is one of the most common ailments that affects long-distance triathletes. Not only is it uncomfortable, it is aerodynamically costly to sit up or come off the aerobars. If you suffer from back pain, there are four things you should consider.

Are you riding enough on the aerobars? You need to build experience with riding long periods on the bars without long breaks. In the final seven weeks before key races, insert long aerobar rides into your training plan. Briefly stretch every 15–20 min. while riding, but aside from that, spend the entire time on your aerobars. Even at an easy pace, these sessions are quite demanding.

How good is your flexibility? Tightness in the hips and pelvis is a leading cause of back pain. When back problems arise, a focused, consistent stretching program will help. This plan should encompass all of the main muscle groups of the hip region (hamstrings, hip flexors, back extensors, glutes, quads, adductors). Flexibility imbalances can be just as troublesome as a lack of flexibility. A simple flexibility progression is described in Chapter 9 (see Figures 9.32–9.42).

How are you treating hills? If you are at risk for back pain, you should always remain seated on climbs. Standing, particularly when pushing a big gear, will increase the strain through your lower back.

How hard do you ride early in the bike leg? The transition from swimming to cycling can be stressful on the body. Following an Ironman-distance swim, it is easy to lock up your hamstrings and irritate your back. Athletes at risk include those who tend to kick very hard when sighting. This places considerable strain on the low back; combine that with some hard early riding, and back pain can be the result.

Keep in mind that there is no right bike or right position. Correct position can vary considerably from one person to the next, even if they appear to be the same size. As the pros and elite age groupers show, a wide range of setups can be both comfortable and powerful. You may notice that many triathletes are very stretched out on their bike frames and have their elbows a long way in front of their shoulders.

■ Bike Fit

Bike fit starts from the feet up. After your cleats are set, adjust the saddle and then the handlebars. Once these three are correctly positioned, you will ride more economically and comfortably, which translates into faster bike splits.

The best way to get your bike set up for racing is to pay a professional bike fitter to do it. Look for one who has a lot of experience working with long-course triathletes, not one who usually fits roadies. If you investigate bike fitting, you will find that there are many opinions on the best way to accomplish an economical position, with several methodologies accompanied by certification. If you are new to Ironman-distance racing, don't get caught up in debate. Simply find someone who is respected by other athletes for his or her bike fitting and make an appointment. Then trust that person to do a good job for you. If you don't have a professional bike-fit specialist where you live and must do it yourself, then you will need to pay close attention to the following issues.

The methods described here are starting points for your eventual correct setup. You may want to experiment with adjustments, keeping in mind that it's best (and biomechanically safest) to make incremental changes. This approach is especially important if you have ridden in one position for a long time. A half-inch change in your saddle height, even though it may eventually improve your position, will feel strange at first and is likely to cause discomfort. You should avoid making more than quarter-inch adjustments every two weeks.

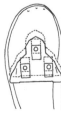
FIGURE *4.1*

Cleat Position

The starting point for cleat position is placement of the pedal axle somewhere between the ball of the foot and the middle of the arch. For long-distance time trials, we recommend that you consider moving the cleat slightly toward the heel (Figure 4.1). As the cleat is moved back, more force is transferred to the pedal and the calf's workload is decreased. This adjustment makes the transition to running easier. The trade-off is that cadence slows, which can result in an ultimate loss of power when sudden changes in velocity are necessary (this is not an issue for long-course triathlon). Start by making a quarter-inch adjustment from the midpoint of the ball of the foot and see how it feels after several rides.

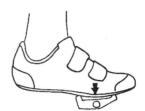

FIGURE *4.2*

Find the ball of your foot with your cycling shoes on, mark it on the side of each shoe, and adjust each cleat individually. On an indoor trainer, clip in to your pedals while someone checks to see if the marks are over the spindles. Aligning the marks with the axles puts you in the neutral position (Figure 4.2).

Saddle Position and Height

For an aero position, the correct saddle fore-aft adjustment depends on the length of your thigh and the flexibility of your hips and lower back. Establish a neutral saddle position by placing your bike on an indoor trainer. If your top tube still appears to be sloping, place a carpenter's level on the top tube or between the wheel axles to make the necessary adjustments. Spin for a few minutes to warm up. Then, with the pedal in the 3 or 9 o'clock position, drop a plumb line from the knob on the outside of your leg just below the knee (head of the fibula). When the line intersects the pedal axle (Figure 4.3), the saddle is neutral.

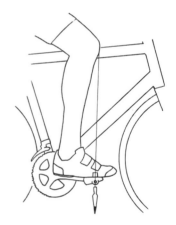

FIGURE *4.3*

Moving the saddle forward of neutral by as much as one-half inch may make you more comfortable and improve your power and aerodynamics. The saddle should be parallel to the floor, or slightly tipped down at the nose, for comfort. If your flexibility is excellent, and you opt for an aggressive handlebar position, then you may find that you slip forward slightly on your saddle. This can be corrected by giving the saddle a very slight upward tilt.

Your saddle height has the greatest effect on power output. The easiest way to make adjustments is to place yourself in the aero position and have your shoes unclipped. Place your unclipped heel on the pedal at the bottom of the stroke, crank arm lined up with the seat tube (Figure 4.4), and set the saddle to neutral position by adjusting the height until your knee is straight. Note that as the saddle goes up, it also moves back, and as it is lowered, it shifts forward slightly. For every 2 centimeters (cm) it moves up, it must also move forward about 1 cm. Likewise, if you lower it 2 cm, move it back by about 1 cm.

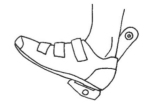

FIGURE *4.4*

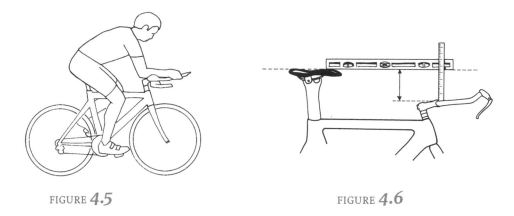

FIGURE **4.5**   FIGURE **4.6**

Handlebar Height, Reach, and Angle

One of the best investments you can make in setup equipment is an adjustable stem. It allows you to make a wide range of small changes in position to produce the most exact position needed for aerodynamics and comfort. It also allows for changes throughout the season.

When the armrests of the aerobars are about 1 inch below the high point of the saddle, you are in neutral position (Figure 4.5). Determine this point by extending a yardstick from the saddle top out to the armrest and leveling it with a carpenter's level. By measuring the distance between the yardstick and the armrest (Figure 4.6), you can set the stem height. Depending on your flexibility, the handlebars can be raised or lowered by an inch. As the handlebars are lowered, you may need to move the saddle forward, opening the angle between the thigh and trunk. Otherwise, you may experience discomfort in your hip region.

Correct handlebar reach, or stem length, places your ear over your elbow in the aero position. A rough gauge is that the distance from the nose of the saddle to the back of the handlebars should be about 1–1.5 inches longer than the distance from the back of your elbow to the end of your extended fingers.

When the up-and-down angle of the aerobars is neutral, the bottom of your hand is below the bend in your elbow, and the top of your hand is above it (refer back to Figure 4.5). As always, small adjustments from neutral may improve your comfort.

The Aggressive Fit

Stronger athletes with superior flexibility, lean bodies, and a good range of motion may want to consider a more aggressive race position. This section lays out a number of areas in which you can increase the race effectiveness of your setup and riding technique. We are grateful to John Cobb of Blackwell Research for his assistance and education.

Body position has a direct impact on power. More specifically, the most aerodynamic position is almost always inferior in terms of power generation. For a quick illustration, you will need an indoor trainer and a power meter. Place your bike on an indoor trainer and ride with the aerobar pads about two-thirds of the way back from your wrists. Increase the resistance to the point where you are putting out 350–400 watts; then move your arms until the aerobar pads are nearly under your elbows (stretching you out and making you more aero). You will instantly lose about 50 watts of power—you're working just as hard, but your watts will simply disappear. To put this in context, 50 watts of power can be up to 30 min. in an Ironman-distance bike leg. If you are a strong rider, learning to get the most out of your setup could be the difference between a podium finish and missing the rolldown.

Why such a clear loss of power? What happens is that the "longer" position takes out the large muscle groups of the upper body (arms, shoulders, and back) as well as reducing the impact of your core strength. You are unable to engage your full muscle mass and therefore lose power. In addition, for a given level of power output, your legs will be working harder. This is a key consideration for long-distance triathlon because you need to run when you leave the bike. Being able to effectively bring the upper body into the cycling leg gives you an advantage.

Remember that you can trade quite a bit of aero for a more powerful position. Powerful riders do not need to be as concerned with aerodynamics. For example, consider the success (and position) of riders such as Greg Bennett and Miguel Induráin.

Many aero positions can rob riders of valuable wattage. It's not so much the frame geometry as how the overall configuration relates to the rider's biomechanics. Experienced riders can sometimes improve their performance simply by changing their positions. For some athletes, this leads to a breakthrough, a new level in their riding. Just as in weight lifting, experienced athletes can overcome plateaus through a radical change in training stimuli.

Riders who change their position on the bike often overcome plateaus, if only because the change stimulates new muscular adaptations. If you have not reached a plateau, you can start with the traditional neutral time trial setup that we outlined in the previous section. A comfortable, traditional setup is probably the best starting point for most age-group triathletes.

Many athletes wonder how flat their backs need to be. What is optimal? Much has been written on the goal of getting the back flat, but remember that your goal should be to get your

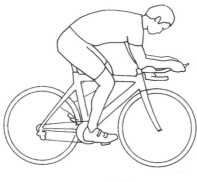

FIGURE *4.7*

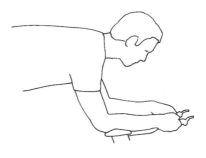

FIGURE *4.8*

scapula as flat as possible, not necessarily to get your shoulders as low as possible (Figure 4.7). The spine sits in a wind shadow behind the head, so as long as any arch in your back is behind your head, it is less important (especially if you are a more powerful rider). The more aggressive your position, the more likely you are to frequently come out of the aero position and the more stressful it will be on your digestion. Given that comfortable eating and drinking are fundamental to long-course race performance, you should be cautious with highly aggressive positions.

Where should you place your elbows? The elbows need only protect the legs. Much has been written regarding aerobar width. Until recently, the conventional wisdom was that the more narrow the elbows, the more aero the position. However, recent wind-tunnel analysis has shown that there is no need to get your pads nearly side by side. The distance between the elbows can be fairly wide so long as they shadow the legs. You can set this position by checking the placement of your elbow relative to your knee when at the top of your pedal stroke (12 o'clock). A wider elbow position opens the chest, with positive impacts on lung capacity and rider comfort.

Set your aerobar angle with reference to the bottom of the forearm (Figure 4.8). Throughout the bike-fit process, the goal is to minimize air disturbance over the body. This implies a forearm position parallel to the ground that avoids pushing any air down toward the legs. Go to any bike rack on race day, and you will see that there is a wide variation in aerobar height and forearm angle. Again, the prevailing belief has been that a slight upward angle (15 degrees) is best because it helps "guide" air down and around the body. The faster the air moves across the body, the better—and trying to "steer" the air is counterproductive.

Now that you've made all those adjustments, you won't want something like a bottle cage catching the air that you've worked so hard to avoid. The best type of bottle cage depends on your bike frame—most are better on the seat tube and behind the saddle. For bike frames where a behind-the-seat cage is superior to a frame mount, models that place the bottles low are the best choice. Ensure that your rear-mount cage doesn't leave your bottles sitting high and exposed to the wind coming off your back.

Ultimately, go with what feels right to you—meaning what is comfortable. Test your setup well in advance of race day, and resist the urge to go for the last few percentage points of aero. There are many stories of elite athletes who DNF key races owing to a little race week tinkering. Optimize your setup early in the season, and stick with it.

Finally, the "cleaner" your frame, the better. Front-end bottle mounts and gear and food bags are useful for novice athletes. However, these products create unnecessary drag. Check out the bikes of the most experienced riders, and you will see that they use as clean a setup as possible. But also bear in mind that if your fuel and fluids are difficult to reach, you may not take in enough on race day.

■ *Gearing*

As coaches, we often hear the question, "What gearing do you recommend?" Many new cyclists spend a lot of time in their big chainrings and use a gear at the top of the cluster. When confronted with a steep hill, they run out of gears and are forced to rapidly switch from the big chainring to the small chainring. Suddenly they are "spinning air" as the gear ratio dives—this is the leading cause of dropped chains in races. Learning how to efficiently shift is an essential skill for all athletes.

The big chainring can quite often seem smoother, which is one of the reasons that novice cyclists use it. However, developing good shifting habits will be an asset in your races. For elite athletes, the little things add up, and you won't want to give away any unnecessary time.

Recommended gearing is individual to each athlete's abilities as well as the topography of each individual racecourse. Before getting into general suggestions, let's first explain the gearing lingo.

The most common gearing on a bike with 700c wheels is 53/39 and 12–25. What does that mean? The first pair of numbers, separated by a slash, describes the number of teeth in the front chainrings. The second pair of numbers, separated by a dash, refers to the range of teeth in the rear cassette. As an example, if the big ring has 53 teeth and the small ring has 39 teeth, the gearing is 53/39. For the rear cassette, if the smallest cog has 12 teeth and the largest cog has 25 teeth, the gearing is 12–25.

To find out what gearing you currently ride, count the teeth on the two front chainrings. Next, count the teeth on the smallest gear and then the largest gear on your rear cluster.

Once you know what gearing you have, it's time to learn about how your gears are combined into an effective shifting pattern. For example, for a flat ride you may prefer the 53/21 with the big ring and the 39/15 with the small ring. By comparing the ratios, you can determine if you are riding the "same" gear. Let's illustrate with an example. Your biggest gear might be 53/11. That gives you a gear ratio of 4.82—for each turn of the cranks, the rear wheel will turn 4.82 times. Your smallest gear might be 39/25, giving you a gear ratio of 1.56—for each turn of the cranks, the rear wheel will turn 1.56 times.

When cyclists talk about "gearing up," they mean moving from a low gear ratio to a high gear ratio. New cyclists can find this terminology confusing because "gearing up" means shifting "down" the rear cluster (i.e., 53/15 is 3.53, and 53/11 is 4.82). Shift down the cluster (from the 15 to the 11) and therefore increase the gear ratio—you have "geared up." Gearing down is the same thing in reverse. Table 4.2 gives a sample shifting pattern for a basic shifting pattern. See the end of this chapter for a Web link to an online gearing calculator.

When it comes to race day, always try to ensure that you have a "bail-out" gear. You may not need or use that last gear, but having it can be your saving grace if your pacing gets off or you blow up late in the bike leg. On most North American Ironman courses, a 50/36 and 12–27 is generally enough gears for age-group athletes. Cyclists in the 5-hour range for an Ironman-distance bike split typically ride an 11–23 on the rear (with 53/39 on the front), and cyclists in the 6-hour range could use a 12–27. These figures are for the average athlete on an average course and refer to bikes with 700c wheels.

TABLE 4.2 STANDARD GEARING TABLE

GEARS ON REAR CASSETTE	SCR RATIOS	BCR RATIOS
23	1.70	2.30
21	1.86	2.52
19	2.05	2.79
17	2.29	3.12
16	2.44	3.31
15	2.60	3.53
14	2.79	3.79
13	3.00	4.08
12	3.25	4.42

SCR (small chainring) = 39 teeth
BCR (big chainring) = 53 teeth

The 53/19 and 39/14 gears are equivalent, so this is the point where the athlete should move between the big and small chainrings.

When gearing up, an athlete would shift from the 39/15 to the 53/19.

When gearing down, an athlete would shift from the 53/17 to the 39/14.

If you are a novice or you expect to be riding longer than 6 hours for your bike split, or if your racecourse is particularly hilly, then compact gearing is likely to prove best for you. With compact gearing, the front chainrings are reduced in size from 53/39 to 50/36 or another combination. When this configuration is combined with a 12–27 rear cassette, the athlete has a much easier time avoiding power and heart rate spikes in hilly terrain.

STANDARD GEARING	WHEEL	FRONT CHAINRING	REAR CASSETTE
Novice/6+ hour cyclist	700c	50/36	12–27
Novice/6+ hour cyclist	650c	53/39	12–27
Experienced/faster cyclist	700c	53/39	12–25
Experienced/faster cyclist	650c	55/42	12–25

■ Other Cycling Equipment

Stationary Trainers

There are several types of stationary trainers—rollers, wind, fluid, and magnetic resistance. Rollers are beneficial in learning proper balance and for spinning, and they are inexpensive. However, they do not simulate road riding and are easy to crash on. Wind, fluid, and magnetic-resistance trainers are more stable because you can lock your bike down on them. These are affordable options for indoor training during long winter months.

CompuTrainer

Although it exceeds most people's budgets, a CompuTrainer is an excellent tool for riders. It is an especially valuable addition to the training equipment for athletes who live in climates with nasty winters, are preparing for an early-season race, or have an excellent base. A CompuTrainer can be used for interval sessions and power testing, giving you immediate feedback that can be adjusted during the workout.

PowerCranks

The main benefit of PowerCranks (PC) is their impact on cycling economy. Economy is a tricky thing to evaluate because improvements in it are often obscured by changes in fitness. However, the major economy improvements come from closing the "dead spot" in the pedal stroke and in timing of the stroke—forcing your leg muscles to learn a correct firing pattern.

Athletes who are using PC should do regular speed-skills workouts to maintain muscular quickness. Athletes who tend to race with low cadences should supplement their PC use with spin-ups (high-cadence drills).

RUNNING EQUIPMENT

■ *Choosing Running Shoes*

After all the money spent on a bike, bike accessories, a wetsuit, and so on, you may tend to overlook running shoes. This is a mistake because good-quality shoes can help you to avoid injury and lost training time.

When choosing your shoes, consider your personal biomechanical issues, such as overpronation, supination, flat feet, and high arches. Next, address comfort. The quality of your fit can make the difference between happy feet and potential injury.

Be sure to go to a running specialty store where the salespeople are runners themselves. A good running store—not your average chain store—will let you run outside in the shoes to see how they feel. A staff member will also watch your gait and make suggestions. Choose the shoes that feel most comfortable to you—if they don't feel good at the shop, they won't feel better later at home.

As when shopping for cycling shoes, try to go late in the day after you've been on your feet a lot, as feet swell naturally throughout the day. Wear the same socks you normally run in to ensure that the shoes fit properly. If you use orthotics, then take them along as well. Ensure that there is a thumb's width between your big toe and the front of the shoe when standing.

Your shoes may be only a few months old or still have a lot of tread, but that doesn't necessarily mean they're still giving you the support you need. Shock absorption and support are usually the first things to go. You will want to ensure that your shoes are working for you because training for long-distance triathlons places a great deal of stress on your feet and body. Many foot and lower leg injuries are caused by poor-fitting or overly worn running shoes.

The general rule of thumb is to replace your shoes at least every six months or after one Ironman-distance race. You can also go by mileage—every 250–300 miles of running. To get the longest wear out of your shoes, it is wise to purchase two pairs and rotate them. Never do strength training in your current training shoes.

The life span of your shoes includes time spent walking in them; however, walking in your training shoes is not recommended. Once your shoes have reached the end of their safe training duration, they can be retired and become gym shoes. Also check with your local running-shoe store because some will buy back old shoes or donate them to charity.

Some athletes believe they need to change to a lighter or thinner shoe, such as a racing flat, for racing. This is acceptable for shorter races but quite risky for ultradistance racing because the risk of injury is far too great. A racing flat will save only a couple of grams in weight and 1 or 2 seconds per mile in pacing—hardly justifiable when the risk of injury and extended recovery time increases substantially. The marathon leg in an Ironman-distance triathlon is not the time to increase the stress on your legs.

Generally, it is best to race in the shoes that you train in. If your training shoe is heavy, then visit your local running-shoe store and experiment with shoes that may be a little lighter for racing. Ensure that your race choice offers you adequate support and comfort.

Be sure to purchase any new shoes well in advance of your A-priority race in order to break them in. We do not recommend running a marathon or half-marathon in brand-new shoes. Some suggest that you should have about 100 miles on new shoes before racing a marathon, although with modern shoes, two long runs is enough. For Ironman-distance racing, you would do well to get new shoes at the beginning of your Peak period. That will be enough time to ensure that they are broken in prior to the race while maintaining their shock absorption and support qualities throughout the race.

RACE WEAR

What to wear on race day is a common thread in triathlon discussions—skinsuits, trikinis, trishorts, regular cycling shorts? What works for one athlete may not necessarily work for another. Clothing should be chosen based on functionality and comfort as well as race climate and fitness levels. The longer the race distance, the more important comfort becomes.

A one-piece skinsuit is suitable for races up to a half-Ironman distance, for Ironman-distance races in hot or humid climates, or for elite athletes. A skinsuit will keep you cooler if you keep it wet by dumping water on yourself; however, it can become somewhat tedious to get in and out of when you make stops at the porta-potties.

A regular cycling jersey is comfortable and functional for long-distance racing. If you make this selection, then choose a material that aids in keeping you cool when wet. Jerseys can be worn under your wetsuit to save changing time in transition (but test before race day). If you plan on getting changed between the swim and the bike, then a full-zip jersey will be far easier to manage than trying to pull clothes over a wet body.

Where conditions are hot, you may want to consider a top with short sleeves (as opposed to a singlet) to reduce the amount of skin exposed to the sun. Recently, arm coolers have come on the market, and these can be useful for cooling as well as sun protection.

Trishorts are the most common choice. They have a slightly thinner chamois pad and can be worn for the entire race. Some athletes prefer regular cycling shorts because they offer more comfort on the long bike ride. Elite athletes often race in no more than a trikini or swimsuit. These have some thin padding; however, they are most suitable for those closer to the front of the pack who finish the bike early.

Whatever you choose to wear on race day, use it extensively in training.

TRAINING AIDS

■ *Heart Rate Monitors*

If there is one gizmo you need, it is a heart rate monitor (HRM). HRMs range in price and functionality from a basic model that simply shows your current heart rate to top-of-the-line models that record multiple variables and let you download all the information to your computer for graphing and further study.

Though the extra features can be fun, especially for the technically minded, the only features you really need are current heart rate, average heart rate, maximum heart rate, and average heart rate by split. A fifty-lap memory option is plenty for training needs.

Chapter 5 explains how to use your heart rate monitor in training.

■ *Power Meters*

Power-Tap

Second only to an HRM, a power-measurement device is very useful. The Power-Tap is a proven power meter. Training by power—or watts—provides more immediate feedback than training by heart rate and lets you know whether your efforts are having an effect on performance.

When combined with an indoor trainer and portable lactate analyzer, a wireless Power-Tap wheel provides the athlete with a mobile physiological testing lab. Training with power is discussed in more detail in Chapter 7.

SRM

The SRM training system is similar to the Power-Tap and is used for collecting and analyzing power data while cycling. The system measures pedal rate, torque, and power output. It also displays and records heart rate, cadence, wheel speed, distance covered, ambient temperature, and energy expenditure. Though it is more expensive than the Power-Tap, the SRM can be used with any wheel configuration.

Ironman Training

PART II

5

TRAINING OVERVIEW

O ur goal for this chapter is to give you a crash course in training. We assume that you have relied on at least a few sources
and experts in your triathlon pursuit thus far, and what follows will
probably sound familiar. Our approach is rooted in the tradition of
periodization, which takes on new meaning and importance when training for an Ironman-
distance triathlon.

> *Be strong at the end.*
>
> —DAVE SCOTT,
> SIX-TIME IRONMAN WORLD CHAMPION

ANNUAL TRAINING PLAN

It is possible to be a successful triathlete racing shorter distances without a formal training plan.
For obvious reasons, this strategy becomes less feasible as you become more competitive and
race in Ironman-distance triathlons. An annual training plan (ATP) will significantly improve
your chances of both finishing and performing to your best abilities if you carefully plan out
every block and period of your training. If you are training for your first Ironman-distance
event, you will find that a race of this length involves different considerations that will cause
your ATP to vary from previous years and races.

In building your ATP, you should always interpret our advice in light of your own experience and personal limiters. Remember that your ultimate success will be built on a platform
of endurance, strength, and skill development. When in doubt, always refer back to the basics.

If you know the basics and put them into practice, you will have a solid foundation for performance and longevity in triathlon.

■ *Preparation Period*

The period of training between the Transition (off-season) and the early Base periods is the Prep period. Most athletes will have a Prep period that lasts from four to twelve weeks. The exact length of your Prep period will depend on the timing of your first A-priority race and your experience in the sport. For Ironman-distance racing, the training done in the Prep and early Base periods is essential because your ability to absorb the challenging sessions that will occur later in the season is directly related to the depth of fitness that you establish early in the season. Without adequate preparation, your late-season training will flatten, rather than lift, your performance.

The main purpose of the Prep period is to ease the body back into structured training, develop a training strategy for the upcoming season, prepare the body for the increasing requirements of the Base period, and improve fundamental and technical skills. The general physiological adaptations that this period is intended to bring about are renewed cardio-respiratory (heart, blood, lungs) fitness through easy aerobic exercise; improved economy of movement through speed-skills development; improved metabolic efficiency; and greater total body strength through weight lifting as well as rubber cords, isometrics, and other resistance exercises.

Athletes who use a shorter Prep period should maintain a training emphasis on session frequency while keeping the duration and intensity of sessions low to moderate. This approach will enable the body to become reacquainted with structured training and ensure recovery from the previous season's efforts. Most athletes find that their bodies take four to six weeks to adjust back to structured training. It is important to remember that you are rebuilding fitness and to be patient with yourself rather than expecting to instantly return to the level of fitness you had achieved by the end of your previous season. In order to develop beyond previous highs, it is necessary to slow down and lay the foundations for continued development.

Athletes who use a Prep period of eight or more weeks may find that they are ready to start some longer endurance sessions after the four- to six-week initial adaptation period. Remember to keep these sessions reasonable in duration and to slowly stretch your endurance abilities.

Athletes with a longer Prep period should consider slowly building their weekly volume to achieve a smooth transition to the Base 1 period. Athletes targeting a late-season peak, novice athletes, and athletes living in climates with severe winters should consider an extended Prep period. The main benefits of this approach are a reduction in the risk of burnout and an increase in skill levels.

Early in the Prep period, sessions should be relatively short and skills-oriented. It's also a good idea to include a considerable amount of cross-training activities, such as hiking, mountain biking, and cross-country skiing. These sessions should gradually stretch your endurance while keeping training intensity low and developing general fitness. Athletes who face climatic challenges (rain, cold, snow, and wind) should feel free to substitute alternative forms of indoor aerobic activity.

Weekly volume should be comfortable, typically two to five hours less than what you believe you can handle. Despite the lower volume, a recovery week is still recommended to maintain mental freshness and ensure continual physical adaptation. Typically just one recovery week, the last week before the Base period begins, is sufficient. This time can be used for testing.

> **HIGHLY MOTIVATED ATHLETES MAY BE TEMPTED** to increase the intensity and duration of their key sessions. Particularly in the first Prep block of the year, training at such levels is counterproductive. It's not possible to maintain race fitness throughout the year. Attempting to do so will only lead to overtraining, burnout, or injury.

Early in the Prep period, testing should be aerobic in nature. Athletes wishing to test functional threshold values should wait until later in the Prep period or until the early Base period. The end of the fourth week of Prep training is a good time to establish your baseline functional threshold data because the results of these tests will allow you to gauge your progress in the months ahead.

■ *Base Period*

Once you have completed the Prep period, you are ready for the Base period. The Base period is the most critical for Ironman-distance racing. It is during this time of year that the athlete develops the three most important elements of performance: endurance, force, and speed skills. If these abilities, especially endurance and strength (force), are underdeveloped in the Base period, then race-specific fitness will suffer and the challenging workouts of the Build period will not lead to better performance. Coaches and athletes often use the analogy of a triangle—the broader the bottom of the triangle (Base), the higher the peak.

TWO THINGS TO REMEMBER
WHEN PLANNING YOUR SEASON:

1. You can race fast on Base alone.
2. Only the strongest athletes are
   able to handle more than one
   Build period.

After this base of fitness is laid down, the Build period begins, with workouts that specifically prepare you for the demands of your event.

■ Build Period

When you are training for an Ironman-distance race, the training in the late Base and Build periods will be essentially the same, but, as the name suggests, volume increases in the Build period. The purpose of the Build period is to specifically prepare for the demands of an A-priority race that will last from 8 to 17 hours. That means a lot of endurance and muscular endurance work plus force training under conditions that mimic the targeted race's course. By this time the training should be focused on race-simulation workouts that target your specific

Finishing Your Build Period

The Build period ends with a race-simulation workout, typically 2.5–3.5 hours on the bike, followed by 90 min. of running. If it's convenient, you may choose to swim before the bike. However, the swim is not essential.

If you are working on improving your endurance or you are a novice, your pace in the race-simulation workouts should begin in Zone 1, building to Zone 2. Increase your volume, planning your workout for closer to 3.5 hours to balance the lower intensity.

If you find yourself with a strong endurance base leading into this race-simulation workout, you should still hold back at the start of the bike. You will be rested and likely think that you can go faster. It is an excellent time to practice the discipline that you will need on race day during

the early part of the bike. After the first 15 miles on the bike, gradually build to a pace faster than Ironman-distance race pace. The last 15 minutes of the bike should be done fast, in Zone 5. Push a big gear and ride fast.

The bike-to-run transition should be a race simulation as well. Get all of your gear in a bag as quickly as possible.

If you rode strong, your legs will be loaded and stiff as you begin your run—just like on race day. For the first 2–3 miles, focus on a high cadence and getting your step back. Then sit in Zone 3 (faster than Ironman-distance pace). Finish the last 30 min. of the run working at the top of Zone 3 to Zone 4.

Post-workout recovery food and stretching are very important in race-simulation workouts.

limiters. We recommend that you hold off on race-simulation workouts until after you are confident in your endurance.

For an experienced athlete, the key physiological limiter is nearly always cycling muscular endurance. See Chapter 7 for a summary of key workouts for the Build period designed to enhance race performance.

When you are in Build period training, it is important to remember that your key focus should be preparing your body to race well over the duration and specific terrain of your A-priority race. You should schedule one or two race-simulation workouts each week. Typically, you will do only four to seven of these key race-simulation workouts, so you should ensure that you are fully prepared for each session.

> **OPEN-WATER SWIMS ARE A USEFUL ADDITION** to your Build period swim program. Do these with a partner, and practice race tactics, including pacing and drafting.

With the approach of your A-priority race, you will likely have the urge to increase your training volume above the levels recommended in this book and "test" your fitness. Remember that your race performance will be dictated by the duration and intensity of your key workouts, not your total weekly volume. In fact, if you are doing your race-simulation sessions properly, you will probably find that you need more recovery time in your Build period than during any other time of the training year.

■ Peak Period

The goal of the Peak period is to start the process of bringing you to a physiological peak for your Ironman-distance race. The two most important elements of this period are intensity and recovery. The Peak period is discussed in detail in Chapter 14. Be sure to resist the urge to do "one last" megaworkout.

■ Race Period

There is one goal for all athletes during race week—to arrive at the start line fit, fresh, and focused. Race week is discussed in detail in Chapter 15.

■ Post-race Recovery

One of the most common mistakes an athlete makes after an A-priority race is to return to long training sessions too quickly. Even at a very easy pace, long sessions can leave you feeling spent.

It is common to start feeling quite strong ten to fourteen days after an Ironman-distance race. You are likely experiencing the tail end of your peak. Don't let your mind trick you regarding the level of deep fatigue that accumulates during a long race. Even if you ended up "going easy" at the end of the race, the likely reason was that you were exhausted. At the end of the season, many athletes have small biomechanical problems from either their race or their training. Rest, unstructured light activity, massage, and flexibility work are the quickest path to a return to normal training.

Most athletes hit a second wave of fatigue the third week after an A-priority race, so there is nothing to be gained from rushing back to training. If you feel great, you could include some 30- to 60-min. sessions (for a total daily volume under 1 hour) of heart rate Zone 1 swimming or cycling, or start with some easy weight lifting.

If you give your body a chance to heal, you will find that it starts rebuilding itself sometime in the first two to four weeks after an Ironman-distance race. At that stage, you will realize just how tired you were. Your mind will try to convince you that you are different from everyone else, that you need less recovery. However, history has shown that almost everyone is best served by resting. Rushing recovery is a false economy. When your body needs to rest, it will take the rest that it needs by any means necessary. Fatigue, illness, burnout, and injury are clues that additional rest is required.

■ Transition Period

After four to eight weeks of unstructured training, you will sense that you are ready to start back on your program. When coming back from a training break, emphasize frequency rather than duration or intensity. Simply put, frequency is your friend. Your aerobic systems will not be accustomed to structured training, and you will be many months away from your next key race. Therefore, you should focus on three simple goals:

1. Stimulate your aerobic pathways.
2. Maintain your skill base.
3. Start the process of rebuilding the strength that you lost over your break.

Even if you are gearing up for another Ironman-distance race, you should keep your focus on these three areas for your first block of structured training.

It is normal to gain some weight in the Transition period, often from a mixture of getting down to race weight and then slacking off on nutrition. The more control you are able to show in your nutrition, the less you will have to lose once you get back on your program. Some athletes gain as much as twenty pounds during this period. However, by following the "Key Three" (which we'll expand on in Chapter 10), you can avoid the difficulties associated with trying to shed your off-season pounds. Athletes who are quick to gain (and slow to lose) weight would be well advised to follow the "Key Three" at all times.

You will lose aerobic fitness during your Transition break. This deterioration is normal, and you should expect to see material losses in strength when you come back. Stay calm—we bounce back quickly, so the slowness and weakness should be temporary.

Long breaks are costly in fitness terms. If you feel sickness or fatigue coming on, it is wise to immediately take off one or two days. There is a real fitness cost if you lose a week owing to illness. Consistent training is the easiest way to long-term improvement. Learn from unplanned setbacks, and consider their root causes. Many athletes will be coming off a lot of racing and more than likely pushed themselves very hard in their final A-priority race. Ironman-distance fatigue is unlike any other sort of fatigue you will have experienced (except maybe in ultra-marathons), and it takes a long time to clear. All athletes face this issue. The more motivated you are, the more you'll need to hold back.

The overall goal of the Transition period is mental and physical rejuvenation. This means if you feel like doing nothing, that is okay.

BALANCED TRAINING

Each period and week of your ATP will vary, emphasizing volume, intensity, and frequency at different times and in different ways to bring about your optimal level of fitness. The ATP periods we've described here map out an approach to periodized training that we've found to be highly successful for triathletes. There are as many different approaches to volume, intensity, and frequency as there are athletes. In general, novice athletes should focus on frequency over volume and intensity. The shorter the race distance, the more important intensity becomes. There are many different approaches to volume as well. There are no hard-and-fast rules, as there are examples of successful athletes using a wide range of protocols.

■ *Volume*

Most competitors will compete in no more than one Ironman-distance race per year, and it's normally timed for the end of their local race season. A few athletes will do two, but they are normally close together (the so-called double), which is effectively the same thing. Only a very small number of athletes actually do two or more Ironman-distance races a year, distributed throughout the year, because these competitions usually involve significant travel and expense. Of that number, the majority are "social" competitors—in it more for the lifestyle than for serious competition. This leaves only a few hard-case "nuts" who actually race Ironman distance every four to six months or so and are thus always building on a retained base.

For most people, doing one major long-course race a year allows them to start from scratch at the end of the off-season, compete in shorter events early in the season, work to pay the bills, and so on. Only at crunch time, having rebuilt the base needed to deal with the next step, do they make the commitment to train for their impending race. The key commitment period is the final eleven weeks of training because the training in this period will have the greatest impact on your ultimate race performance. The more thorough your preparations leading up to this period, the higher the quality of your final preparations, and therefore the greater the probability of superior race performance.

The volume that is appropriate for you depends upon your base, the time of year, your nontriathlon obligations, and your physiology. Each year, construct your plan with a little less volume than you think you can handle. Once you have eight to twelve weeks of training behind you, take a second look at volume and adjust it based on your recovery experience. When you are operating at the limits of your recovery abilities, even one or two extra training hours can push you over the edge.

Be particularly careful with your running volume. Many athletes run far too much for Ironman-distance racing. Remember that the best place to build endurance and aerobic fitness is on your bike. Running beats you up, and the greatest challenge for most folks training for Ironman-distance racing is how fast they can recover. There should be a specific purpose to each run session. Remember that there is no such thing as a "recovery run." Recovery sessions should be non-impact-oriented.

When training at high volume, most athletes can handle only one high-intensity session a week. High intensity will vary for everyone according to experience and fitness, but for most people it means threshold or above-threshold (anaerobic) work. You will find that threshold and anaerobic exercise greatly increase your recovery needs. This type of training also increases the risks of burning out, illness, and injury. The deeper your base, the better your recovery, and the lower your nontraining stress, the higher your tolerance to intensity will become.

For your first Ironman-distance race, you should build gradually toward a target of three key sessions each week (one for each sport): one long swim of 75–100 min., one long ride of 4–6 hours followed by a 20- to 30-min. transition run, and one long run of 90–150 min. Everything else is filler.

Training on a four-week cycle, your schedule may look something like this:

WEEK 1	BIKE AND SWIM EMPHASIS

Include one extra swim and one extra ride; for your running, the key workouts would be a transition run, a long run, and an aerobic run that ends with a strides session.

WEEK 2	RUN EMPHASIS

Include an extra run this week, and have the additional session focus on your greatest running limiter—for most athletes, that would be a moderate-duration endurance session. As the season progresses, this session could include some muscular endurance training.

WEEK 3	BIKE AND SWIM EMPHASIS

Repeat week 1.

WEEK 4	RECOVERY

Maintain your workout frequency, but at 50 percent of training week volume, and schedule some testing toward the end of the week (see Table 5.4 and also refer to Appendix B).

▪ *Time Versus Distance*

When scheduling your weekly workouts, think in terms of total training time, not distance traveled. To illustrate, an 8-mile run could be an aerobic maintenance session for an elite athlete, whereas the same distance would be a tough endurance session for a novice. Distance is even less relevant for cycling, where terrain, wind, and road surface all have an impact on the nature of a ride. Tables 5.1 and 5.2 provide suggested daily and weekly training hours for riding and running. Do the time, and the miles will fall into place come race day.

You will find that you get the best results by separating your longest run from your longest ride. Avoid the monster weekends that many people recommend. Put your long run midweek and your long ride on the weekend for effective recovery. Scheduling a long ride on Sunday, a long swim on Friday, and a long run on Wednesday will give you plenty of recovery time.

IF IN DOUBT, LEAVE IT OUT. Most first-timers spend the majority of their training year tired. The focus should be on your key workouts and recovering. Success is correlated to the duration and intensity of your key sessions, not your total volume.

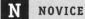 **NOVICE**

Remember that your greatest time gains will come from focusing on your limiters. Your endurance requirement is to be able to swim 4,000 m, bike five to seven hours, and have the ability to run a marathon. Until you have the aerobic fitness for this task, "going hard" is a wasted opportunity for further endurance training.

TABLE 5.1 DAILY TRAINING HOURS							
WEEKLY HOURS	LONGEST RIDE			May be two-a-day workouts			
3:00	1:30	0:45	0:45	off	off	off	off
3:30	1:30	1:00	1:00	off	off	off	off
4:00	1:30	1:00	1:00	0:30	off	off	off
4:30	1:45	1:00	1:00	0:45	off	off	off
5:00	2:00	1:00	1:00	1:00	off	off	off
5:30	2:00	1:30	1:00	1:00	off	off	off
6:00	2:00	1:30	1:00	1:00	1:00	off	off
6:30	2:00	1:30	1:00	1:00	1:00	off	off
7:00	2:00	1:30	1:30	1:00	1:00	off	off
7:30	2:30	1:30	1:30	1:00	1:00	off	off
8:00	2:30	1:30	1:30	1:30	1:00	off	off
8:30	2:30	2:00	1:30	1:30	1:00	off	off
9:00	3:00	2:00	1:30	1:30	1:00	off	off
9:30	3:00	2:00	1:30	1:30	1:00	0:30	off
10:00	3:00	2:00	1:30	1:30	1:00	1:00	off
10:30	3:00	2:00	2:00	1:30	1:00	1:00	off
11:00	3:00	2:00	2:00	1:30	1:30	1:00	off
11:30	3:00	2:30	2:00	1:30	1:30	1:00	off
12:00	3:00	2:30	2:00	2:00	1:30	1:00	off
12:30	3:30	2:30	2:00	2:00	1:30	1:00	off
13:00	3:30	3:00	2:00	2:00	1:30	1:00	off
13:30	3:30	3:00	2:30	2:00	1:30	1:00	off

continued >

TABLE 5.1 CONTINUED

WEEKLY HOURS	LONGEST RIDE	May be two-a-day workouts					
14:00	4:00	3:00	2:30	2:00	1:30	1:00	off
14:30	4:00	3:00	2:30	2:30	1:30	1:00	off
15:00	4:00	3:00	3:00	2:30	1:30	1:00	off
15:30	4:00	3:00	3:00	2:30	2:00	1:00	off
16:00	4:00	3:30	3:00	2:30	2:00	1:00	off
16:30	4:00	3:30	3:00	3:00	2:00	1:00	off
17:00	4:00	3:30	3:00	3:00	2:00	1:30	off
17:30	4:00	4:00	3:00	3:00	2:00	1:30	off
18:00	4:00	4:00	3:00	3:00	2:30	1:30	off
18:30	4:30	4:00	3:00	3:00	2:30	1:30	off
19:00	4:30	4:30	3:00	3:00	2:30	1:30	off
19:30	4:30	4:30	3:30	3:00	2:30	1:30	off
20:00	4:30	4:30	3:30	3:00	2:30	2:00	off
20:30	4:30	4:30	3:30	3:30	2:30	2:00	off
21:00	5:00	4:30	3:30	3:30	2:30	2:00	off
21:30	5:00	4:30	4:00	3:30	2:30	2:00	off
22:00	5:00	4:30	4:00	3:30	3:00	2:00	off
22:30	5:00	4:30	4:00	3:30	3:00	2:30	off
23:00	5:00	5:00	4:00	3:30	3:00	2:30	off
23:30	5:30	5:00	4:00	3:30	3:00	2:30	off
24:00	5:30	5:00	4:30	3:30	3:00	2:30	off
24:30	5:30	5:00	4:30	4:00	3:00	2:30	off
25:00	5:30	5:00	4:30	4:00	3:00	3:00	off
25:30	5:30	5:30	4:30	4:00	3:00	3:00	off
26:00	6:00	5:30	4:30	4:00	3:00	3:00	off
26:30	6:00	5:30	5:00	4:00	3:00	3:00	off
27:00	6:00	6:00	5:00	4:00	3:00	3:00	off

continued >

TABLE 5.1 CONTINUED

WEEKLY HOURS	LONGEST RIDE	May be two-a-day workouts					
27:30	6:00	6:00	5:00	4:00	3:30	3:00	off
28:00	6:00	6:00	5:00	4:00	3:30	3:30	off
28:30	6:00	6:00	5:00	4:30	3:30	3:30	off
29:00	6:00	6:00	5:30	4:30	3:30	3:30	off
29:30	6:00	6:00	6:00	4:30	3:30	3:30	off
30:00	6:00	6:00	6:00	4:30	4:00	3:30	off
30:30	6:00	6:00	6:00	5:00	4:00	3:30	off
31:00	6:00	6:00	6:00	5:00	4:00	4:00	off
31:30	6:00	6:00	6:00	5:00	4:30	4:00	off
32:00	6:00	6:00	6:00	5:30	4:30	4:00	off
32:30	6:00	6:00	6:00	5:30	4:30	4:30	off
33:00	6:00	6:00	6:00	5:30	5:00	4:30	off
33:30	6:00	6:00	6:00	6:00	5:00	4:30	off
34:00	6:00	6:00	6:00	6:00	5:30	4:30	off
34:30	6:00	6:00	6:00	6:00	5:30	5:00	off
35:00	6:00	6:00	6:00	6:00	6:00	5:00	off

TABLE 5.2 WEEKLY TRAINING HOURS

		ANNUAL HOURS									
PERIOD	WEEK	200	250	300	350	400	450	500	550	600	650
Prep	All	3.5	4.0	5.0	6.0	7.0	7.5	8.5	9.0	10.0	11.0
Base 1	1	4.0	5.0	6.0	7.0	8.0	9.0	10.0	11.0	12.0	12.5
	2	5.0	6.0	7.0	8.5	9.5	10.5	12.0	13.0	14.5	15.5
	3	5.5	6.5	8.0	9.5	10.5	12.0	13.5	14.5	16.0	17.5
	4	3.0	3.5	4.0	5.0	5.5	6.5	7.0	8.0	8.5	9.0
Base 2	1	4.0	5.5	6.5	7.5	8.5	9.5	10.5	11.5	12.5	13.0
	2	5.0	6.5	7.5	9.0	10.0	11.5	12.5	14.0	15.0	16.5
	3	5.5	7.0	8.5	10.0	11.0	12.5	14.0	15.5	17.0	18.0
	4	3.0	3.5	4.5	5.0	5.5	6.5	7.0	8.0	8.5	9.0
Base 3	1	4.5	5.5	7.0	8.0	9.0	10.0	11.0	12.5	13.5	14.5
	2	5.0	6.5	8.0	9.5	10.5	12.0	13.5	14.5	16.0	17.0
	3	6.0	7.5	9.0	10.5	11.5	13.0	15.0	16.5	18.0	19.0
	4	3.0	3.5	4.5	5.0	5.5	6.5	7.0	8.0	8.5	9.0
Build 1	1	5.0	6.5	8.0	9.0	10.0	11.5	12.5	14.0	15.5	16.0
	2	5.0	6.5	8.0	9.0	10.0	11.5	12.5	14.0	15.5	16.0
	3	5.0	6.5	8.0	9.0	10.0	11.5	12.5	14.0	15.5	16.0
	4	3.0	3.5	4.5	5.0	5.5	6.5	7.0	8.0	8.5	9.0
Build 2	1	5.0	6.0	7.0	8.5	9.5	10.5	12.0	13.0	14.5	15.5
	2	5.0	6.0	7.0	8.5	9.5	10.5	12.0	13.0	14.5	15.5
	3	5.0	6.0	7.0	8.5	9.5	10.5	12.0	13.0	14.5	15.5
	4	3.0	3.5	4.5	5.0	5.5	6.5	7.0	8.0	8.5	9.0
Peak	1	4.0	5.0	6.0	7.0	7.5	8.5	9.5	10.5	11.5	11.5
	2	3.5	4.0	5.0	5.5	6.0	7.0	7.5	8.5	9.0	10.0
Race	All	3.0	3.5	4.0	4.5	5.0	5.5	6.0	7.0	7.0	8.0
Tran	All	3.0	3.5	4.5	5.0	5.5	6.5	7.0	8.0	8.5	9.0

continued >

TABLE 5.2 CONTINUED

		ANNUAL HOURS										
PERIOD	WEEK	700	750	800	850	900	950	1,000	1,050	1,100	1,150	1,200
Prep	All	12.0	12.5	13.5	14.5	15.0	16.0	17.0	17.5	18.5	19.5	20.0
Base 1	1	14.0	14.5	15.5	16.5	17.5	18.5	19.5	20.5	21.5	22.5	23.5
	2	16.5	18.0	19.1	20.0	21.5	22.5	24.0	25.0	26.0	27.5	28.5
	3	18.5	20.0	21.5	22.5	24.0	25.5	26.5	28.0	29.5	30.5	32.0
	4	10.0	10.5	11.0	12.0	12.5	13.5	14.0	14.5	15.5	16.0	17.0
Base 2	1	14.5	16.0	17.0	18.0	19.0	20.0	21.0	22.0	23.0	24.0	25.0
	2	17.5	19.0	20.0	21.5	22.5	24.0	25.0	26.6	27.5	28.8	30.0
	3	19.5	21.0	22.5	24.0	25.0	26.5	28.0	29.5	31.0	32.0	33.5
	4	10.0	10.5	11.5	12.0	12.5	13.5	14.0	15.0	15.5	16.0	17.0
Base 3	1	15.5	17.0	18.0	19.0	20.0	21.0	22.5	23.5	25.0	25.5	27.0
	2	18.5	20.0	21.5	23.0	24.0	25.0	26.5	28.0	29.5	30.5	32.0
	3	20.5	22.0	23.5	25.0	26.5	28.0	29.5	31.0	32.5	33.5	35.0
	4	10.0	10.5	11.5	12.0	12.5	13.5	14.0	15.0	15.5	16.0	17.0
Build 1	1	17.5	19.0	20.5	21.5	22.5	24.0	25.0	26.5	28.0	29.0	30.0
	2	17.5	19.0	20.5	21.5	22.5	24.0	25.0	26.5	28.0	29.0	30.0
	3	17.5	19.0	20.5	21.5	22.5	24.0	25.0	26.5	28.0	29.0	30.0
	4	10.0	10.5	11.5	12.0	12.5	13.5	14.0	15.0	15.5	16.0	17.0
Build 2	1	16.5	18.0	19.0	20.5	21.5	22.5	24.0	25.0	26.5	27.0	28.5
	2	16.5	18.0	19.0	20.5	21.5	22.5	24.0	25.0	26.5	27.0	28.5
	3	16.5	18.0	19.0	20.5	21.5	22.5	24.0	25.0	26.5	27.0	28.5
	4	10.0	10.5	11.5	12.0	12.5	13.5	14.0	15.0	15.5	16.0	17.0
Peak	1	13.0	14.5	15.0	16.5	17.0	18.0	19.0	20.0	21.0	21.5	22.5
	2	10.5	11.5	12.0	13.0	13.5	14.5	15.0	16.0	16.5	17.0	18.0
Race	All	8.5	9.0	9.5	10.5	11.0	11.5	12.0	13.0	13.0	13.5	14.5
Tran	All	10.0	10.5	11.5	12.0	12.5	13.5	14.0	15.0	15.5	16.0	17.0

■ *Intensity*

It is important to remember that training at the highest intensities year-round is ultimately detrimental to performance because you will wind up sick, injured, burned-out, or overtrained. Intensity levels during the bulk of your training should be devoted to building or maintaining endurance and strength. There are many ways to measure intensity when you train, and the best approach is probably a combination of two or three methods, made more effective by a good understanding of your past training as well as the other factors that affect performance.

Heart Rate

Heart rate monitors have been a standard training tool since the 1980s. In spite of the value a heart rate monitor lends to training, athletes should avoid relying solely on it because heart rate by itself does not tell you how well you're performing in a workout or a race. However, many athletes do try to draw conclusions from that one number. For example, many believe that if they can't get their heart rate up, they should stop the workout. A low heart rate could be bad, but then again, it might be good. One of the physiological side effects of improving aerobic fitness is an increased heart-stroke volume—more blood is pumped per beat. Simply put, you need to work harder to get your heart rate up owing to your increased fitness. So a low heart rate in a workout or race may be telling you that your fitness is high and that you should keep going—not that you should stop.

Many athletes also use the heart rate monitor number to draw incorrect conclusions about their state of well-being. They believe they are overtrained if their resting heart rate is high. It is not possible, however, to reach an accurate conclusion by looking at resting or exercising heart rates. To have meaning, the number must be compared with other measures such as RPE, power, and pace (as discussed later in this chapter).

Heart rate training zones are best tied to the standard of functional threshold. Often maximum heart rate is used to determine zones; however, exercising at such intensity may not be safe for some athletes. Functional threshold is a better indicator of what the body is experiencing, as percentages of maximum heart rate are not as precise as basing zones on FT. Using the testing protocols discussed in Appendix B, find your FT and use Tables A.1–A.3 to establish your heart rate training zones for each sport (see Appendix A).

Rate of Perceived Exertion

Perceived exertion is one of the best measures of intensity, particularly for experienced athletes. One of the most important skills for a novice athlete to acquire is the ability to link RPE to the other indicators of training intensity. As you increase or decrease pace, your RPE will also change, reflecting greater or lesser stress. RPE used in conjunction with other intensity indicators can help you decide whether or not to push harder or back off. For example, a low heart rate and high RPE are a sign that your fitness and well-being are probably good. A high heart rate and low RPE suggest that something isn't right. Think your way through the various possibilities.

For an example of when to ignore heart rate and rely on RPE, let's consider an athlete who lives at an elevation of 5,000 feet climbing to 14,225 feet. The athlete would use heart rate early in the event but would change to RPE as he progressed higher. If he stuck exclusively with heart rate, then he might have slowed unnecessarily because elevation and reduced oxygen cause the heart to work harder to get the same amount of oxygen. In other words, a higher heart rate relative to RPE is normal at high elevations. Another example is an athlete under increased heat stress. In hot and humid conditions, heart rate can be 5 to 10 bpm above normal. In these situations, the use of RPE is critical for success. The Borg Scale of Perceived Exertion (Table 5.3) is applicable to any sport and is used by sports scientists to determine at what level a subject is working.

Power

In the same way that heart rate monitors revolutionized training methods in the early 1980s, power meters have changed the way athletes train. When it comes to cycling performance, comparing heart rate with power is an excellent way to measure changes in fitness. If heart rate is low and power is normal to high when compared with previous performances, then fitness is high. If heart rate is high and power is high, then you are probably still building aerobic fitness. If heart rate is low and power is also low, then you may be experiencing fatigue, lifestyle stress, or even overtraining.

When doing interval work, even though heart rate and RPE will be higher, the actual work done—power output—will likely decline as you become fatigued. With power, the heart rate profile will be less steep, but the work done will be steadier. When doing intervals based on heart rate, athletes are, in reality, working much harder than heart rate alone would appear to indicate. Training by power is discussed further in Chapter 7.

TABLE 5.3 TRAINING ZONES AND BORG SCALE OF PERCEIVED EXERTION

ZONE		RATE OF PERCEIVED EXERTION (RPE)	DESCRIPTION
1	Recovery	6	
1	Recovery	7	Very, very light
1	Recovery	8	
2	Extensive endurance	9	Very light
2	Extensive endurance	10	
2	Extensive endurance	11	Fairly light
3	Intensive endurance	12	
3	Intensive endurance	13	Somewhat hard
3	Intensive endurance	14	
4	Subthreshold	15	Hard
5a	Threshold	16	
5b	Anaerobic endurance	17	Very hard
5b	Anaerobic endurance	18	
5c	Power	19	Very, very hard
5c	Power	20	Kaboom!

Pace

Prior to 1980, training intensity was based primarily on pace. Today, swim and run pace on established courses may be used in conjunction with heart rate, just as power is used on the bike. For example, after you run or swim a given distance at a given heart rate, your resulting time may be compared with previous such tests to gauge progress.

For the experienced athlete, pace is the best gauge for swimming intensity; however, it is less of a consideration for running and least beneficial for cycling owing to changes caused by such variables as wind and hills.

As with the five heart rate training zones, there are five levels of pace. The steady pace usually forms the bulk of your training program. This is the pace at which you train your oxygen-processing mechanisms, relevant for health and fitness as well as performance.

The following is a five-zone pace scale designed by Dr. John Hellemans of New Zealand.

1. *Easy.* Easy pace is mainly used for a warm-up or as a main part of a longer session. The pace is very comfortable. Heart rate corresponds to Zone 1 intensity.

2. *Steady.* Steady pace is one gear up, with the heart rate corresponding to Zone 2 intensity. This is a pace at which you can still have a conversation but you are slightly out of breath. For most athletes, the bottom half of this effort corresponds to the intensity at which maximum rates of fat oxidation are achieved.

3. *Moderately hard.* This pace requires concentration to maintain the intensity, although when you are fit, you can keep it up for a longer period. Heart rate corresponds to Zone 3 or Zone 4 intensities. The oxygen supply still keeps up with the oxygen demand, and therefore your metabolism is still efficient as all the lactate produced is being cleared.

4. *Hard.* At this pace, your muscles will rapidly deplete your glycogen stores. Heart rate intensity is threshold.

5. *Very hard.* This is close to maximum pace, also called sustained speed or VO_2max pace. Most athletes can sustain this pace for approximately 6 min.

High-intensity training is powerful medicine that should be used sparingly and treated respectfully. As coaches, our greatest concern with threshold work (close to, at, or above threshold) is that if an athlete is injured, sick, or tired, then he or she quickly loses the endur-

Cardiac Drift

Cardiac drift is a condition in which the heart rate increases as the workout progresses despite no increase in pace or power. A lot of factors can cause this effect. Fatigue and hydration status are probably the most common contributors. Heat stress will elevate heart rate, but probably more from the beginning of a workout than over time. However, heat stress speeds the onset of fatigue, thereby contributing to drift.

Most people talk about cardiac drift in terms of a rising heart rate. In endurance events, you may also see a declining heart rate over time. As athletes move toward their endurance, or fueling, limits, the ability to elevate heart rate is reduced. In other words, fatigue and depletion inhibit the ability to place a demand on the cardiovascular system. This effect is seen in nearly all athletes at the latter stages of an Ironman-distance race.

ance gains that we have spent months building. Although high-intensity work is essential for elite athletes, 90 percent of the field in any race consists of average age groupers. There is too much emphasis on intensity in training, and newcomers can get the wrong impression when elite competitors start talking about their quality sessions. Consistency beats intensity in nearly all age-group situations.

The most challenging workouts of the year should be limited to the Build and Peak periods because high-intensity workouts are the most potent stimulus for both improving and maintaining fitness. Your top-end fitness can be optimized in a relatively short period of time. Even during this time, the majority of your workouts should be no more intense than slightly above the effort level at which you expect to race.

▣ *Frequency*

How often you work out is the most basic element of training for long-distance triathlon. Novice athletes typically work out five or six times per week, whereas an elite athlete may work out twelve to eighteen times in a week. The appropriate frequency varies for each level of athlete.

As your fitness improves, you will see increased benefits in active recovery instead of total rest days. Active-recovery workouts are just that—an easy spin on the bike, an easy technique swim, or some other form of nonimpact light aerobic exercise.

Frequency varies throughout the season. It should be increased early in the season to add training stresses on the body, and decreased prior to and during race season to allow more time for recovery. That said, consistent frequency throughout the year is the most effective way to maintain fitness, and high-frequency running is the safest way to build mileage.

▣ *Testing*

The most critical data for you to memorize are your key training data, such as pace, power, and heart rate zones. In order to get the most out of your training sessions, schedule frequent physiological tests. The second half of a recovery week is the preferred time to undertake sport-specific testing. Because of the important role played by the FT value, we recommend that you reconfirm your sport-specific FT every eight to twelve weeks. Testing protocols are detailed in Appendix B.

> **NOVICE ATHLETES WILL NEED TO TEST MORE FREQUENTLY** than experienced athletes. When an athlete is new to a sport, his or her threshold values can rise 5–15 bpm per annum for the first several years of focused training.
>
> **N**   **NOVICE**

Once reliable baseline data have been recorded, you may benefit from substituting races to reconfirm test data. When interpreting race data, consideration should be given to the terrain, temperature, and duration and intensity of your effort. Races are most effectively used in the late Base and Build periods.

Remain conscious of the relationship among all training variables, such as heart rate, pace, power output, and RPE. When heart rate data appear to contradict other variables (most particularly RPE, pace, or power), consider the possible causes. Don't limit yourself to what your heart rate monitor is telling you.

As mentioned earlier, heart rate by itself tells you little about performance or well-being. It must be compared with other factors to have meaning. For example, if heart rate and RPE are low while pace and power are normal to high, then fitness is likely high. If heart rate and RPE are high when pace and power are low, it could be a sign of inadequate recovery. You may be experiencing fatigue, lifestyle stress, or even overtraining. Depressed or elevated heart rate is often an indicator of fatigue or impending illness. There are other possibilities as well, so all we really know is that something is not right.

If you see a large change in threshold values (10 bpm or more) between tests, you should consider the validity of the test results. If you believe the test to be valid, then gradually, over a series of weeks, adjust your training zones toward the new values. When adjusting training zones, increase the attention you pay to RPE indicators.

Refer to Table 5.4, a sample testing program for an experienced age-group athlete. Note the mixture of aerobic, FT, and VO_2max testing. (For details on testing protocols see Appendix B.) The protocols shown in square brackets in the table would be undertaken only if an athlete felt that confirmation was required. Most athletes would test no more than two sports in any one recovery week. If you have access to power-based testing, then you need to build critical power testing into your test schedule. Such sessions are stressful, so resist the urge to stack these workouts.

Remember that there are no "right" answers for any test. Testing merely provides you with useful data, which you may then use to guide your training and to track progress. Seasonal, climatic, and other external variables will influence your results.

Laboratory testing is most useful for offering insight into athletic economy, metabolic efficiency, and tracking fitness over time. Determining endurance training zones based on maximal testing is prone to error, so use these data carefully, if at all. You will do your training in the field, so we recommend that you do most of your testing in the field.

TABLE 5.4 SAMPLE TESTING SCHEDULE

	TIMELINE	SWIM	BIKE	RUN	NOTES
Prep 1	October	FT	[FT]	FT	
Prep 2	November	500s	[FT]	Aerobic step	500s: 5 x 500 on 30 sec. rest, each one slightly faster
Prep 3	December	Best average	Max aerobic	FT	Best average: 12 x 100 on greater of 2 min. and 30 sec. rest
Base 1	January	30-min. TT	[FT]	Aerobic step	
Base 2	February	FT	Max aerobic	VO₂max Pace /10K TT	Run: 10K TT on weekend; VO₂max pace test early in week
Base 3	March	Racing	Racing	Racing	Olympic-distance race: Check data against bike and run FTs
Build	April	FT	Race simulation	Race simulation	
Peak	May	Best average	None	None	
Race	May	Racing	Racing	Racing	Half-Ironman race
Base 2	May/June	Choice	Choice	Choice	Choice: No testing or aerobic testing
Base 3	June/July	Racing	Racing	Racing	Half-Ironman race
Build	July/August	FT	Max aerobic	Aerobic step	
Peak	August	Best average	None	None	
Race	August	Racing	Racing	Racing	Ironman race

Note: Testing in brackets would be done only if the athlete felt it necessary to confirm threshold. Protocols for FT, aerobic, and VO₂max tests can be found in Appendix B.

Northern Hemisphere athletes who experience harsh winter conditions should perform indoor tests for correct winter training zones and outdoor tests to establish outdoor training zones. Nearly all athletes will have a variation in intensity zones between an indoor and an outdoor situation. This variation is most noticeable for cycling zones.

Testing Tips

Athletes should always undertake a *thorough warm-up* before any testing session. The warm-up should last between 20 and 75 min. and include short efforts that build to target intensity and/or pace. For nonmaximal tests, experienced athletes will likely benefit from building these efforts to slightly beyond target intensity and/or pace. For all athletes, efforts of 15 to 90 sec. in duration are appropriate. As a rule, the higher the intensity of the test, the shorter the duration of the warm-up efforts. Typically, four to eight efforts are sufficient. Avoid the accumulation of high levels of lactate during your warm-up.

The **initial pacing** of any test effort should be slightly slower than what you believe is achievable for the test as a whole. It is far easier to recover from a start that is slightly slow than from one that is slightly fast. This is critical in threshold and maximal testing, where high early lactate levels will distort test results. Build into all tests, and aim for a pace that will enable you to finish strong.

Although most athletes are able to perform best in the afternoon and early evening, we recommend that testing be done at the same time as the majority of your training sessions. For example, if you always swim or run in the morning, then these tests should be performed in the morning.

Do your best to ensure that tests are performed in as **consistent conditions** as possible. Although external factors such as temperature, humidity, and wind are impossible to control, you should note such conditions and consider them when interpreting data. For factors under your control, do your best to ensure consistency. The key variables that you can control are recovery, hydration, nutrition, session timing, and pacing.

Occasionally, testing may indicate that you have lost fitness. When this disappointing result occurs, consideration should be given to the reasons behind it. The answers normally lie in the approach that has been taken with volume, intensity, and/or recovery. For most endurance athletes, a lack of recovery is the leading cause of reduced performance. Inability to control the many variables that affect a field test is also a consideration—weather, fatigue, diet, mental stress, tire pressure, course, running shoes, and so on. Full details of the testing protocols can be found in Appendix B. Also see the "Testing Tips" sidebar.

■ *VO$_2$max, or Anaerobic Endurance Training*

The toughest part of VO$_2$max training is the initial time trial (TT) or lab test, which is in Appendix B. Most athletes find that the training pace determined from the TT is actually a comfortable pace (for anaerobic work).

You must have an excellent endurance base before starting any high-intensity training. It is best to wait until you are seven to eleven weeks out from your first A-priority race before starting these kinds of sessions. Most new endurance athletes will benefit more from training endurance and muscular endurance than from VO_2max training. For example, in the first two years of cycling, your lactate threshold may rise 5 bpm per annum just from your muscles learning how to cycle. It may not be until your third season of focused bike training that high-intensity work is appropriate—and even then it should likely be muscular endurance work, not VO_2max work.

We recommend that you train your skills and endurance, then muscular endurance, and finally anaerobic endurance. Not only is this the safest way to progress, it also mirrors the requirements of long-distance triathlon.

Anaerobic endurance sessions are biomechanically stressful and require extra recovery time. Although many athletes believe that this kind of work is beneficial, research shows that greater results are achieved from endurance and muscular endurance work. These types of workouts are also less risky and are subject to quicker recovery.

Certain athletes find VO_2max sessions fun, so small amounts of high intensity can be useful to maintain mental freshness. However, the heavy-duty VO_2max sessions should be attempted only by strong, experienced athletes who are biomechanically sound. These sessions are risky. Remember that the most valuable intensity is one gear up from average Ironman-distance race effort.

OVERLOAD TRAINING

When sensibly incorporated into your regimen, "overloading" can lead to improved fitness. Overloading introduces higher volume, frequency, or intensity for a specific workout or a short period of time. Both novice and elite athletes must be cautious in how they apply the overload principle because it can quickly lead to overtraining and undo the valuable progress made. The following are some of the ways you might opt to overload your training.

■ *Breakthrough Workouts*

A breakthough (BT) workout is any workout or group of workouts that requires more than thirty-six hours to recover from. The nature of your BT workouts will vary throughout the year. Early in the season, or in your career, a four-hour easy ride could be considered a BT workout, but as your endurance increases, such a session could become an aerobic maintenance workout.

Breakthrough (BT) Workout and Recovery Tips

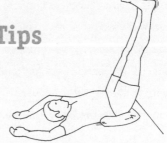

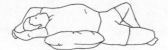

FIGURE **5.1**

FIGURE **5.2**

BT WORKOUT TIPS

Timing is an important consideration in scheduling your BT workouts. Most athletes find they have higher-quality BT sessions when they are able to complete their key sessions in the afternoon. Next best would be in the morning.

Some athletes will benefit from a cup of regular coffee taken 60 to 90 min. prior to the start of a BT session. Athletes who use caffeine should consume it cautiously, as it is most effective in low to moderate doses.

All longer BT sessions should begin with a low-intensity warm-up to allow your body to build into the session. This is particularly important for the longest BT sessions as well as those that incorporate high-intensity workloads.

BT sessions are an excellent opportunity to practice mental skills such as focus, pace, fatigue management, and cue words.

Pain, specifically during high-intensity sessions, should be carefully monitored. Build period BT sessions are difficult, and late in the workout athletes will be training through fatigue. The ability to train through fatigue is an important skill to learn. However, you should never train through pain. All athletes should be conservative during the Build period, when an injury can be costly in terms of race fitness. As a general rule, "if in doubt, leave it out."

BT RECOVERY TIPS

After a BT session, have a quick snack, shower, put on some comfortable clothes, and eat your main recovery meal. Then, sit on the floor cross-legged with one or two pillows directly behind your back, and lean backward over the pillows (Figure 5.1). You will be doing a mild back bend and should feel your hip flexors and pelvis open. Relax into the stretch, then sit up slowly and reverse the upper and lower crossed legs. Lean backward over the pillows for the same length of time. This will ensure a balanced hip stretch.

Between this recovery exercise and the next one, walk around for 4–8 min.

Now move your pillows against a wall, lie on your back with the pillows under your lower back, and place your legs up against the wall (Figure 5.2). The amount of support that you will need under your lower back will depend on your hamstring flexibility. Leave your legs against the wall for 5 min. for each hour of your workout. When you have finished your wall time, roll gently onto one side. Stay on your side for a few minutes to ease the transition back to vertical.

This exercise helps get blood to your vital organs, allowing you to recover more quickly. If you are tired, then you may get sleepy. This exercise, combined with some deep breathing, is an excellent way to relax prior to a nap or bedtime.

Because your focus will change from one training period to the next, the reverse is also possible: After twelve weeks of base training, you may recover quickly from strength training, but at another time of year, strength training could require forty-eight hours of recovery.

BT workouts should be designed to focus on your A-priority race limiters. These are different for each athlete. Your role is to design appropriate BTs and allow enough recovery time. Most self-coached athletes tend to stack too many BTs into a block, and as a result, they do not get the recovery that they need in order to take their fitness to the next level. This is the primary cause of sport-specific and overall performance plateaus.

Novice Ironman-distance athletes should schedule no more than two BT workouts per week. Experienced or elite athletes who recover quickly may schedule three BT workouts in a week. Stronger athletes may also be able to stack two or three workouts into a "BT day." However, you need to have a clear view of your goals and the key sessions within your days, weeks, and blocks.

Your easiest days should follow your toughest days. In other words, the best place for a rest day is after your toughest day of the week. However, this is a general rule, and there are situations in which it makes sense to vary it.

In the race season, BT quality is most important. Most athletes find that they require additional recovery periods after their toughest sessions. It is far better to recover from a limited number of high-quality sessions than to push the volume up and do lots of moderate sessions. This issue of quality becomes more important as your A-priority race approaches. Superior race performance results from what you do, not how much you do.

■ *Crash Cycles*

Overcompensation (the same thing as overloading) is a standard training method—after a training stress is applied and the body is given ample recovery, fitness will begin to develop at a higher level. When these training stresses are closely spaced over an extended period followed by a long recovery phase, the level of overcompensation is enhanced. This supercompensation is called "crashing."

Crash cycles appeal to Ironman triathletes, but they are often inappropriate because they are highly risky. There are significant mental and physical benefits from this kind of training; however, it should be attempted only by the strongest athletes who are completely biomechanically sound. It is important that you meet the following criteria before attempting a crash cycle:

- You have no recent injury history.
- You recover quickly from tough sessions (four to five days in a recovery week, normally).
- You are at the top of your age group (or an elite athlete) and want to take it to the next level.
- You are willing to accept injury in your life.

An example of a crash cycle follows:

CRASH WEEK

Monday	Swim endurance, bike endurance
Tuesday	Run endurance, bike active recovery
Wednesday	Swim endurance, bike endurance
Thursday	Off
Friday	Swim endurance, run speed skills, bike active recovery
Saturday	Bike endurance
Sunday	Swim endurance, bike endurance

RECOVERY WEEK

Monday	Off
Tuesday	Bike active recovery, swim active recovery
Wednesday	Run active recovery, bike active recovery
Thursday	Strength, swim active recovery
Friday	Run active recovery, bike active recovery
Saturday	Bike endurance, swim endurance
Sunday	Run endurance, swim active recovery

IF YOU THINK A CRASH CYCLE IS FOR YOU, watch closely for the typical signs of overtraining because the risk rises dramatically during such a buildup. Crash cycles shouldn't be attempted more than once per month and should end no later than four weeks prior to your goal race.

E | **ELITE**

This is only one example of a way in which a crash cycle may be organized; however, it is preferable to crash only one sport at a time. Crashing running is too risky and should be avoided. Crashing swimming with good stroke mechanics is highly effective. For Ironman-distance racing, crashing volume is the way to go. Be very cautious with the use of Zone 3 and higher intensities when seeking to extend your volume. For ultradistance triathlon, the most useful adaptations flow from overloading with Zone 1 and Zone 2 training. Just as in your BT sessions, it can be useful to probe your limits at times. World champion triathlete Mark Allen says, "Push your limits rarely; when you push them, push them hard." This can be an effective strategy for elite and experienced athletes.

■ *Challenge Workouts*

A safer way for you to push your limits is through challenge workouts. These workouts are tougher than what we would normally recommend and go a little beyond BT sessions. They are fun, keep training fresh, and provide athletes with motivating goals.

The early Base period is the best time for challenge workouts that have an endurance component. These are workouts that push your endurance, but not your muscular endurance. Here are some examples:

- Rim to river on the Grand Canyon
- Easy open-water swimming, 3 miles
- Double metric centuries, all on the small chainring
- All-day hiking
- Mountaineering
- Riding to the next state, county, or city
- Multiday hiking trips
- Multiday bike tours
- Mountain bike tours

Allow plenty of time for recovery, and remember that the main goal of these sessions is to have fun while building endurance.

■ *Back-to-Back Workouts*

Crash cycles and challenge workouts are a bit extreme, and that could explain their appeal. Another overload technique that can be used safely, and more often, is back-to-back workouts. This technique provides race-specific overload without deep fatigue. As you will see, the main goal is to overload steady-state endurance rather than intensity.

A simple example would be running 6–10 miles on Tuesday evening and repeating the workout on Wednesday morning. This would give the athlete 12–20 miles of running within a short window of time. However, by splitting the distance into two workouts, the biomechanical risks are reduced and the likely recovery period is shortened. Another example would be 60 miles of riding on both Saturday and Sunday. Most athletes will find that their average work rate will be higher if they split the endurance overload across two days.

Like the sample schedules in the "Crash Cycles" section, here are some examples that can be used to create a sport-specific overload block. In our experience, combining more than two back-to-back days is counterproductive. Be particularly cautious when using these techniques with run training. You will notice that the running block example has two easy days between the back-to-back sessions. An easy day can be either a very light day or a day off from that particular sport. Note that you should not try to crash both volume and intensity simultaneously.

SWIMMING BLOCK

Day 1	Muscular endurance	70–90 min.
Day 2	Endurance swim (continuous)	50–75 min.
Day 3	Easier day	0–30 min.
Day 4	Endurance swim (threshold)	70–90 min.
Day 5	Muscular endurance	50–75 min.

CYCLING BLOCK

Day 1	Endurance, flat terrain	3–4 hrs.
Day 2	Muscular endurance, hills	4–5 hrs.
Day 3	Easier day	0–30 min.
Day 4	Muscular endurance, hills	60–90 min., followed by max aerobic test 1 hr.
Day 5	Race-simulation ride	

RUNNING BLOCK

Day 1	Flat tempo run	60–90 min.
Day 2	Hilly endurance run	75–105 min.
Day 3	Easier day	0–30 min.
Day 4	Easier day	0–30 min.
Day 5	Easy to steady-paced flat run	60–90 min.
Day 6	Long, slow distance (hills, then flats)	2–2.5 hrs.

Avoid using single-sport overload all the time, and remember that your greatest gains will arise from moderate, balanced training over time. However, when an athlete is seeking safe, race-specific overload, this technique is highly effective.

SKILLS

Among endurance athletes, perhaps the most overlooked aspect of performance is skills. Most athletes know the intricacies of interval sessions, hill repeats, tempo workouts, and the like, but many leave movement proficiency to chance.

This is an important point because improving economy of movement means less energy is wasted, allowing for faster times and greater duration in training and races. In fact, scientists have demonstrated that three physiological variables are key to endurance performance—aerobic capacity (VO_2max), functional threshold, and economy. Of these three, the one with the most room for improvement in experienced athletes is nearly always economy.

It's possible for an already fit and experienced athlete to improve economy, and therefore performance, by 5 percent or more in a year by working on skills a little bit every week. This level of economy enhancement has been accomplished even with world-class athletes. For the rest of us, there is tremendous room for improvement.

The intelligent athlete is constantly thinking about form; however, a particularly good time to work on skills is easy training days. There may be three or four such sessions a week, with each devoted to one or more skills in which you have a personal limiter.

■ *Fundamental Skills*

Fundamental skills provide the building blocks upon which proper sport-specific technique rests. Many long-course athletes come to triathlon from a nonathletic background, so building and strengthening fundamental skills is one way to increase economy and reduce susceptibility to injury.

With respect to triathlon, the key fundamental skills can be broken down into two subcategories: movement and awareness skills.

Movement skills, such as walking, running, skipping, jumping, hopping, leaping, and bounding, assist in the ability to move the body from one place to another. Nonmovement skills, also known as stability skills, consist of balancing, turning, and twisting.

Awareness skills relate to movement of the body within the athletic arena. These skills include spatial awareness, depth perception, proprioception, and rhythm as well as the abilities required to process visual, tactile, and auditory feedback. As children, it is likely that we developed these skills through play—games such as tag, dodgeball, soccer, and baseball develop a range of fundamental skills. Hence, the triathlete who supplements his or her Prep and early Base periods with crosstraining activities gains an added benefit.

Athletes can benefit from incorporating a range of fundamental skills into their training programs. What follows are drills that target fundamental skills. The first three are stability skills, so they are best performed without shoes.

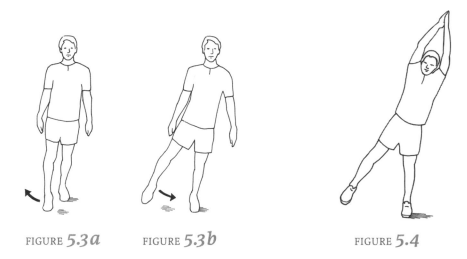

FIGURE 5.3*a*   FIGURE 5.3*b*   FIGURE 5.4

ALPHABETS. Stand on your left leg and trace large letters of the alphabet with your right foot (Figures 5.3a and 5.3b). Change your support leg and repeat. Close your eyes to increase difficulty.

LEANING TOWER. Start with two legs as support. Lean forward, backward, and sideways. As skill level increases, move your feet closer together, then try with a single support leg (Figure 5.4). Once that is mastered, try with your eyes closed.

SINGLE-LEG SQUAT TOUCHES. Perform a single-leg squat and touch the ground (Figure 5.5a). Touches should be to the front, side, and rear. Use either hand for touching. Touches that involve crossing over the body (Figure 5.5b) increase difficulty. When squatting, bend at the ankle, knee, and hip. You can position your suspended leg forward or backward (see Figure 5.5c) to balance. Movement should be slow and controlled. Once this is mastered, close your eyes for increased challenge.

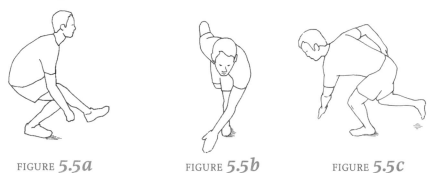

FIGURE 5.5*a*   FIGURE 5.5*b*   FIGURE 5.5*c*

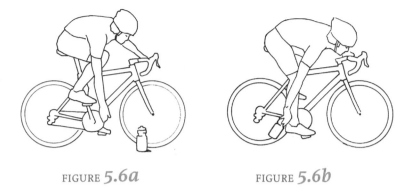

FIGURE *5.6a*   FIGURE *5.6b*

LINES. On a bicycle, ride a straight line—edges of roads and parking lots are good places to find these lines. Drill difficulty can be increased by looking down, looking over one shoulder, or reaching for a water bottle (Figures 5.6a and 5.6b). As skill level increases, try to stay on one edge of the line. This drill should never be attempted in traffic.

In Chapters 6, 7, and 8, we'll explore more sport-specific skills and introduce myriad drills to improve your form and economy.

In addition to specific drills, activities such as yoga, jazz dance, scrambling, trail running, mountain biking, cross-country skiing, body surfing, and rock climbing as well as team sports such as softball, basketball, and soccer can contribute to your inventory of fundamental skills.

Give consideration to this inventory. If a particular skill is lacking, the early season is the perfect time to close the gap. When learning any new skill, we recommend following this progression:

1. Learn the proper movement pattern for the skill.
2. Learn to perform the skill at speed.
3. Increase the load under which the skill is performed.
4. Increase the situational stress under which the skill is performed (i.e., do it in front of a crowd).

■ *Flexibility: The Benefits of Yoga*

When you combine a strong aerobic engine with good bike position, you get cycling speed. If you want to have a long and successful career, a commitment to a structured flexibility program such as yoga is essential. The fastest elite athletes in our sport have outstanding bike positions.

To achieve this takes only time—not genetics, not hard miles, not volume. It is relatively free speed. As well, a flexibility program has clear benefits for recovery, strength, and economy.

If possible, try to find an instructor who is familiar with multisport or endurance athletes. Discuss what you are trying to achieve and have him or her develop a personal program for you involving a fusion of various styles. When you are tired, stick to mainly floor work. As you learn and become more flexible, begin adding more traditional poses; however, be sure that you are ready for the progression. A few exercises in isolation might not be best for most people.

One to two hours per week is the minimum amount of time that you need to devote to see results. As with other aspects of your training, the results are related to dedication and consistency. As little as ten minutes per day of flexibility training goes a long way toward reducing the risk of injury and increasing economy.

Your yoga should focus on restorative poses. Avoid strenuous poses. Standing poses can be quite tiring for many people and interfere with recovery. Do a lot of floor work, and keep it mellow.

Tips for getting started:

- Start slowly.
- Learn the fundamentals.
- Take your time.
- Maintain a smooth, relaxed breathing pattern.
- Focus on the seated postures first.
- Never force a pose.
- Focus on frequency—this is very important.

Many athletes tend to drop yoga sessions unless they schedule them. The first thing they drop is stretching. However, experience has shown that this is a big mistake. Stretching has one of the largest rates of return (per hour invested) of all training activities for an athlete with a reasonable level of flexibility. An inflexible athlete has an even greater rate of return.

For working athletes, we recommend a regular flexibility routine rather than a full-on yoga regimen. One session a week is acceptable, but you should supplement with at least two solo sessions of a minimum of 20 min. These sessions should focus on employing the stretching techniques that cover the parts of your body where you hold tension. See the hip progression in Chapter 9 for a simple flexibility routine.

PLANNING YOUR BASE AND BUILD WEEKS

Now that we have reviewed the structure of the annual training plan; the careful balance among volume, intensity, and frequency; the common ways to manipulate or overload volume, intensity, and frequency for improved fitness; and the role of skills in improving economy, it's time to put it all together.

In classic periodization, there are two training periods that precede the first A-priority events of the season: the Base and Build periods. In the Base period, the workouts are not necessarily similar to the stresses that will be encountered in the race. The exception is that for ultraendurance events, such as an Ironman-distance triathlon, endurance workouts are similar to what is expected in the race because long, slow distances and hill strength are common to these types of races and to Base training.

In the Build period, the workouts become increasingly similar to racing, culminating in the Peak period, when the workouts are essentially miniraces at levels of intensity greater than those reached on race day. Often, actual races of lower priority may be substituted for workouts in the Build and Peak periods to better prepare for A-priority events.

■ *Base Week Structure*

Your primary goals in the Base period are to develop aerobic endurance, strength, and skills in each individual sport. The Base period is commonly split into three phases—Base 1, Base 2, and Base 3. Depending on your limiters, it may make sense to extend your base training right up to your goal race. You can have an excellent race experience by focusing your training on the fundamentals of endurance, strength, and skills.

The goal of Base 1 is to improve endurance and maximum strength. During this period, endurance workouts are longer, and the focus on technical skills increases. To balance the maximum-strength phase, frequent skills-oriented workouts are important to maintain your quickness.

For most athletes, we recommend reducing the duration of BT workouts in Base 1. Swimming is the exception. You may choose to increase volume, but not intensity.

The Base week for the novice stays the same through the entire cycle:

BASE WEEKS	
Monday	Endurance brick and strength training
Tuesday	Long run (BT) and easy swim (technique)
Wednesday	Second-longest swim workout (endurance)
Thursday	Second-longest bike workout (muscular endurance focus) with short transition run
Friday	Key swim workout (endurance) and easy run (endurance)
Saturday	Key endurance day: long ride or big day training
Sunday	Family day: Easiest day of the week, completely off or light aerobic training

N   NOVICE

For an experienced or elite athlete, a typical Base 1 week might be the following:

BASE 1 WEEK	
Monday	Masters swimming, aerobic ride, yoga
Tuesday	Endurance swimming, bike BT (muscular endurance focus)
Wednesday	Endurance run (including skills work), yoga
Thursday	Masters swimming, aerobic brick
Friday	Skills swimming, skills running, strength training, skills cycling
Saturday	Day off
Sunday	Endurance ride

I/E   INTERMEDIATE/ELITE

With the completion of the higher-intensity strength training, sport-specific muscular endurance work is introduced in Base 2. Muscular endurance workouts should be done at moderate intensities in the initial stages to give you time to convert "gym strength" to sport-specific muscular endurance. Endurance workouts continue to increase in duration.

For most athletes, swimming will start to take a slight backseat as your focus moves toward bike, run, and brick sessions.

Base 2 is tricky because you will likely feel ready for some higher-intensity work. However, patience must be practiced to avoid peaking too soon. Therefore, we recommend that you continue to include plenty of endurance training to help channel your energy into a productive area of training. This approach will help you exercise the necessary control.

For an experienced or elite athlete, a Base 2 week might look something like this:

BASE 2 WEEK	
Monday	Masters swimming, skills cycling, yoga
Tuesday	Endurance swim, skills cycling
Wednesday	BT ride with transition run, yoga
Thursday	Technique swim, skills running, strength training, easy spin
Friday	BT swim, skills cycling, massage
Saturday	BT run
Sunday	Strength training, aerobic ride

I/E INTERMEDIATE/ELITE

Your weekly volume reaches a peak in Base 3. Intensity also rises slightly with the addition of more muscular endurance training. Athletes need to be very careful with intensity during their BT workouts, as individual tolerance for this kind of training varies tremendously. C-priority races can be used during this period as tempo or intensity sessions.

For an experienced or elite athlete, a Base 3 week may be structured like this:

BASE 3 WEEK	
Monday	Masters swimming, aerobic ride, yoga
Tuesday	Endurance swimming, BT ride (muscular endurance focus)
Wednesday	Endurance run (including muscular endurance work), yoga
Thursday	Day off
Friday	BT swim (muscular endurance focus), skills running, strength training, skills cycling
Saturday	Masters swimming, aerobic brick
Sunday	Endurance ride

I/E INTERMEDIATE/ELITE

Designing a week of training in the Base period is fairly simple when compared with the more complex Build period.

■ *Build Week Structure*

The Build period is not a requirement for success in Ironman-distance triathlon. The critical success factors are superior endurance, pace control, and the ability to fuel yourself across your event. Race-simulation workouts are an essential part of your preparations and should be included. Many athletes ruin six months or more of patient preparation by inserting far too much Zone 4 and 5 training into their final preparations.

To properly schedule workouts for the Build period, it's important to know two things: what the demands of your key races are and how your athletic strengths compare with these demands. Build training must focus on areas where there are gaps. In other words, concentrate your training on your key race limiters (see Chapter 3).

Build period planning is not recommended until your limiters have been identified and you have the skills, endurance, and strength to complete your race distance. Many athletes fail to consider their limiters and train blindly. Such pointless training is common and prevents even the very talented from achieving their potential.

Once your limiters have been established, it's a good idea to focus your training on them once or twice each week. Assuming you are doing three BT workouts weekly, that means you will have at least one other weekly session dedicated to maintaining your strengths. If your scheduling or recovery considerations mean that you can complete only two key sessions a week, then you should maintain your strengths within one of your BT sessions.

When planning a Build week, it is also necessary to know how quickly you recover from BT workouts of various types. If your recovery is good (diet, rest, low stress, massage, active-recovery sessions, etc.), then it is possible to schedule multiple BT workouts in a week. If recovery is slow, which is often the case with veteran athletes and novices, it may be possible to complete only one or two such sessions in a week of training. Remember that the quality of the BT workouts is far more important than the quantity.

Separate your BT workouts by at least thirty-six hours. For most, forty-eight to sixty hours set aside for recovery is optimal. If your BT session quality suffers, you should extend your recovery time. The majority of each BT session should be done at an intensity that mimics Ironman-distance race pace. For most athletes, it is not usually necessary, and may be counter-productive, to train at intensities that are greater than 110 percent of goal-race intensity. In other words, one of the purposes of training in the Build period is to prepare for the exact stresses expected in the race. The closer you get to the race, the more critical this pacing becomes.

With all of this in mind, a typical Build period week of training may look something like this:

BUILD WEEK	
Monday	Rest, active recovery, or weights
Tuesday	Key-limiter BT
Wednesday	Active recovery, speed skills, and/or rest
Thursday	BT to maintain key strength
Friday	Active recovery, speed skills, and/or rest
Saturday	Key-limiter BT
Sunday	Aerobic maintenance (endurance, force, speed skills)

As the Build period progresses, it is a good idea to combine limiters and strengths into single workouts. After all, a race is not composed of just one element, such as muscular endurance. Typically, many physical abilities are challenged within a race. Combining several elements into one session makes training even more racelike.

Elite and experienced athletes may schedule multiple sessions on a given day, but such planning should never compromise recovery. Some athletes may be able to handle two or even three workouts on a recovery day so long as the intensity and duration are low relative to their training load. If training performance is substandard, question your recovery strategy. The all-too-often-chosen solution is to make the easy days a little harder in a poorly thought-out attempt to raise the average training intensity of the week. Keep your hard days challenging and your easy days easy.

Most athletes place too much training load in their Build period. Remember that the goal of your tougher sessions is to lift, rather than flatten, your performance. If you challenge yourself specifically to the demands of an Ironman-distance race, then two to four BT workouts in a fourteen-day period are enough. Long, continuous, steady-state training is the most specific to your race demands.

The last consideration for this period is the nature of the recovery week that completes each two- to three-week period of race-specific training. The first few days of each of these recovery weeks should be dedicated to rest by including downtime and fewer, shorter, and easier workouts than usual. Near the end of the week, after you are positive that your body is rejuvenating, is a good time to test progress with a time trial or a race. It's a good idea to get in two or more races before the first A-priority events of the season. Not only will these serve as tests of progress, but they will also allow you to practice the strategy and tactics you are considering for the A-priority races.

If all goes well in the Build period, you should come into the Peak period feeling significantly more fit and confident than you did at the end of the Base period, but first let's consider training in more detail.

CHAPTER 6

TRAINING FOR THE SWIM

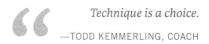
> *Technique is a choice.*
> —TODD KEMMERLING, COACH

Because the swim is the shortest of the three events in an Ironman-distance triathlon, many athletes are tempted to do the bare minimum in their swim preparation. Although this strategy can make sense for strong swimmers as well as severely time-constrained athletes, swim training provides a range of benefits to the endurance athlete.

In addition to becoming a better swimmer, the benefits associated with swim training are:

Nonimpact aerobic work. Swimming provides aerobic training in a low-impact environment. This combination enables most athletes to achieve a greater volume of aerobic work without compromising their recovery from their other training.

Recovery. Because it promotes overall circulation, swimming can be used for active-recovery sessions. In addition, many athletes find water to be a calming influence that reduces their overall stress levels.

Improved race efficiency. For slower swimmers especially, the reduction in time spent in the water means that in a race situation, they are able to start refueling themselves sooner. Although greater time savings can often be found in focused bike and run training, decreasing the time spent in the water has clear nutritional advantages for an Ironman-distance athlete.

STAGES OF SWIMMING DEVELOPMENT

■ *Stage 1: Building Endurance and Technique*

There is no point in swimming hard before you are able to swim well. For most triathletes, swimming is the weakest of the three sports. Even if their endurance is adequate for the race distance, they don't have the technique that would improve their efficiency in the water. For this reason we will devote the better part of this chapter to technique, or how to swim well.

Triathletes who come from a nonswimming background must remember that they have no competitive experience to carry them through the first part of their important races. In order to reach your swimming potential, you must build your fundamentals. This means a commitment to improving your body position in the water. Building a bigger engine does not help if you are dragging your hips. Technical improvement comes through a commitment to incorporating different drills into your workouts, but more importantly, you must constantly think of your stroke mechanics and work to make stroke improvements during each and every interval and set.

Focusing on bilateral breathing can greatly increase swim economy and help you learn to relax in the water. However, you need to be willing to endure the Transition period, during which you may slow as your body adjusts to the new movement patterns. By having patience, you will become a more efficient swimmer. In triathlons, efficiency may not always translate to improved swim times; however, reduced energy expenditure in the water will translate to more energy for your bike and run.

Given that swimming is a very technique-intensive sport, workout frequency plays an important role. Specifically, it is difficult to achieve a material improvement without a minimum of three 60-min. swims per week. Increase frequency before you increase distance. With your longer workouts, it is best to slow down and focus on maintaining form.

Technique and the ability to maintain stroke mechanics over a long period of time are the most important aspects of swimming for all athletes. Only after these aspects are established should you focus on increasing your endurance and, ultimately, adding muscular endurance sessions. Remember that in an Ironman-distance swim, economy dominates power.

THERE ARE ESSENTIALLY TWO WAYS TO SWIM FASTER:

1. Decrease drag by streamlining body position.
2. Increase propulsion by improving aerobic and anaerobic fitness.

Of these two, scientific studies have found that reducing drag has the potential to produce the greater gains. Drag is the retarding force created by turbulence around the body as it moves through the water. The more streamlined the body, the lower the resulting drag force.

■ *Stage 2: Building Muscular Endurance*

Muscular endurance is the ability to maintain a steady pace for long periods. Many athletes can swim fast 50 and 100 m sets, but they find it challenging to bring that speed into 400, 800, and 1,500 m distances. This is where muscular endurance comes into play.

As you enter your Build period, work in a moderate amount of focused muscular endurance swimming to mimic the demands of your key races. Specific workouts are highlighted later in the chapter.

■ *Key Stroke Issues*

For the novice swimmer, the tendency is to push the arm down as the first movement following entry—this habit is particularly common in swimmers with weak deltoids and shoulder rotators. Pushing the arm down lifts the upper body and drops the hips. This position feels comfortable because the head comes out of the water and the face is exposed for the breath. Although the swimmer is comfortable, he or she slows greatly at every breath.

Learning to keep your face in the water will help you keep your hips higher and make you faster. If you have trouble breathing, force yourself to rotate your hips, then your chin, a little farther. Two good cues for this technique are to "breathe from your hips" and "chin up, chin down."

The following paragraphs discuss the major technical challenges facing triathletes and some ideas for addressing them. How do you know if these issues apply to you? The quickest and most effective way to find out is to have a friend videotape you from the front, back, and side while you are swimming freestyle. If you have never seen yourself swim, it will likely prove to be a shocking experience. Take heart in the fact that the more technical issues you have with your stroke, the easier it will be for you to improve—so long as you are committed to technical improvement.

Balance. Improved balance and high hips are the quickest way to faster times. Side-kicking drills can be very useful to

---

ELEMENTS OF MODERN FREESTYLE

- Body is horizontal with no vertical shoulder movement on entry.
- Stroke begins with immediate catch with vertical alignment of hand, wrist, and forearm—minimal downward pressure post-entry and rapid transition to horizontal pull. This is a clear limiter for virtually all triathletes. The pull pattern should have your fingers and forearm pointing straight down as if you were trying to touch the bottom of the pool.
- Face is in the water looking down, except when breathing look to the side.
- Hips and shoulders rotate together and to the same degree.
- Legs are kept within the body shadow.
- Kick rotates with hips.
- Upper arm is aligned with shoulders for pull and recovery (tough for swimmers who have inflexible shoulders).
- Feet are streamlined.

improve your overall balance as well as your comfort in the water. These drills are discussed in more detail later in this chapter.

Head position. It is natural to want to have your whole head out of the water when you breathe. It is also instinct to want to be completely vertical when breathing. Both of these urges are present in all swimmers; the difference is the magnitude of stress required to make them apparent. When you are swimming, your head should be steady, in line with the spine, with your face looking down at all times. The breath cycle is initiated by the hips and shoulders rotating together and completed with a slight head rotation led by the chin. Focus on keeping your face in the water, as this position will keep your hips up. If you lift your head when you breathe, correcting this error should be your sole objective until you have mastered the technique.

When breathing, remember to swivel your head and rotate your chin up for air, then turn your chin back down to swim and exhale, always keeping your face in the water. Hips lead your chin. By starting at the hips, you get a solid rotation and also engage your trunk and back in the stroke.

Exhale underwater. If you find that you don't have enough time to breathe or that you are not getting a full breath, then ensure that you are exhaling in the water. If you try to exhale and then inhale with your face out of the water, you may get only a partial inhalation. As soon as you are able to get a full breath, the urge to lift your head will be reduced.

Offside arm. In an attempt to push their head out of the water, many swimmers will push down with their offside arm when breathing. Remember to let your leading hand glide for a little bit when breathing. Bilateral three-stroke breathing patterns are very helpful in correcting this problem, which is best identified by underwater video analysis.

Pressing the T. If you have a tendency to drag your hips through the water (uphill swimming), keep your face down and focus on pressing your chest down in the water while maintaining a long body line (think about a T with the top running between your shoulders). Many swimmers think they are pressing the chest downward when they are really leaning their heads, so watch for this mistake. When the head tips forward and drives underwater, there isn't any real change in body position; in order to lift the hips, the T needs to be pressed while the head is in a neutral position looking down (for most) or slightly forward (for fast swimmers).

Distance per stroke. Focus on a full, relaxed, smooth style. Count your strokes and try to maximize distance per stroke.

Hand entry. Hand entry should be shoulder width apart, with the ring and pinkie fingers entering first.

Legs together. Swimmers typically split their legs when they are uncomfortable rotating or breathing. Improving your in-water comfort through balance drills can quite often eliminate this challenge. Another useful technique is to create a set of "shackles" from rubber tubing. The ankles are given enough room to kick, but the tubing prevents a large split in the legs. Finally, you can correct a scissor kick by learning to touch your big toes together every time you breathe.

■ *Bilateral Breathing*

Bilateral breathing is one of the quickest ways for an experienced swimmer to increase swimming efficiency. Bilateral breathing refers to breathing on an odd stroke count, typically every third stroke. Experienced athletes will find that they can breathe bilaterally quite comfortably up to a heart rate Zone 3 level of intensity. Although extensive use of bilateral breathing is recommended for training, breathing every cycle is recommended for racing.

When you start bilateral breathing, it can be very difficult to relax. If you are having trouble, keep the interval length short and stick with it. Eventually you will be able to extend the interval. Remember your goals—if you are training to relax or to build base endurance, keep the pace easy. It is far easier to relax when the aerobic stress of the exercise is low. It is very difficult to improve your economy (in any sport) when there is tension in your body. Pay particular attention to your face, neck, and shoulders.

Following is a discussion of some of the principal benefits of learning to master bilateral breathing.

Improved technique. With bilateral breathing, you will initially be forced to slow down, giving you the opportunity to work on your stroke mechanics. For long-distance athletes, it can be quite beneficial to use longer interval distances (400–1,500 m) that include faster segments combined with bilateral, active-recovery segments.

Offside improvement. Nearly every athlete can improve the efficiency of his or her "away" arm when breathing. Swimming bilaterally helps you even your stroke. When you are completely comfortable with bilateral swimming, try some swimming while breathing every cycle on your offside. Not only will you learn a lot about your stroke, you will also gain the ability to swim comfortably on your offside. This can be very useful in a race situation in which you may need to breathe away from swells, splashing, or waves. It also lets you check out your competition and spot landmarks located on your offside.

Improved stroke and balance. Stroke imbalances are very easy to detect when swimming bilaterally. Once these areas are discovered, it is easy for you to correct them. For example, you may notice your hand pulling wide when you are breathing onside and not breathing offside. Your offside now becomes a role model to correct your onside stroke more quickly.

Improved timing. Bilateral breathing has a smooth rhythm and helps develop stroke and kick timing. It is also beneficial to the timing of flip turns because it offers you the opportunity to breathe on either side coming into the turn.

Improved breath control. The breath control that you learn from bilateral swimming will enable you to improve your flip turns. Why are turns important? Because they enable you to swim with stronger swimmers, maintain your workout momentum (particularly when swimming short-course), draft faster swimmers in group time trials, and improve your streamlining and balance. Being comfortable with a moderate amount of "breathing stress" is very useful for race starts, rounding marker buoys, and bridging forward to a faster group of swimmers.

Improved rotation. Many athletes find that they rotate well to their breathing side, then "flatten out" without rotating at all to their offside. A flat stroke can increase the load on your shoulder and result in swimmer's shoulder. With more rotation to both sides, you are able to pull through your stroke much more easily and increase the power of your stroke.

Confidence. The feeling of breathlessness that you may experience in the water is not a lack of oxygen; rather, it is a buildup of carbon dioxide. Learning to live with this sensation is an important skill for swim starts, turns, and pool swimming. Knowing that you can swim bilaterally is a real confidence-booster if you miss a few breaths during a race. It will also help your threshold performance when swimming hard and breathing every cycle.

There is some discussion in swimming circles regarding whether or not bilateral swimming improves lung capacity. There is no substantial research to support the concept of bilateral breathing as a technique to improve lung capacity or lung function. However, it does increase an athlete's carbon dioxide tolerance and breath control. Both of these skills transfer to other sports.

Rather than training the body to get more oxygen out of each breath, bilateral breathing teaches the athlete to breathe fully while maintaining a relaxed focus on stroke mechanics.

THE PROGRESSION

There is a natural progression most swimmers can follow to better performance:

1. Develop an efficient body position by focusing on balance, relaxation, and smoothness through all aspects of the swimming cycle.

2. Increase the effectiveness of each stroke by improving your catch-and-pull mechanics.

3. Using superior balance and stroke mechanics, increase stroke rate while maintaining technical excellence and distance per stroke.

The drills that follow in the workout section of this chapter will help you improve your balance, setting the stage for continued improvement. In our opinion, these drills are best mastered in order and done frequently. The first two things for any swimmer to master are balance and body rotation. For any time of the year, sets that include bilateral breathing, single-stroke change, and triple-stroke change are beneficial. A complete (and highly recommended) explanation of many of these drills can be found in Terry Laughlin's Total Immersion series of books and videos. Terry's teaching methods have helped thousands of adults become better, more confident swimmers.

Remember that the most important part of these drills is learning to improve your balance, body position, and in-water comfort. A pull-buoy gives you an artificial aid for achieving better body position and for this reason is not recommended when drilling. When learning these drills, many athletes will benefit from the use of short fins. As your technical competence improves, you should perform the drills without fins.

SWIMMING DRILLS

■ *Balance*

Most triathletes have balance as a limiter. How do you know if your balance is not a limiter? If you can swim all but your toughest main sets with three-stroke breathing, you are comfortable with five-stroke breathing, and you can swim hard with offside, two-stroke breathing, then you are likely a well-balanced swimmer. Until you are at this stage, you are likely to gain materially from working to improve your balance. As we need to be relaxed to learn any new skills, you should always do your drills at a comfortable pace.

It is best not to use any swim gear, such as fins or kickboards, for balance drills; however, you can begin the side-kicking drills with short fins. Most athletes will find that after a few

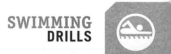

**SWIMMING
DRILLS**

weeks, they do not need fins. In fact, being able to comfortably do these drills without fins is a clear indication of improved balance.

Drills to improve balance consist primarily of learning to balance and breathe while kicking and moving through different orientations. Most athletes will find the following progression beneficial to improving their balance; all of these drills are done while maintaining a relaxed kick.

BACK-KICK. Start by kicking on your back with your hands at your sides. Kick at a relaxed pace and breathe calmly. Push your shoulders down and your belly up, and feel your hips lift. Become comfortable with having your goggles slightly underwater, with only your mouth and nose out of the water.

BACK-KICK TWIST. Again kicking on your back, keep your head still and face pointing up at all times. Rotate your hips and shoulders together so that your body moves to a 45-degree angle. Pause for at least three breaths on each side and when you return to the middle. Keep your arms tight to your body with your hips and shoulders coming out of the water with each rotation.

BACK-KICK TWIST-DOWN. Establish a relaxed position on your back, rotate to your side, and stabilize; now swivel your chin so that you are looking straight down at the bottom of the pool; swivel your chin back up, stabilize, and move back to the middle. Now do the same thing on the other side.

BACK-KICK CHANGE. This is the same drill as the preceding one, but now you change sides by rolling across your front (rather than onto your back). If you have trouble with the transition, then pause on your front and slow the movement down.

Once you have mastered these drills, you will be ready to move on to the more difficult side-kick drills.

SIDE-KICK. With both arms at your sides, kick on your side for an entire length of the pool. Rotate your chin to breathe while keeping your head aligned with your spine and your body in alignment (think surfboard rather than noodle). When you are well balanced, you will be able to spend the majority of the time with your face down in the water. Your goal is to increase your comfort until you need to swivel only your chin to breathe.

SIDE-KICK EXTENDED. Extend your lower arm outward, and keep it aligned with your body (6 to 8 inches under the water). If your arm is at the surface, your hips are likely low in the water. This drill is easier than the preceding one. Remember that you will get significant balance benefits from the arms-at-side version before progressing.

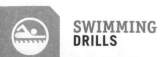

SWIMMING DRILLS

Tips for Swimming Drills

Make sure you are doing transitions in both directions. You will quickly notice that you have a side and a rotational direction that feels more comfortable. Work to improve your limiting side for the most technical gains.

Remember that your goal is to become balanced at all times of the rotation. Your speed down the pool is meaningless.

Keep your intensity down and rest periods long. You want to have absolutely perfect technique. You may think that the intensity is too low, but the concentration required for perfect swimming will leave you fatigued. Let your bike and run training take care of your cardiovascular needs. Successful long-distance swimming is about having the lowest energy consumption for a given pace.

Relax your face and neck, particularly when you are breathing. Muscular tension lowers economy of movement.

If you find that you are not traveling in a straight line, then you are likely curving your body toward the direction that you are going. In other words, you have a banana shape, with your hips being pushed away from your body.

■ *Body Rotation*

Triathletes are overachievers and set high expectations for themselves. Be aware that you will have a tendency to rush your skills work. Slow down, enjoy the sessions, and master the previous section before continuing.

SINGLE-STROKE CHANGE. Start as you did for side-kick extended and change sides by doing a single stroke. Transition as if you are moving between two rails. Settle, take at least three breaths, and transition back. Repeat as you move down the pool.

THREE-STROKE CHANGE. The same as single-stroke change except that three transitions are made between sets of breaths.

With the two preceding drills, start by keeping the face down during the transition, pausing, then taking three (or more) breaths to settle (using the chin-swivel method and keeping the face in the water). Once you are comfortable with this technique, transition directly to a breath and follow with two additional "swivel breaths." Once you are able to do three-stroke change with a single breath on each side, you have achieved three-stroke bilateral breathing. Congratulations! More detailed notes on bilateral breathing appear earlier in this chapter.

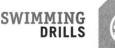

SWIMMING DRILLS

It is easy to spot athletes who have mastered the side-kick drills. They have excellent balance, are relaxed in the water, and achieve good distance per stroke. At this stage in your development (and not before), it makes sense to begin to focus on your overall stroke mechanics as well as your muscular endurance. What about endurance? You may not have realized it, but you will have been building it throughout your balance and body-rotation drills.

PROPULSIVE SWIMMING

Rich Strauss was kind enough to contribute his views on Propulsive Swimming in this section.

Once you are comfortable and aligned, you are ready for some "Propulsive Swimming." Athletes often wonder when they should begin doing fewer drills and more swimming. There is a pace that is the line between swimming for technique and swimming for speed and fitness. This pace is about 18.5 to 19 min. per 1,000 m (long-course), or about 1:51 to 1:54 per 100 m. If you want to express it as a "swim golf" score, the goal would be sub-90, or fewer than 45 strokes (for 50 m) and about 45 sec. In other words, if you are slower than these times, there are far more gains to be made by focusing on technique than on fitness. Once you cross this threshold, your performance becomes more a function of propulsive skills and swimming fitness. This is not to say that once you break 18 min. for a 1,000 m time trial, you have a pass to never do drills again. Rather, you would be justified in doing an increasing amount of fitness-oriented swimming in place of dedicated drill work.

Before this point, you should focus on balance skills to develop a good horizontal body position and on "side swimming"—spending as much time as possible on your side and presenting less surface area to the water. After you have become proficient with these drills, it is time to learn how to get the most power out of your stroke.

■ *The Catch*

When your hand enters the water, your palm is down toward the bottom of the pool. If you start pulling now, without doing anything else, you will be directing force downward and lifting your body rather than moving your body forward. This movement continues until the natural sweep of your arm eventually directs forces rearward.

The correct idea is to get your palm from "down" to "facing rearward" (and thus pushing you forward) as quickly as possible. The proper way to do this is by bending the elbow, or "catching" the water as soon as possible. This would be analogous in cycling to "rolling the barrel" at the top of your pedal stroke and beginning to apply power at noon rather than waiting until 2 or 3 o'clock.

To further illustrate the proper catch, sit at a table or a desk and stick your left arm out directly in front of you, parallel to the table, palm down.

Now bend your left elbow (without moving your upper arm) and touch your left fingertips to the desk in front of you. Your forearm is probably at a 45-degree angle from your upper arm. Notice three things:

- Your elbow is high and has not moved significantly.
- Your elbow is directly above your hand (relatively speaking).
- Your "paddle" essentially includes your hand and your forearm. This is very important.

With your fingers still on the desk and elbow up high, now just let your elbow drop. This is referred to as a poor catch, dropping the elbow, or slipping the front of your stroke.

■ *Combining the Catch with Your Pull*

Now put your arm out directly to the left, parallel to the ground, palm down. Turn your head left so that you are looking at your hand. Without moving your elbow or upper arm, bend your elbow and forearm as you did before. This position combines the elements of:

- An aggressive shoulder roll—the shoulder is pointing down at the bottom of the pool, belly facing the side wall
- Proper head position—looking down
- Aggressive catch

■ *Mastering the Catch*

Here are a few ideas on how to master the proper catch.

FIST DRILL. Swim with a closed fist, normal to fast arm speed, no fins. Visualize a barrel on top of the water and imagine that you are trying to reach over and around it, to carry it in your arm. This will help you keep your elbow high. Next, imagine that your forearm is a paddle. Swim with your forearm, not your hand.

Perform this drill for two to three lengths, then open your hand in the middle of the pool. You should feel the increase in power.

After you have done this drill a few times and return to normal swimming, these two ideas will help you maintain your high-elbow, aggressive catch.

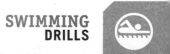

SWIMMING
DRILLS

OVER THE BARREL. Maintain the feeling of reaching over a barrel as you swim.

FINGERS DOWN. Put your left arm out in front of you, palm down. Now point your hand downward, bending at the wrist while the rest of your arm remains in place. Duplicate this in the pool by pointing your fingers to the bottom as soon as possible. The rest of your catch will fall into place.

Beginning to practice these skills is the line between balance swimming and propulsive swimming. If your body position and balance are not correct, it doesn't make sense to develop propulsive skills. However, if your body position is dialed in, then this aggressive catch is where the money is. Swimmers spend years refining this one small aspect of their strokes.

■ Stretch-Cord Exercises

When you are ready to start Propulsive Swimming, you are likely to find that your catch is your key limiter. The more quickly you are able to rotate your shoulder and set up the pull, the better. All athletes can afford to be stronger in the initial phase of their catch. If you are already swimming three times per week, then you will likely benefit from one or two stretch-cord sessions of 10–15 min. per week.

You must use perfect form at all times with these exercises (or any technical drill, for that matter). Focus on technique before trying to move quickly or under load. The learning progression for any new skill or movement pattern is the same:

- Learn the movement pattern slowly.
- Add speed.
- Add resistance.
- Perform under stress.

When learning the half pull, keep the movement slow and controlled with very light resistance. Then add speed to the half pull. Then add resistance to the half pull. Then add the full pull and slow it down again. Then add speed, then add resistance. Maintain the same pattern for all the exercises. Your long-term goal should be to train the muscles so you can bring the quickness of the catch into your swim stroke. Also, remember to control the "negative" portion of the exercises. Work your muscles in both directions.

Start with light-resistance stretch cords. You can always make the exercise harder (if needed) by moving away from the tie point. In addition to strength, the cords give you the benefit of being able to train your muscle-firing patterns without having to worry about balance

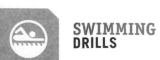

SWIMMING DRILLS

and breathing. You can find stretch cords at the sports shops of most large swimming pools, at sports medicine clinics, at sporting goods stores, and through mail-order vendors.

The first two stretch-cord exercises are the most important for swimmers. Full pulls should not be attempted until the half pulls are mastered.

HALF PULLS. Tie cords slightly above waist height and extend your arms until the cords are just tight. The elbow stays perfectly still while the forearm rotates forward and down. The elbow stays high and still; the hand remains aligned with the forearm; the arm, forearm, and hand all rotate slightly inward. The elbow does not move back; all movement is done by rotating the forearm. The goal is to build front-end strength. Look down with a neutral head position and maintain hand and forearm alignment.

Figures 6.1a and 6.2a demonstrate the half pull starting position. The goal is alignment of hip, shoulder, and wrist at the start. Figures 6.1b and 6.2b demonstrate the half pull ending position.

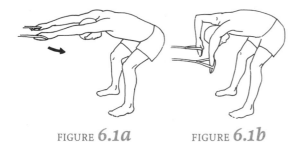

FIGURE **6.1a**   FIGURE **6.1b**

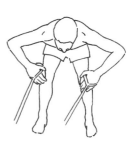

FIGURE **6.2a**   FIGURE **6.2b**

FORWARD ROTATIONS. Kneel or stand with your back to the cords. Cords should be tied at the same height as shoulders. Arms are extended straight out, bent at the elbows, and the forearms are perpendicular to the shoulders and upper arms, making an "L" on each side. The elbows stay perfectly still while the forearms rotate forward through 90 degrees. Figure 6.3a demonstrates the starting position, and Figure 6.3b demonstrates the ending position.

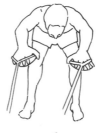
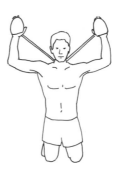

FIGURE **6.3a**   FIGURE **6.3b**

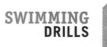

SWIMMING DRILLS

FULL PULLS. This is a catch simulation with pull-through. Tie cords slightly above waist height and face the tie. Bend at the waist. With both arms, catch, pull, and push through. The pull should be straight back with the elbows above the wrists. Focus on a quick catch.

Repeat the first two positions, as in half pulls. Figures 6.4a and 6.5a demonstrate the pull-through. Figures 6.4b and 6.5b demonstrate the final position of the full pull. Throughout this exercise, the hands and forearms are always pointing straight down and the palms are always facing straight back.

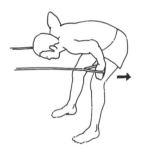
FIGURE **6.4a**

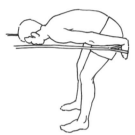
FIGURE **6.4b**

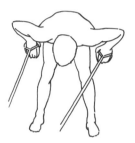
FIGURE **6.5a**

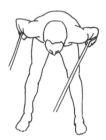
FIGURE **6.5b**

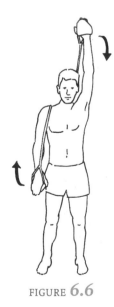
FIGURE **6.6**

STANDING STRAIGHT ARM. Face away from the tie point, both arms straight with hands overhead; alternating arms, move each arm in a semicircle from 12 to 6 o'clock. See Figure 6.6.

TRICEPS EXTENSION. Face away from the tie point, elbows high and in close, and extend hands to do a triceps extension. The goal is to keep the elbows high and tight. Do three sets: 60 sec. on, 60 sec. off, 50 sec. on, 50 sec. off, 40 sec. on, 40 sec. off. Those with a limited range of motion in their hips and back may benefit from a higher tie point. Athletes must hold 100 percent perfect form at all times. It is most important to maintain high elbows. Figure 6.7a demonstrates the starting position of the triceps extension; Figure 6.7b demonstrates the ending position of the triceps extension.

RECOVERY DRILL. Face away from the tie point, bend at the waist, and look into a mirror. Strengthen your recovery by "swimming" while using the cords to create resistance on the recovery portion of your stroke. This drill is

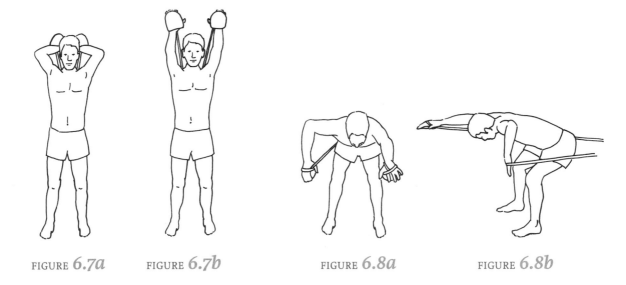

FIGURE *6.7a*   FIGURE *6.7b*   FIGURE *6.8a*   FIGURE *6.8b*

particularly effective for athletes (commonly female) who become fatigued when swimming in wetsuits. Figure 6.8a shows a front view of the recovery drill; Figure 6.8b shows a side view of the recovery drill.

"Sock swimming" is an alternative to swim cords for dry-land training. Start by placing 8–24 ounces of fishing weights into two athletic socks and tying a loop into the top of each sock. Bend at the waist and "swim" freestyle while watching your form in a mirror. Maintain a high elbow throughout the swim stroke. Sock swimming can be done in sets lasting 8–20 min. Maintain your cadence throughout the "swim." Lift your cadence for the final 20 sec. of each minute and for the final minute of each set. This workout is surprisingly tough and an effective way to maintain your swimming muscles when you are unable to get to a pool.

KICKING

Many triathletes believe that in order to swim faster, they need to kick harder. For nearly every triathlete body type, the kick is secondary. The muscles used for kicking are big muscles that consume large amounts of oxygen and energy relative to their propulsive benefit. In addition, the limited ankle flexibility in most triathletes further limits the effectiveness of their kicks. For most of us, increased speed comes from technique, balance, and stroke mechanics, not the kick.

However, using your kick during technique swims can be beneficial to learn balance and comfort in the water. Through focused-technique swims on form, balance, and comfort, your

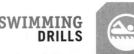

SWIMMING DRILLS

THE MAIN BENEFITS OF SWIMMING WITH FINS are improved body position, better ankle flexibility, and better speed. Kick sets with long fins are also an opportunity to work on core stability, especially the fly kick done on your back. For all swimmers, particularly novice swimmers, fins are useful in the following situations:

- Balance drills for swimmers with weak kicks—short fins are best; try to go fin-free as soon as possible.
- Front-end stroke drills—fins will help you relax and focus on the front end of your stroke. No more than 50 percent (maximum) of drilling should be done with fins.
- Fly-kick sets—done on the front, side, and back, this is an excellent core workout.
- Recovery sets—200–400 m of easy swimming between harder sets.
- Long-axis-stroke drills for advanced swimmers.

If balance is your key limiter (as discussed earlier), avoid fins and pull-buoys.

kick will naturally improve, as will your body position. You can also work on ankle flexibility and kick sets—both are the keys to improved kicking. Belly kicks with long fins and a kickboard will help with ankle flexibility—as will stretching.

There is a portion of the triathlon population who will benefit from a strong kick. These athletes are typically male, below average height, and muscular, with very low body fat. For these athletes, a solid kick is essential to swim at a high level. The lean, large legs of this body type cause the hips and legs to drop, and an effective kick is therefore a prerequisite for effective non-wetsuit swimming.

Depending on your Ironman-distance swim times, a stronger kick might knock a minute out of your swim. Most triathletes will likely have a better return on investment by working on their bike and run instead.

Kick sets can be most useful when they are used to rest the upper body—for example, following a long pull set—or to improve balance—for example, the side-kick drills.

KEY TRAINING SESSIONS

■ *Endurance*

See Appendix C, "Swimming Glossary," for definitions of terms. Endurance swims should be technique-oriented sessions that build your base endurance. They are best done in a long-course pool.

To get the most benefit from your endurance swims, always work on a technical limiter. Plan in advance which items will be worked on during which swims. Hold perfect form the whole way.

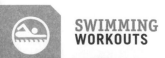

ENDURANCE 1

W/U

Build to a peak based on length of desired warm-up
  50/100/150 b/l build (:05–:10 RI)
  150/100/50 b/l descend (:05–:10 RI)

MAIN SET

Up to 8 x 400
  Odd sets: 4 x 100 (:15 RI) | 1st and 2nd steady, 3rd mod-hard, 4th easy
  Even sets: 400 b/l (:20 RI) | Easy to steady

C/D

  200 nonfree

ENDURANCE 2

W/U

| 300 choice | Easy |

PULL SET

| | Pull-buoy/band (odd), paddles (even) |

2–4 x
  150 pull (:10 RI) | Long and smooth
  3 x 50 pull (:10 RI) | Faster and smooth
  Rest 20 sec. between sets

KICK SET

Fins are optional
  3 x 200 descend (:30 1st RI, :45 2nd RI) | 100 kick with board, 50 swim, 50 kick

MAIN SET

| 100s on T(1) + :05 (:10 RI) | Swim 30 min. Focus on maintaining stroke mechanics. Hold the same split for each 100. |

C/D

| 200 mix of strokes | Easy |

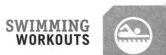

SWIMMING
WORKOUTS

ENDURANCE 3

W/U

300 b/l 3 (:10 RI)
400 IM, no fly, head up free to start (:10 RI)
100 kick (:10 RI)
4 x 50 w/c (:10 RI)

DISTANCE SET

6 x [4–6 x 100]	Set 1: Pull f/g b/l 3 on T(1) + :15 per 100
	Set 2: Pads only b/l on T(1) + :10 per 100
	Set 3: Swim on T(1) + :10 per 100
	Set 4: Fin kick on T(1) + :15 per 100
	Set 5: Swim on T(1) + :10 per 100
	Set 6: Swim on T(1) + :15 per 100

C/D

200 choice

ENDURANCE 4

W/U

| 800 DPS (:10 RI) | Easy to steady pace |
| 4 x 100 kick/dr (:10 RI) | Alternate kick and drill |

MAIN SET

3–5 x	
300 pull b/l 3 on T(1) + :15 per 100	Steady
100 on T(1) + :10 per 100	Fast

FIN SET

200 bk	Easy
2 x	
2 x 50 (:10 RI)	Fast
4 x 25 (:10 RI)	Fast

C/D

| 200 choice | Easy, fins optional |

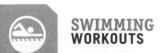

ENDURANCE 5

W/U

400 free (:15 RI)	Every 4th length nonfree, easy
300 b/l 5 (:15 RI)	Steady
200 bk kick (:15 RI)	Mod-hard
100 IM (:15 RI)	

SPEED SET

2 x 100 easy swim recovery	
5 x 100 (:20 RI)	25 polo, 25 easy free, 50 free
Descend the final 50 to fast effort	
2 x 100 easy swim recovery	

MAIN SET

400 pull b/l 5 steady on T(1) + :10
2 x 200 swim b/l 3 fast on T(1) + :10
4 x 100 swim b/l 3 fast on T(1) + :15
2 x 200 swim b/l 3 fast on T(1) + :10
400 pull b/l 5, steady on T(1) + :10

C/D

200 mix of strokes	Easy

ARE YOU READY FOR PULL SETS? Stroke mechanics are more important than speed. A swimmer with huge power, poor form, and excellent speed is likely to reinforce poor form by doing pull sets. Slower swimmers with excellent form, on the other hand, can use pull sets to build strength and muscular endurance.

For these sets, your gear includes a pull-buoy, paddles, and a band. The pull-buoy goes between your legs, the band around your ankles, and the paddles on your hands (remove the wristbands). You can mix and match the equipment for various levels of intensity (refer back to Table 4.1). Pull sets with "full gear" means using all three pieces of equipment. Swimmers with a history of shoulder problems should be very careful using paddles and bands.

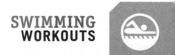
SWIMMING WORKOUTS

■ *Muscular Endurance*

These workouts will challenge your ability to tolerate pace changes and higher-effort swimming. You should swim only to the limit of your ability, keeping technique intact. Be wary of reinforcing poor technique when you are increasing training load.

MUSCULAR ENDURANCE 1

W/U

600 free	Build, steady for last 200–300
5 x 200 (:15 RI)	25 fly, 175 free, steady

MAIN SET

4 x 300 (:30 RI)	Set 1: Band only, mod-hard
	Set 2: Free, steady
	Set 3: Pull-buoy/band, mod-hard
	Set 4: Free, steady
100 back (:20 RI)	Easy
2 x 50 free (:10 RI)	Fast

Coach's tip: It is very important to be able to maintain form when doing this type of work; otherwise it is counterproductive.

C/D

200 free	Easy

MUSCULAR ENDURANCE 2

MAIN SET

12 x 200	
3 x 200 pull-buoy, b/l 5 (:10 RI)	Set 1: Steady
3 x 200 pull-buoy/band, b/l 3 (:20 RI)	Set 2: Mod-hard
3 x 200 pull-buoy/band, descend (:30 RI)	Set 3: Fast
3 x 200 no gear (:30 RI)	Set 4: Build, finish mod-hard

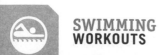

MUSCULAR ENDURANCE 3

W/U

500	Long and steady

PULL SET

1–2 x	
200 (:30–:40 RI)	Fast
4 x 50 (:05 RI)	Fast, hold split
Rest 1:00 between sets	

KICK SET (WITH FINS)

3–4 x 200 descend (:40 RI)	100 kick with board, 50 kick no board, 50 swim

SPEED SET

2 x (3 x 50)	Sprint 1: First 3rd max, rest easy
All on greater of 1:20 SI and :20 RI	Sprint 2: Second 3rd max, rest easy
	Sprint 3: Third 3rd max, rest easy

MAIN SET

2–5 x (3 x 100)	Odd sets: 1st and 2nd 100 fr, best average pace (:45 RI); 3rd 100 IM
	Even sets: :10 RI at 50 mark, :20 RI at all 100 mark

C/D

200	Easy

MUSCULAR ENDURANCE 4

W/U

400	Easy, every 4th length bk

PULL SET

100 (:30 RI)	50 easy, 50 fast
200 (:30 RI)	100 easy, 100 fast
300 (:30 RI)	150 easy, 150 fast
400 (:30 RI)	200 easy, 200 fast

SPEED SET

10 x 50 (:20 RI)	Odd swims easy, even swims fast

MAIN SET

100 choice	Very easy
3–6 x 200 best average pace	Leave on T(1) + :10 per 100

C/D

200 mix of strokes	Easy, fins okay

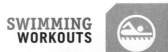

SWIMMING WORKOUTS

MUSCULAR ENDURANCE 5

W/U

2 x 300 b/l 3 or 3/5 (:15 RI)	Easy

KICK SET

2 x	
3 x 50 descend 1–3 (:15 RI)	Kick/swim by 25
No extra rest between sets	

MAIN SET

6–12 x 150 (:15 RI)	50 build/50 fast/50 DPS easy, hold split
200 choice	Very easy
15 min. pull-buoy b/l 3/5	Continuous swim, easy pace

C/D

200	Easy

MUSCULAR ENDURANCE 6

W/U

2 x 400 mix of strokes	Easy

DRILL SET | Focus on catch

No pads, no band, focus on front end of stroke	
2–3 x (4 x 50) fist drill (:10 RI)	1st 50: All fists
	2nd 50: 75 percent fists, then swim
	3rd 50: 50 percent fists, then swim
	4th 50: 25 percent fists, then swim
	25 kick, 25 swim
2 x (3 x 50) kick/swim (:10 RI)	

KICK SET (WITH FINS)

8 x 100 descend (:20 RI)	Odds: Kick with board
	Evens: Kick/swim by 50
Descend every 2nd swim	Swims 7 and 8 are fastest

MAIN SET

1–2 x (6 x 200) descend 1–6	Send-off is T(1) + :30 per 100 to start;
	reduce total send-off by :10 per interval
	(this implies T[1] + :5 per 100 for 6 and 12)
	No extra rest between sets

Coach's tip: The long rest will tempt you to go hard early, but show discipline. If you can swim T(1) pace the whole way, then you are doing very well!

C/D

200 mix of strokes	Easy

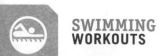

■ *Technique*

Remember that you should always use your best technique when swimming. The purpose of swim drills is to make you a better swimmer, not to make you great at drills. Know why you are doing each drill and incorporate what you learn into all of your swimming.

TECHNIQUE 1—FREESTYLE TECHNIQUE

PART 1

4 x 50	Set 1: Side-kick, arm at side
	Set 2: Side-kick, arm extended
	Set 3: Side-kick, one stroke, three breaths
	Set 4: Side-kick, three strokes, three breaths

Coach's tip: This is a challenging session. Focus on duration for this type of swimming. Distance guidelines are given for each component of the swim workout. Mix and match components to suit your time and swim limiters.

TIPS ON THREE-STROKE SWIM

- Fins can be used for all side-kick drills, but no fins is a superior workout for experienced swimmer.
- If swimming short course, stop every 25 or 50, change at each 12.5.
- If swimming long course, stop every 50, change at each 12.5 or 25.

- You must stay relaxed: Pace should be easy; rest interval is whatever is required to stay comfortable and relaxed. Beyond this point, if you feel fatigued or if your stroke starts to go, then you should stop and repeat the "Side-kick, three strokes, three breaths" (SK33) for 200 m of easy pace, pausing every 25 to 50.

PART 2

| 4–6 x 100 b/l free | Perfect form (at 50 :05–:10 RI; at 100 :15–:20 RI) |

Coach's tip: If technique starts to decline, return to SK33 drill. Rest interval should be as long as is required to maintain perfect, relaxed form. You will speed up naturally over time; have patience.

PART 3

| 2–6 x 50 bk (:15–:20 RI) | Perfect form |

Coach's tip: Focus on quick recovery: Stroke can be easy, with quick, straight arms. Keep head perfectly still, with shoulder opposite stroking arm coming out of water.

STILL HEAD POSITION on this drill (part 3) is very similar to the progression drill, where you drop alternating shoulders while kicking on back/side. Just as in freestyle, this stroke is done from side to side and requires comfortable balance with side-kicking.

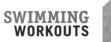
SWIMMING WORKOUTS

PART 4

4–8 x 50 b/l 3 count (:10–:20 RI)	Easy pace

A GOOD COUNT WOULD BE 40 STROKES when swimming long-course meters (LCM) of 40 to 50 sec. If your stroke count is above 50, then you want to focus on DPS—this can be achieved through better stroke finishing, improved balance, and comfort in the water. If your stroke count is below 40 strokes per LCM 50 and you are swimming longer than 50s, then you may be gliding too long, and you may benefit from increasing your hip drive to generate more efficiency. Your stroke rate should climb only slightly, but you will get a lot more speed and power. The increase in stroke rate will feel very fatiguing, as your body will be used to lots of rest. This tip is appropriate only for well-balanced athletes who swim with a normal stroke that essentially looks like catch-up drill.

PART 5

2 x 600 swim limiter	Swim 25s or 50s, working exclusively on personal limiter

Short course: Stop every 25 or 50, change at each 12.5
Long course: Stop every 50, change at 12.5 or 25
Rest as needed to be comfortable and relaxed

CHOOSE YOUR PERSONAL TECHNIQUE LIMITER (e.g., stroke finish, balance through rotation, catch and pull straight back, enter in front of shoulder and pull straight back). It is essential that you remain relaxed for this drill. Advanced athletes can swim 100s or 200s—however, you must be able to hold perfect form and work on limiter for entire time.

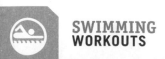

SWIMMING WORKOUTS

PART 6

2–6 x 50 3/4 drill (:10–:20 RI)

PART 7

4–8 swims count (:10–:20 RI)   Swim either 50s, 100s, or 200s
Short course: Count your even-length strokes
Long-course 100s: Count your return-length strokes
Long-course 50s: Count all strokes

PACE SHOULD BE COMFORTABLE AT ALL TIMES. If you feel winded, then swim a shorter interval. If you require more than 20 sec. of recovery, slow down and swim a shorter interval.

If balance and comfort in the water are your limiter, then interval distance and speed are not important. Rest a lot, and keep interval distance short. If you are a 70-min.-plus Ironman-distance swimmer or if your T(1) pace is 1:50 per 100 m LCM or slower, then you should assume that this is the case. T(1) LCM of 1:50 per 100 would be about 1:40 per 100 short-course yards (SCY).

If stroke endurance is your limiter (the likely issue for 70-min. or faster Ironman-distance swimmers), then your goal is to increase your interval distance while holding perfect form. For this type of swim, it is not necessary to go much beyond 200s—unless you are comfortably under an hour for an Ironman-distance swim. Then some mod-hard stroke endurance work at distances up to 400 m can be beneficial.

Once you can swim 1,000 m total with perfect form, increase your pace from easy to steady; note what happens to your stroke count. We want to see only a small increase in stroke count; a total increase of 5 percent is reasonable. As a guide, until you are under 50 strokes per LCM length, it doesn't make sense to speed up.

TECHNIQUE 2—STROKE TECHNIQUE

W/U

500, mix of strokes	
5 x 100 free	Easy

KICK SET (WITH FINS)

4 x 50 IM order (:30 RI)	

PULL SET

4 x 200 (:15 RI)	Easy pace; breathing by 50 is b/l 3, 5, 7, 9

Coach's tip: If you have trouble with 9, then use 7; if you have trouble with 7, then use 3, 5, 7/3, 7/5.

MAIN SET

5 IM swims (:45 RI)	10 fly strokes, 20 bk strokes, 10 br strokes, 20 free strokes
	Goal is maximum distance on each swim
3 x 100 IM count (:45 RI)	Hold good DPS
200 IM	Relaxed, smooth

C/D

200 choice, with fins	

TECHNIQUE 3—SHORTER RECOVERY SWIM

MAIN SET

300–600 free	Every 4th length bk
3 x 200 b/l	b/l 3, 5, 7, 5 by 50
400 straight b/l 5	Focus on offside arm mechanics
3 x 100 b/l 3	
100 bk	
100 br	

Coach's tip: This swim would be appropriate for an active-recovery day or following a strength training session. Rest intervals are as required to keep heart rate well down.

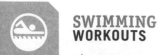

SWIMMING WORKOUTS

Other Swim Strokes

As you approach the fitness and skills required for, say, a 60-min. Ironman-distance swim, you will find the other strokes to be a useful addition to your training. By "other strokes" we mean backstroke, breaststroke, and fly.

Of the four strokes, improving your backstroke is the most useful in improving your freestyle. The primary reason is the similarity in critical success factors, most importantly long-axis balance and smooth body rotation.

When swimming backstroke, the ideal entry point is at 11 and 1 o'clock. However, more important than entry location is a quick, straight-arm recovery. A quick recovery with the hand entering pinkie finger first will nearly always result in a straight arm. Drive your arm deep, bend your elbow, and push as much water as possible straight back toward the far wall.

Very strong swimmers, those with sub-60-min. Ironman-distance swim times, are likely to benefit from adding the fly stroke to improve their power and muscular endurance. Fly is beneficial because it builds swim-specific power. Also, in conjunction with individual medley swimming, fly is beneficial because it improves an athlete's ability to recover from a strong effort while swimming.

Breaststroke is beneficial because the catches of breaststroke and freestyle are similar. Athletes with a history of knee problems should substitute a fly kick for the traditional whip kick.

Mastering all four strokes improves your swimming agility and strength, leading to improved economy.

PROS AND CONS OF SQUAD TRAINING

There are many advantages to swimming with a squad or masters group. Squad training offers a structured workout for athletes of all levels as well as having a coach on deck to ensure that you are swimming correctly. Your squad or masters coach is the best person to evaluate the impact of technical changes because he or she can see what is happening with your overall stroke and form. As well as having a coach to oversee and recommend drills for improvement, squad training is beneficial when you wish to train at a higher intensity level. Leading a lane with other swimmers is a good incentive to help you push your efforts. A little friendly competition can make training more fun and mentally easier. Keep in mind, however, that you should go only as fast as your ability to maintain good form allows.

The power of demonstration is also a powerful learning tool, and swimming with technically proficient swimmers gives you a visual picture to mirror. However, the opposite can be true when swimming with novice swimmers.

This point leads to the drawbacks of squad training. Swimmers nearly always swim too hard, and many masters coaches (and athletes) have no interest in working on technique. This attitude makes it difficult for you to learn and master correct form before adding speed to the equation. Novice swimmers are better off sticking to a slower lane and developing solid skills before advancing.

Remember that any session with others always includes an element of compromise, and the temptation to sacrifice form for the sake of speed can be great. Control and maturity are needed to avoid overdoing it. Hammering each workout will quickly lead to a performance plateau. Although all-out 50s and 100s on short rest intervals are fun, to reach your swimming potential, balance the mixture of technical, endurance, and faster work.

TRAINING FOR THE BIKE

 ycling accounts for roughly half of your race day, and it forms the core of an effective training strategy for all long-distance triathletes. A deep love of cycling is a fundamental requirement for successful long-distance racing. This chapter will discuss training strategies in detail, but first we'll take a look at a typical year of training for the bike leg.

> *Cycling is a blue-collar sport.*
> *You gotta do the miles.*
>
> —JONAS COLTING,
> SWEDISH CHAMPION TRIATHLETE

STAGES OF CYCLING DEVELOPMENT

Before we discuss the details of how to train for an Ironman-distance bike leg, it is essential that you understand our bike training philosophy as well as the physiological requirements for long-course cycling success.

In our experience, the bike is the biomechanically safest and most effective place for an athlete to build his or her aerobic base. Most athletes will be able to safely tolerate weekly cycling volume that is double or triple their run volume. Overall race endurance is the key limiter for the majority of long-course athletes, which implies a lot of riding.

There are three physiological components required for success in the "average" Ironman-distance bike leg:

1. *Race endurance:* The ability to complete the swim and bike legs and to run for a long time

2. *Climbing:* The ability to minimize the energy cost of riding (not racing) all climbs as efficiently as possible

3. *Time trialing:* The ability to push a big gear for a long time in flat and rolling terrain

Each of these components is best addressed by a different training focus, and most athletes will be addressing them to varying degrees throughout their athletic careers. We have found that most athletes achieve the greatest gains by eliminating these potential limiters in the order of endurance, force, and then muscular endurance. These three physiological attributes relate directly to race endurance, climbing, and time trialing, respectively.

The following sections describe the overall life cycle of a novice cyclist and the seasonal periodization of an experienced cyclist. Even speedy, experienced athletes need to revisit the basics each season. Especially for Ironman, the largest part of every season's training needs to focus on establishing/building cycling endurance. The more experienced you become as a cyclist, the more your training should focus on your personal race limiters.

■ *Stage 1: Endurance and Skills*

The most important component in your cycling development is building the endurance necessary to complete your race distance. Your triathlon season begins with concentration on easy endurance cycling, or low-intensity riding. Endurance rides should be supplemented with skills sessions and a focused strength training program. The overall goal is to increase cycling economy, enhance overall aerobic fitness, and prepare the body for the tougher work to come later in the season. This period will last three to six months. If

---

IF YOU HAVE SOME EXPERIENCE WITH LONG-DISTANCE BIKE RACING, here are some of the ways you can expect the cycling leg of an Ironman-distance race to be different.

Anaerobic endurance. If you are dropped during a bike race, your chances of success are greatly reduced. Road cyclists need to be able to endure, and recover from, frequent bouts of high-intensity riding well above their functional threshold. In contrast, triathlon cycling is a steady-state, subthreshold event. The patience and maturity to avoid high intensity are a limiting factor for many athletes.

Pacing. Although a single rider can have an impact on the pace of a long-distance cycle race, the overall pace of a bike race is governed more by group dynamics than by the personal decision of any one rider. In triathlon, the intelligent athlete is typically the one who is able to avoid the temptation of dueling with the athletes around him or her.

Finish line. Although this reminder may seem obvious, remember that you will be running a marathon when you get off your bike. Triathletes who "race" the bike leg tend to walk the marathon, which is very costly in terms of overall time.

N   **NOVICE**

you are new to Ironman-distance racing, this type of training can form up to 65 percent of your annual training volume. Until you are confident about your ability to complete the race distance, your training should be heavily biased toward endurance-based cycling. A strong cycling endurance base is the platform upon which your entire season will be built.

Volume

The core of your week is your longest steady-state endurance session, and you will want to plan on building your ride up to five to six hours. Build your session and overall volume slowly: two or three weeks of focused training, one week of recovery, and then repeat. A good rule of thumb is to limit increases to 10 percent in terms of long workout duration and/or weekly volume. The body will not be rushed, and even if you are racing early in the season, you will have plenty of time to prepare yourself.

You will receive a lot of advice on appropriate workout distances and durations. Listen to your body, and be conservative about the long stuff. This approach will enable you to recover quickly, maintain consistency, and avoid injury. The two most likely times for injury are during high-intensity training and when you run long after a long ride. We recommend avoiding these kinds of sessions.

Long, Slow Distance

Long, steady-state endurance cycling is the most effective way to improve general endurance, giving you the base fitness required to compete at the Ironman-distance level. The less experience you have with the distance, the more importance you should place on endurance training. For experienced athletes, the best time to build endurance is through the winter months into spring. Summer is generally the time for more focused muscular endurance cycling work.

"How long is long?" is a frequent question. For cycling, "long" starts at two hours. Your goals and experience should guide your decisions on bike volume. A novice athlete with a goal to finish will have different "longs" than an experienced athlete who is trying to place in his or her age group.

For athletes who are new to long-course training, it is best to slowly build the long ride up to five to six hours. The reason for building up slowly is that numerous physiological benefits accrue from a gradual increase in your endurance abilities. A tip for going "really long" on the bike is that you want your backside to give out before your legs. In other words, you are doing a workout in which intensity and average speed do not matter. Your goal is to train the physiological systems involved in going very long.

Endurance rides start in heart rate Zone 1 and will sometimes end in heart rate Zone 2 owing to cardiac drift. For a fit athlete, the entire ride will quite often be in heart rate Zone 1. Table A.2 in Appendix A will help you identify your heart rate zones based on your functional threshold. (See Appendix B for instructions on determining your functional threshold.) During your Base period (and throughout the year), do a portion of your endurance training at an easy pace. When you head into the late Build and Peak periods, you can increase the pace as you prepare your body to go faster.

In the early and middle Base periods, build your endurance with rides that focus on easy to steady pacing. Experienced and elite athletes should take this seriously—frequent racing (formal and in training) in the early sea-son will limit your endurance gains and greatly increase your risk of burn-out. Limit your "megarides" to two or three per month. Keep them slow, and gradually increase your boundaries. Consistent weekday rides are superior to an extra couple of hours on the weekend.

Cycling Economy

At the same time that you are building your aerobic engine, you can be improving your ped-aling and bike-handling skills. Technical improvements have a direct benefit on your cycling economy and lead to more successful long-distance racing.

In the exercise physiology lab, economy is a rating of submaximal work output in relation to oxygen consumed. For example, if we tested two riders with the same VO_2max and discovered that Rider A used less oxygen at 200 watts than Rider B, we would say that Rider A was more economical. Since Rider A wastes less energy in pedaling a bike, we could also surmise that Rider A is capable of riding longer at any given speed before becoming fatigued. That's quite an advantage in long-course racing. The longer the race, the greater this advantage becomes.

Economical pedaling comes from the split-second timing of muscle contractions and relax-ations. Throughout the pedal stroke, scores of muscles must fire, some for longer than others, and then relax. These muscle recruitment patterns are initiated by signals from the central nervous system and are automatic, but can be improved. When the nervous system is enervating muscles in intricate harmony, it's like the New York Philharmonic Orchestra: elegant. A nervous system firing muscles at the wrong times is more like a junior high school band: amateurish.

More than likely, your pedaling economy is somewhere between elegant and amateurish. To improve your skills, you need to think while you pedal. This means drills (see specific drills later in this chapter). Winter is a great time to develop your pedaling skills because winter weather is often not suited to outdoor riding.

There are two keys to improved economy. One is to refine the movements that take place at the top and bottom of the stroke, when the leg must shift from "up and back" to "forward and down," with the reverse situation at the bottom of the stroke. At the top of the stroke, the foot should feel as if it is pushing forward in the shoe. At the bottom, you should get the sense that mud is being scraped from the shoe.

The other key is to focus on the relaxation part of the pedal stroke. Tensing more muscles than are needed to apply force to the pedals is wasteful and uneconomical. Start with the muscles you have the most control over—the face and fingers. Once you can relax them, try relaxing your calves and toes while spinning. The idea is to activate only the muscles needed when they're needed. No more, no less.

The following equipment may help you become a more economical rider.

Spinning bikes. The bikes used in health clubs typically have a heavy flywheel with adjustable resistance. The flywheel minimizes leg-speed variations while pedaling and keeps your stroke smooth. Although you can get some benefit from using these bikes, be careful with spinning workouts; they can be a training disaster under the guidance of an overenthusiastic leader. You don't need to be in race shape in February (unless you live in Australia). Keep the intensity in check and work on your pedaling economy.

Fixed-gear bikes. To set up a fixed-gear bike, remove the derailleurs and shifters from an old frame. Have an older-style freewheel body welded, or buy a track-hub wheel. Select a gear that puts you at about 90 rpm on the flats when riding easily—this is probably in the range of 39–42 × 15–19 gearing. Ride only on flat to gently rolling courses. Be cautious at first—you'll have to unlearn old coasting habits, such as standing on the pedals to stretch and pausing to sit back down.

CompuTrainer SpinScan. If you are fortunate enough to have a CompuTrainer to train on, you can use the SpinScan mode to improve economy. By pedaling in this mode while watching the monitor, you can vary left-right leg output and force application to the pedal and see the result immediately. Isolated leg training, with one leg at a time doing all of the work, is an excellent drill with this equipment. The idea of drills with the SpinScan is to lower the peaks and raise the valleys of your power curve.

Of course, all of these ideas have only one purpose: to make your pedaling more economical in the real world of the road. It doesn't matter how proficient you become at any of these exercises if the gains don't translate to your bike in a race. During the winter months, think about what you're doing on the road. Is your pedal stroke relaxed even when the tempo picks up? Are you making smooth transitions at the top and bottom of the stroke? Are you pedaling at the high end of your cadence comfort range? By spring you should be answering yes to all of these questions.

■ *Stage 2: Overall Strength*

As you begin to establish your endurance base throughout the training year, you will want to begin increasing your muscular endurance using hills and steady long rides in heart rate Zone 2. It is a common mistake for experienced riders to believe that they need to train more intensely, but even the more experienced riders need plenty of Zone 2 riding.

On the bike, muscular endurance is best described as the ability to push a big gear for a long time. Because it can take four to eight weeks to reap the full benefits of your higher-intensity strength work, the transition to sport-specific strength work (muscular endurance training) is normally planned for no later than eleven weeks prior to an A-priority race. For athletes from the middle of the pack forward, cycling muscular endurance is typically their most significant limiter.

Elite and stronger cyclists may benefit from the higher-intensity workouts and training strategies addressed later in this chapter. Novices and midpack athletes are best served by narrowing their focus to building endurance in all sports and muscular endurance in cycling. It is possible to put together a very fast race with the right combination of this kind of training.

> **REMEMBER, THE TRANSITION FROM ENDURANCE TO MUSCULAR ENDURANCE IS GRADUAL.** If you have any doubts about your overall endurance, it is best to postpone (or cancel) the transition to muscular endurance training. It is pointless to be able to ride hard if you lack the overall endurance for the entire event. Ironman-distance racing is about having the ability to sustain a moderate speed for a very long time. Top-end speed and anaerobic endurance are not requirements for success—at either end of the field.
>
> **N** NOVICE

Warming Up

Prior to any time trial, race, or test, you will generate the best results if you are able to complete a thorough warm-up. An effective warm-up for a time trial of any duration follows:

Step 1: Ride 40 min., easy to steady pace. While riding, survey the course and build to 80–100 percent of threshold perceived effort on some short rollers. Ensure that there is no significant lactate accumulation during this period of the warm-up.

Step 2: Take a short bathroom break and if it is a hot day, have a good drink.

Step 3: Ride 20 min., steady pace. While riding, insert four or five efforts on long recoveries.

The efforts should be done in time trial position, roughly twenty pedal revolutions that build to a cadence of 100–120 rpm and power output of 150–165 percent of hard to very hard perceived effort. Again, ensure that there is no material lactate accumulation. Efforts should last just until you notice a change in your breathing pattern.

Step 4: Following the completion of the final effort, take a 2- to 5-min. break. During the break, focus on goals for the test or race. If the session is to last longer than 15 min., eat a small, highly glycemic snack and have another drink. Once the drink and snack have settled, start the session.

Muscular Endurance in Hilly Terrain

The goal of a hilly ride is typically to build muscular endurance. Novice athletes should begin these sessions on routes that offer an hour of easy terrain to warm up and then move to gentle rollers. You will want to work over these rollers keeping your heart rate in Zone 2 and your cadence low, around 60 rpm. Dropping your cadence any lower than 60 rpm can add excessive load on your knees, which can lead to injury or inflammation. Experienced athletes should incorporate longer, steady climbs maintaining heart rate Zone 3. In the Base period, the downhill and flat terrain in these rides is typically done at an easy pace. The key focus is building climbing-specific strength.

Group Rides

As the racing season approaches, many athletes benefit from riding in a group. Some athletes may avoid group rides because they feel they aren't up to group speed, lack group skills, or prefer to ride solo. For those who are new to group riding, the best way to learn is to start with a smaller

Basic Guidelines for Group Riding

- Always ride single file.
- Never half-wheel the person in front of you. Half-wheeling is when the leading edge of your front wheel is in front of the trailing edge of the leader's back wheel. It is highly dangerous because you can clip wheels. Even if you are riding in fierce crosswinds and trying to set up an echelon (riding to the side and back of the leading rider to sit in his or her wind shadow), it isn't worth the risk until you have excellent bike-handling skills.
- When riding at the front, increase and decrease speed gradually. Always continue to pedal when going downhill.
- Even if you think you are speeding up when you come out of the saddle, you are likely slowing down at first. This change has implications for athletes on your wheel.
- When drafting, the safest place for your hands is on your brake hoods. If you are team time trialing (riding on your aerobars), you need a very safe course and a lot of confidence in the other athletes in the group as well as in your own skills. It is highly risky to draft without your hands on the brakes.
- When you peel off the front, peel into the wind. The next rider in line should build into his or her turn gradually.
- If you are riding with stronger riders, don't feel that you have to take a turn. If you are going to sit in, make it clear to the others what your plans are and work out whether you are going to cycle through the group or simply stay at the back. Having a weaker cyclist cycle through can slow down the ride; some riders may prefer that you simply stay at the back and out of the way. Leave your ego behind if you have doubts about your stamina. It is far better to draft than to blow to pieces halfway through the ride.
- If you are much stronger than the rest of the group, take longer turns at the front, or even ride the whole time at the front. There is a huge difference between being at the front and sitting in the group. You can get a solid ride by leading, and the riders behind you will need to match only 60–70 percent of your power output.
- If you are riding with roadies, it is polite to leave your aerobars at home.

group of friends. Have your experienced training buddies explain what you need to know. When riding with a new group, it is best to be conservative and work just like everyone else.

Those who prefer to ride solo will find that riding with another athlete or small group enables them to maintain their focus as they get stronger. Four to five hours of steady riding is much easier when you have someone pushing you from behind, or if you are sitting on the wheel of a much stronger rider. Whichever you choose, you will benefit from both types of rides.

■ *Stage 3: Time Trial Strength*

To review, athletes must first train for the ability to complete the distance and ride efficiently (Stage 1). Second, they must train for the ability to climb hills and add muscular endurance work (Stage 2). Third, they must train for the ability to tolerate pace changes, push larger gears, and ride at a higher average intensity (Stage 3).

Most strong cyclists will find that time trial strength is their key limiter. The best sessions to address this limiter are muscular endurance interval sessions, big-gear work, and cruise intervals (periods of faster, subthreshold riding during a longer workout). The workouts in this chapter can be used as bike-only muscular endurance workouts or as brick workouts (Appendix D offers further brick options).

Novices are unlikely to get to Stage 3 because they will have their hands full building endurance. For experienced athletes, a portion of this type of training will be appropriate in late Base and the Build period.

Which workout to choose? Here are some tips suitable for athletes at all levels.

- Early in the season, interval duration and intensity should be shorter and lower.
- If focus or endurance is your limiter, then high-intensity intervals should be avoided; you will reap greater rewards from steady rides that incorporate cruise intervals.
- To improve your economy, practice interval training at the limits of your comfortable cadence range (both high and low).
- As the season progresses, most athletes will benefit from building toward longer, subthreshold intervals.
- Athletes who are force-limited will benefit from intervals that incorporate large-gear, low-cadence work. When doing muscular endurance intervals, keep your heart rate down and focus on making smooth, powerful circles.
- If your greatest limiter is the ability to focus, ride 5 to 25 km subthreshold time trials.
- The most effective interval session for Ironman-distance racing is a series of moderate intervals incorporated into an endurance-oriented BT workout. Examples of these sessions are included later in this chapter.

CYCLING SKILLS

Bike-handling skills are perhaps the most neglected single aspect of cycling. Triathletes with superior bike-handling skills will complete their bike legs faster, more comfortably, and with lower energy consumption. This leaves them with more energy for the run. Those who have difficulty cornering, descending, and handling the bike in the wind should address those specific areas over the off-season and early Base period. Here are a few basic cycling skills and how to go about developing them.

■ *Pedaling*

Pedaling a bike seems simple, but few triathletes are really good at it. When you ride with someone who pedals efficiently, there is an obvious difference, but it is difficult to describe. To improve your pedaling skills, it's important to smooth out the leg's directional changes at the top and bottom of the stroke.

The best place to practice pedaling skills is on an indoor trainer, as there will be no distractions such as traffic, dogs, or other riders to break your concentration. The sound of the indoor trainer can also provide valuable feedback for an athlete seeking to smooth his or her pedaling stroke. Here are a few pedaling drills.

HORIZONTAL PEDALING. Don't think about the pedal stroke as being up and down or even circular. Think of it as horizontal; at the top and bottom of the stroke your legs are transitioning to go the other direction—either forward and down or back and up. An increase in energy output here decreases the need for a very high effort at 3 o'clock.

There are several elements of the stroke you can focus on to develop this horizontal-pedaling skill. The best mental focus for most riders involves driving the toes toward the ends of their shoes at the top of each stroke. Another mental cue that works for some is scraping mud off at the bottom. Yet a third focus involves imagining that you are throwing your knees over the handlebars. Concentrate on only one of these at a time.

ISOLATED LEG TRAINING (ILT). While riding on an indoor trainer, place a chair on either side of the bike. Place one foot on a chair and pedal with the other for 30 sec., focusing on your critical-stroke mental cue from above. Then switch legs and pedal for 30 sec. with the other, still focusing on your technique. Keep your cadence at around 90 rpm throughout. After working both legs, pedal normally for another minute with both legs, sustaining the same sensation of proper technique. Repeat several times.

DOMINANT LEG. It's not safe to do ILT on the road, but the dominant leg drill can be done anywhere you ride. While pedaling with both feet clipped in to the pedals, use one leg to do

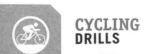

CYCLING
DRILLS

almost all of the work for 30 sec. while the other leg is "lazy." Otherwise, this drill is just like the ILT drill. Pay attention to the road—don't watch your feet.

INCREASED CADENCE. Mashing (pedaling a large gear with a low cadence) is not economical. Continually working on raising your cadence improves your economy. Each of us has a comfortable cadence range. Anytime we get outside it, we feel sloppy. By discovering your range and staying near the top end of it several times each week, you can shift your comfortable range upward. One way to do this is to buy a handlebar computer with a cadence monitor and check it during your rides.

SPIN-UPS. This drill helps you become more economical at higher cadences. Either on the road or on an indoor trainer, while riding in a low gear, gradually increase your cadence over a 30-sec. period until you begin to bounce on the saddle. Then slow the cadence until you are no longer bouncing and hold it for a few more seconds. The key to this drill is relaxation. Relax your toes, your grip on the bars, and your face. Make it seem almost effortless. Do several of these within a ride, separating them with a few minutes of "normal" cadence.

PEDAL RECOVERY. What you do with the leg that is on the recovery side of the stroke is critical to your economy. If this leg rests on the pedal, the other leg will have to work harder to lift it. Be careful not to pull up with the recovery leg (except when climbing or sprinting) because it will cause a tremendous waste of energy. Instead, try to simply "unweight" the recovery pedal. In other words, if you weren't clipped in, the weight of that leg would be taken off the pedal as it came back up. In reality, this won't happen because of the centrifugal force of pedaling, but we can move closer to this ideal.

■ *Balance*

You probably learned to balance a bike as a child, and how to do it never crosses your mind while riding now. It's pretty simple. However, situations may arise during a race or ride that challenge your balancing skills. For example, you might need to avoid a crash that happens unexpectedly right in front of you, or a dog may run onto the road and hit your wheel. These situations require more balance skill than simply riding a straight, unobstructed line down the road.

Some drills can help you become more adept at balancing the bike. Always do them away from traffic and obstructions that may cause an accident. Seldom-used parking lots are often a good choice. Here are a few examples.

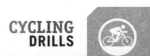

CYCLING
DRILLS

BOTTLE PICKUP. Place your water bottle on the pavement while riding slowly. Then turn around and come back to pick it up. To make these moves, you will need to stop pedaling and keep your foot low on the side you lean to while ensuring that the front wheel stays straight with the frame. Go slowly at first, and as you get the hang of it, gradually go faster. A tall bottle will help you get started, but then progress to a shorter bottle. When this starts to feel easy, try placing the bottle on its side so that you have to reach lower to pick it up.

SLALOM RIDE. Set up four or five water bottles about 8 feet apart in a straight line. Practice riding a slalom course through the bottles by leaning the bike—not your body—to the inside of each turn. Take one or three pedal strokes between bottles so that the inside pedal is always up. It should feel like a rhythmic dance when done smoothly. As you get better, try riding faster.

BOTTLE JUMP. Lay an empty plastic water bottle on its side on the pavement. Ride at it fast several times and attempt to jump the bottle without touching it. Try it in both the upright and crouched positions.

■ *Aero Position*

When it comes to riding a bike on a flat, level course, aerodynamic drag is the greatest challenge. At speeds greater than about 12 mph (20 kph), more than half of the total mechanical work done by the rider is spent overcoming air resistance. Air resistance increases exponentially rather than linearly relative to velocity, as you might expect. In other words, as you speed up, air resistance increases at an ever greater rate. At 25 mph (40 kph), penetrating the air makes up 82 percent of the total resistance that must be overcome. When riding into a headwind, the rider's resulting velocity is essentially increased by the speed of the wind, requiring even greater effort to overcome drag. On cold days, the air's resistance is greater yet because cold air is denser.

Most of this air resistance is a result of the frontal area presented to the wind by the rider's body. The greater the frontal area, the greater the air resistance. Compared with sitting upright on the bike with the hands on the tops of the handlebars, a standard aero position reduces frontal area by more than 21 percent on average.

Though aerodynamics is an important consideration for long-distance triathlon, the criteria of safety, comfort, and power production tend to dominate the position. Athletes should remember that the most aerodynamic position is seldom the optimal position for long-course racing.

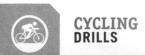

CYCLING DRILLS

◼ *Braking*

To control speed, the rear brake is used more often than the front. This brake is often "feathered," meaning that pressure is applied gradually and in small amounts to reduce speed, as when preparing for a corner. In an emergency situation where an immediate stop is needed, both brakes are applied, with the front brake given the most force. In such a situation you should also slide back on the saddle to weight the rear wheel to prevent it from skidding and losing control. This position also helps to prevent an "end-o," as in end over end.

When descending a hill, you must be careful when using the front brake. Pulling it aggressively can easily result in a crash. Apply the rear brake primarily on a fast descent, feathering the front brake only if more slowing power is needed. It is most stable to do the majority of braking before heading into a turn; braking in the middle of a turn can unbalance a bike and result in a crash.

◼ *Cornering*

One of the most dangerous times in a ride, especially a fast one, comes when negotiating corners. The first rule of cornering is not to brake in the corner. If the turn is free of gravel and water, you should be able to take it at full speed by leaning. If it's necessary to slow down, brake before you get into the turn. Then let go of the brake levers as the turn begins.

The most important time in taking a corner is the early part. If the critical speed and line you have selected are right, then you will have no problems. Practice approaching corners repeatedly at various speeds. Make it second nature to judge how fast to take them. The line you select depends on your speed. A fast speed requires a more gradual and sweeping turn than does slow cornering.

Sit in the middle of your saddle, not on the nose or back end of it. This position will help you better maintain balance. As the turn starts, stop pedaling so that the inside knee is high, put most of your weight on the outside pedal, and lean to the inside. The lean of the bike should be greater than the lean of your upper body. To accomplish this, keep your head upright so that the line of the eyes is parallel to the surface of the road. Never lean your head into a corner.

When the bike becomes more upright as you come out of the corner, begin to pedal again. It is common to stand up out of a corner and accelerate.

Many athletes are afraid to corner. Given that confidence is essential for good cornering, these athletes will benefit from a pre-race reconnaissance in which the technical aspects of the bike leg are reviewed, ridden, and practiced. Large time savings can easily be achieved from a detailed review of technical sections. These time savings require no additional fitness, merely an investment of time. Race week is an excellent time for undertaking these activities, particularly when a friend is willing to offer car support.

■ Climbing

Body mass has a lot to do not only with how well you climb but also with how you climb. Smaller riders (less than 2 pounds of body weight for every inch of height) usually climb best when out of the saddle, whereas bigger riders (more than about 2.3 pounds per inch) climb more effectively seated. Top riders between these extremes often alternate between sitting and standing when climbing but spend more time seated. The standing position is less economical on a moderate grade, but on a steep hill standing reduces the feeling of effort.

When starting a long, steady climb, select a lower gear so that the cadence is relatively high. As you progress up the hill, shift to higher gears. This helps to prevent fatiguing muscles early in the climb, allowing you to finish strongly. Doing it the other way around—going from a high to a lower gear—is associated with slowing down. In a high gear, your cadence may be as low as 60 rpm. The lower your cadence, the greater the strain on your knees and muscles. Even if you spin at 100 rpm on the flats, you'll likely find that a slower cadence is more effective when climbing.

If alternating between sitting and standing positions during the climb, shift to a higher gear while standing and back to a lower gear for sitting down, especially near the bottom of the climb, when your gear is somewhat lower. You can't spin as fast when standing, so a higher gear is necessary then. Near the top of the climb, you may not need to shift up because the gear will already be high.

When standing, allow the bike to sway gently from side to side without weaving off-line. Do not exaggerate this movement. It should happen naturally as the pedal goes down and the hand on the same side pulls to counterbalance the leg force.

When seated, scoot back on the saddle and place your hands on the brake hoods or bar tops rather than on the drops. This position will keep your head up so you can better see what's ahead and open up your chest to allow for easier breathing. Upon standing, grip the brake hoods to better balance the bike. Keep the grip light. Squeezing the bar does nothing to improve climbing and only wastes energy. Bernard Hinault, one of France's greatest riders, used to say that when climbing he kept his fingers as loose as if he were playing a piano.

If the front wheel veers off-line with every stroke due to using too high a gear, locking the elbows, or choking the handlebar, the rolling resistance increases by up to 30 percent. Don't make climbing any harder than it already is. Pay close attention to maintaining a straight line.

■ Descending

Coming back down a hill at high speed requires concentration and trust. You must concentrate on the road ahead, potential dangers on the side of the road (pedestrians, dogs, deer, cars), and other riders and traffic around you. You must also trust your bike and your handling skills. If these are questionable, slow down. It's better to lose a few seconds in a descent than to make a trip to the emergency room.

Most riders have a fear threshold—a speed above which they feel out of control. As you become more experienced at descending, your threshold will rise, but it will never go away. When the threshold approaches, the tendency is to grab the brakes and hang on for dear life. This could make matters worse because the heat buildup from the friction of brake pad against rim may cause the brakes to begin to fail.

Slowing down on a descent is an art form based on using your body as a sail to control speed, evenly distributing your weight between the front and rear wheels, and briefly and repeatedly applying the brakes, primarily using the rear brake. This system allows the brake pads and rim to cool between applications.

If speed is your goal on a descent, the tucked position with the hands on the aerobars, the back flat with head close to the hands, the knees in, and the cranks parallel with the road surface will let you fly. If your skills are solid and you have confidence in them, you can descend on the aerobars provided there are no side streets, blind corners, traffic, or other potential dangers.

■ Drafting

Although draft-legal racing is changing the way elite athletes are training, drafting applies only to short-course triathlon. However, solid drafting skills are beneficial even for long-course triathletes when riding in large groups and for overall bike-handling skills. In addition, drafting the wheel of a stronger rider can increase the quality of specific goal workouts. Drafting can also save your workout if your energy begins to run low, because the power requirement when drafting can be reduced by as much as 39 percent, depending on how many riders are ahead of you.

When drafting, follow the other rider's wheel, staying 6–24 inches behind and a couple of inches to the side so you can see ahead. The side you're on should be slightly downwind. Don't look at the other rider but rather at the hub of your lead rider's wheel or his or her hip. Sighting on the hip keeps your eyes a little higher so you can see down the road and also be aware of the lead rider's slowing cadence. Use your peripheral vision to see what he or she is doing. Never overlap the leading wheel.

An effective way to learn to draft is to ride with road racers on their weekly club rides. Be sure to leave your aerobars at home.

If you are a tentative rider, then you need to realize that you must face your fears to overcome them. The fastest way to improve is to build your skills and confidence gradually. Practice your personal technical limiters in safe, comfortable environments at low speed. As your confidence improves, increase drill difficulty and riding speed. Always remember to breathe when feeling nervous; this reduces the tension in your body and will enable smoother movement patterns. All of the above skills are areas in which a skilled rider can pick up "free speed" in an Ironman-distance race (with the exception of drafting, of course!).

INTERVAL GUIDELINES

As heart rate significantly lags behind effort, those of us who like to use our heart rate monitors for training have to learn to incorporate rating of perceived exertion when doing intervals—or purchase a power meter. Probably the most common mistake with interval (muscular endurance) work is going too hard. An overenthusiastic athlete can blow the entire set by starting too fast.

■ *Interval Pacing*

Most strong cyclists have an inbuilt sense of what pace they are going. They don't need a clock or heart rate monitor; they just know. Different-paced intervals are excellent for helping learn this sense of pace. It can be quite beneficial for all athletes to do pace work on measured courses. Intervals are the perfect way to develop your sense of different paces.

To get the best results, build into each interval and each set. If you are aiming for a heart rate target, then you will need to be patient at the start of each interval and each set. Control your effort and build toward the target at the end of the interval. Pushing extremely hard early in the set or interval is unnecessary. Just as in a race, split the work effort into quarters, as shown in the following list:

1. In the first quarter, your body is fresh and free of lactate; the goal is to hold back.
2. In the second quarter, maintain your goal interval pace and effort.
3. The third quarter is when most people have a dip in output, so this is where you should focus on maintaining your effort while holding perfect form.
4. The final quarter can be tough if the interval intensity is high. However, for Ironman-distance racing, you are rarely doing very high-output intervals. If you have paced yourself through the first 75 percent of the repetition, then the quiet satisfaction of a solid repeat should bring you home.

Interval Intensity

If you are like most triathletes, deep down you probably think that 10×7 min. (flat out) on 5 sec. rest is "better" than 6×5 min. (build to threshold) on 75 sec. rest. Note that the "better" set has longer interval duration, higher intensity, and shorter rest.

Many sports scientists have analyzed the optimal mix of intensity, duration, and recovery. The good news is that you do not have to endure all-out intervals to get the physiological adaptations you desire. This is particularly true for Ironman-distance training, where most athletes are close to their recovery limits. Feelings of nausea and deep fatigue are signs that you have pushed too hard. High-intensity sessions all too often result in extended recovery periods and poor technique.

Mental Strength in Interval Training

Intervals are a great way to get a look at how you are likely to perform in a race situation. Ask yourself these questions:

- Do you fade toward the end of the main set? You will need to focus on mental toughness or better front-end pacing.
- Do you consistently fry yourself in the first few repeats? You will need to leave your ego at the race start.
- Do you want to quit in the middle, struggle through, then feel great at the end? You will likely benefit from visualizing strong performance in the middle of a race.

Many athletes have suffered from going too hard too early in a race. Learning to control yourself in training is an important part of hitting the right effort levels on game day.

■ Nutrition

Drink 1.5 liters of a sports drink before a 40K time trial, and you'll have an idea of how your stomach will fare with the same drink on race day. Ever wonder what it is like to eat solid foods at the end of an Ironman-distance bike? Insert 5 × 3 min. fast on 1-min. recovery at the three-hour mark of a steady-state endurance ride. As soon as your breathing has slowed after the intervals, start eating and see how you feel. These are extreme examples, but they will help you adjust your regular training nutrition for the demands of racing.

KEY TRAINING SESSIONS

Given cycling's low-impact nature, you will have a much better tolerance for cycling intensity than for running intensity.

When incorporating higher-intensity riding into your training plan, remember that most self-coached athletes do too much intensity and volume, tend to keep themselves in a constant state of overreaching, and flirt periodically with overtraining. Often they train at intensities that are inappropriate for Ironman-distance training. You should seldom be at heart rates in Zones 4–5a, even on your hardest rides.

In fact, learning to control intensity and using heart rate to prevent going over FT during a race, especially on hills, is one of the keys to successful racing. If you spend significant time over functional threshold while racing, there is an increased chance that your stomach will shut down. Arousal control needs to be rehearsed in training so that pacing discipline becomes routine.

■ Muscular Endurance Training Sessions

For building early-season muscular endurance, we recommend indoor trainer sessions, starting after the completion of the highest-intensity phase of your strength program. The eight-week protocol outlined in Table 7.1 can be used for these sessions and should be adjusted to your own personal limiters or race-season goals. Athletes who live in temperate climates can do these sessions outdoors. Refer to Appendix D for indoor and outdoor brick options.

Safety Concerns for Outdoor Intervals

Riding at high speed on the aerobars is risky, which makes hard bike intervals outdoors probably the most dangerous activity that we do as triathletes. The following are a few pointers to remember:

- Always wear a helmet. It is amazing that otherwise sane athletes leave their helmets at home (or even take them off). To illustrate this point, drop a cantaloupe from a height of 6 feet onto the road. Now picture the same scene with the cantaloupe starting at a speed of 20–45 mph.

- Never do intervals in the dark, and if you are riding in the dark, use lights and wear reflective clothing. The right equipment will improve your chances of being seen. Once you get used to riding safely, you'll feel naked without your protective gear. High-quality light-emitting diode flashers are inexpensive and greatly increase your visibility.

- Assume that you are invisible. A triathlete moving at high speed on the aerobars doesn't present a lot of frontal area for a driver to see. Always assume that the person in the car doesn't see you. It's better to lose a bit of a repeat than to spend weeks recovering from a Superman impersonation across someone's hood.

- Keep your head up. This advice may seem obvious, but you often see cyclists riding with their heads down. It's not just cars that can get you—it's also joggers, pedestrians, potholes, ditches, other cyclists, and many other possible obstacles.

- Review your route in advance. Warm up by riding through the entire interval route. That way you will be able to spot any potential trouble spots in advance.

- Be aware of the location of all traffic, particularly cars that are approaching you from behind, and know what all the vehicles in your area are doing.

- Start intervals easily, and build into each effort. Be particularly careful with the first 45 sec., as legs will be relatively lactate-free and heart rate lags behind effort.

- Use RPE in conjunction with power and heart rate value. The goal of these sessions is to build toward threshold (FT) efforts. Maximum-effort intervals are not required.

- The goal should be to increase intensity through the session. Finish strong; save a little for the last part of the session. Focus on the third and fourth intervals of each set.

- Rest interval should be easy spinning. Maintain form.

- Never push into deep pain. Learning to tell the difference between normal "training discomfort" and "pre-injury pain" takes time. Back off if you have any uncertainty.

- Alternate between a "climbing" and an "aero" bike position. The appropriate mix of positions will depend on the nature of early-season racecourses and your personal limiters.

- Hold perfect form—relaxed face, jaw, and shoulders; proper back alignment; neutral head position; smooth leg drive; and eyes open. You want to train with perfect form so it will translate to the road and races.

- Intervals are best done after a 20- to 40-min. warm-up that includes several 15- to 30-sec. pickups to threshold effort (not heart rate).

- Follow your interval session with some easy spinning and a stretching session (at least 10 min.).

- Use your own judgment on the cadence guidelines. For example, Athlete A, who is a good spinner, might use 90–95 rpm as normal, whereas Athlete B, who is a grinder, would use 80–85 rpm as normal. Riders with force as a limiter will benefit from lower-cadence intervals, and riders seeking to lift their comfortable cadence will benefit from higher-cadence intervals.

- Be reasonable with all guidelines, in particular heart rate and cadence guidelines.

TABLE 7.1 MUSCULAR ENDURANCE TRAINER SESSIONS

WEEK	MAIN SET		INTENSITY	CADENCE
1	5 x 3 min. on 1-min. RI	A	1. End at low heart rate Zone 3	1. Normal
			2. End at middle heart rate Zone 3	2. Faster
			3. End at upper heart rate Zone 3	3. Slower
			4. End at lower heart rate Zone 4	4. Faster
			5. Build to heart rate Zone 4 in first 45 sec. and hold	5. Normal
2	5 x 3 min. on 1-min. RI	B	1. End at middle heart rate Zone 3	1. Normal
			2. End at upper heart rate Zone 3	2. Faster
			3. End at lower heart rate Zone 4	3. Slower
			4. End at upper heart rate Zone 4	4. Faster
			5. Build to heart rate Zone 5a in first 45 sec. and hold	5. Normal
3	Two sets of 5 x 3 min. on 1-min. RI Repeat with 15+ min. of heart rate Zone 1/2 riding between sets		Both sets at intensity A	1. Faster
				2. Slower
				3. Faster
				4. Slower
				5. Normal
4	Heart rate or power testing			
5	2 sets of 5 x 3 min. on RI 15+ min. of heart rate Zone 1/2 riding between sets		1 at intensity A 2 at intensity B	1. Faster
				2. Slower
				3. Faster
				4. Slower
				5. Normal

continued >

TABLE 7.1 CONTINUED

WEEK	MAIN SET	INTENSITY	CADENCE
6	2 sets of 5 x 3 min. on 1-min. RI	Both sets at intensity B	1. Faster
			2. Slower
	15+ min. of heart rate Zone 1/2 riding between sets		3. Faster
			4. Slower
			5. Normal
7	5 x 5 min. on 90-sec. RI	All sets at intensity B	1. Faster
			2. Slower
			3. Faster
			4. Slower
			5. Normal
8	Heart rate or power testing		

ENDURANCE WORKOUT

Goal: Build muscular endurance, define race strategy

W/U

Ride 60–90 min. at easy pace

MAIN SET

2–4 x

40 min. steady	IM race pace
20 min. mod-hard	Half-IM race pace

Be sure to save plenty of energy for the final 2 hours.

Coach's tip: Ride at a steady pace on flat to rolling terrain, using your aerobars as much as possible. Try to stay down on the bars even when riding uphill grades. The overall intensity is likely to be greater than what you will use on race day, but your observations throughout the ride will help you begin to form an appropriate race strategy. Focus on your effort for this entire ride. Note your heart rate and RPE changes through the session. There may be wind, and it will affect your pace. Stay mentally focused, and control effort rather than riding to a set speed. Eat and drink at race levels.

C/D

If a transition run is scheduled, run easy off the bike, no more than 3 miles.

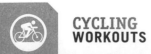

CYCLING WORKOUTS

CLIMBING WORKOUT

Goal: Build climbing strength
Note: Novice and less experienced cyclists should consider building strength in rolling terrain before attempting a ride of this nature. Distance traveled and average pace are not important for this workout. Your aim should be to complete some solid climbs. Include some lower–heart rate strength work where you ride with a low cadence.

W/U	
Ride 60–90 min. at easy pace	
MAIN SET	
Long climbs, 15–40 min.	Building to mod-hard in early season
	Building to threshold as key race approaches
	Build power toward top of climb
C/D	
If a transition run is scheduled, run easy off the bike, no more than 3 miles.	

■ *Late Base and Build Period Muscular Endurance Sessions*

After the previous eight-week program, athletes will be ready to start their race-specific preparations. The purpose of these sessions is to build subthreshold cycling power and prepare you for the specific demands of your A-priority race. These sessions should begin seven to eleven weeks out from your first A-priority race of the season.

Most athletes will benefit from a transition run after these sessions. Novices and athletes who take longer to recover should run for only 10–20 min. while focusing on cadence and smooth running form. Experienced athletes can turn these sessions into race-simulation workouts by adding 45–90 min. of running following the bike sessions. Elite and very strong athletes should build to a tempo finish (heart rate Zone 3) for the run.

CYCLING WORKOUTS

TIME TRIAL STRENGTH WORKOUTS

Goal: Build subthreshold power

Note: These workouts are useful for athletes who have excellent endurance but lack the strength (whether mental or physical) to fully tap their TT potential.

TIME TRIAL 1

W/U
Ride 45–75 min., deep warm-up

MAIN SET	
Ride 30 km, solid tempo	Build to mod-hard pace in the first 3–4 km and hold for the rest of the TT
Coach's tip: This is not an all-out TT, simply solid tempo work.	

C/D
Ride 30–60 min. at easy to steady pace
Brick option: Transition to run, 30 min. at steady pace.

TIME TRIAL 2

W/U
Ride 45–75 min., deep warm-up

MAIN SET	
2 x 20 km (30 min. RI)	1–5 km, build to mod-hard to threshold effort; 5–20 km, hold effort Set 1: 85–90 percent effort Set 2: 90–95 percent effort—in the final 5 km, build to slightly over FT effort
Spin at least 30 min. between TT efforts	

C/D
Ride 30–60 min. at easy to steady pace
Brick option: Transition to run, 30 min. at steady pace.

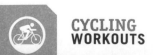

RACE-SPECIFIC MUSCULAR ENDURANCE

Goal: To build time trial fitness within an endurance training session
Note: If your ride time exceeds 4 hours, replace the long run with a cool-down on the bike.

W/U

Ride 60 min., easy

MAIN SET

2–5 x 40 min., steady, followed by 20 min. threshold or strength intervals
Threshold intervals:

5 x 3 min. on 1 min. rest	Build to threshold effort

Strength intervals:

5 x 3 min. on 1 min. rest	Low-cadence, big-gear work
20 min. mod-hard	

C/D

Quick transition to a 60–90 min. run. Split the run into thirds: 1st third focus on relaxed, comfortable cadence; 2nd third run at steady pace; final third should build to a tempo finish (mod-hard pace).

OTHER CYCLING MAIN SET IDEAS

These main set ideas can be mixed and matched. Start easier than directed when you first try them out.

TRIPLE 3s

Goal: Ride steady to mod-hard for duration of main set

30–90 min.	Continuous 3-min. cycles of standing at 60 rpm, seated at 75 rpm, seated at 90 rpm

STANDING

Goal: To learn how to be relaxed while standing and riding at a steady effort
Note: Intensity level is not important; rest intervals are easy spinning.

15–30 min.	Continuous standing in mixed terrain

CHANGE-UP INTERVALS

Goal: Start at a steady effort/power; sustain or build effort/power, depending on time of year and session goals
Note: Rest intervals are easy spinning.

5–10 x 5-min. intervals on 30 sec. rest	20 sec. at 92–94 rpm; 90 sec. at 70–75 rpm; 30 sec. at 92–94 rpm; 60 sec. at 92–94 rpm

continued >

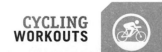

CYCLING WORKOUTS

OTHER CYCLING MAIN SET IDEAS continued

UP-DOWN INTERVALS

Goal: To hit a range of cadences and train muscular recruitment as well as the ability to clear lactate at Ironman race effort level (steady)

2–6 x 15-min., continuous intervals	1st 5 min.: Big gear, low cadence, steady to mod-hard for power, heart rate builds to steady 2nd 5 min.: Normal race cadence, mod-hard or threshold wattage (depends on time of year), heart rate builds to mod-hard 3rd 5 min.: Taper off wattage and heart rate—steady wattage, heart rate comes down gradually to steady

POWER SINGLES

Goal: Fast minutes should start subthreshold and build toward VO_2max effort/power by end of main set
Note: Cadence low or normal; most athletes will benefit from pushing a big gear.

10–30 cycles	1 min. fast, 1 min. easy

RACE SIM 1

Goal: Ride anticipated bike-leg duration or 6 hours, whichever is shorter
Note: Divide the ride into thirds based on duration, not distance.

MAIN SET

3 x 60–120 min.	First third: Easier than goal race effort Middle third: Goal race effort Last third: Slightly higher than goal race effort

C/D

If a transition run is scheduled, run easy off the bike, no more than 3 miles.

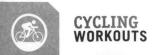

RACE SIM 2

Goal: Ride 100+ miles
Note: Divide the ride into thirds based on distance. Middle- and back-of-pack athletes should exercise caution when riding more than 100 miles.

MAIN SET

Ride 100–120 miles	First third: Easier than goal race effort Middle third: Goal race effort Last third: Slightly higher than goal race effort

C/D

If a transition run is scheduled, run easy off the bike, no more than 3 miles.

RACE SIM 3

Goal: Ride 4–5 hours
Note: Until the start of the main sets, ride easier than goal race effort.

W/U

Ride 1–2 hours, depending on planned duration

MAIN SET

3 x 60 min.	Set 1 (3 hours prior to workout completion): Ride 40 min. on aerobars, in flat to rolling terrain, steady effort; recover Set 2 (2 hours prior to workout completion): Ride 3 x 15 min. continuous; 12 min. at IM effort, 3 min. at half-IM effort; ride the second cycle standing; recover Set 3 (1 hour prior to workout completion): Ride 30–40 min. at just above half-IM effort; recover

C/D

If a transition run is scheduled, run easy off the bike, no more than 3 miles.

CYCLING WORKOUTS

RACE SIM 4	
Goal: Ride at goal race effort **Note:** Ride a measured course that will take approximately 40 min. to complete. Note average heart rate, power, speed, and RPE.	
W/U	
Ride 60 min.	
MAIN SET	
Ride 3–4 hours	Set 1: Ride course at goal race effort; recover at easier than goal race effort Set 2 (2 hours prior to workout completion): Ride 10 x 5 min. (30 sec. RI) slightly more than goal race effort Set 3 (1 hour prior to workout completion): Ride course at goal race effort
Note changes in average heart rate, power, speed, and RPE	
C/D	
If a transition run is scheduled, run easy off the bike, no more than 3 miles.	

CYCLING WITH A POWER METER

With the advent of portable power measurement devices, the field of "power training" has undergone a transformation as athletes and coaches learn the best way to use this unique training tool.

This section focuses on techniques and methods that work in the field. Our goal is to present a methodology that is effective and applicable across a wide range of athletes and abilities. Undoubtedly, these methods will be refined and replaced by superior techniques in the years to come. In order to make this topic easier to interpret, we have simplified certain technical and physiological aspects of power-based training.

The principal benefits of heart rate training are that the equipment is readily available, easy to operate, and affordable. Indeed, a heart rate monitor and a set of aerobars are probably the two best investments for novice triathletes—once they have goggles, a bike, and running shoes! Like all training methods, heart rate training has its limitations, and often we may find that we are a little too focused on our numbers.

One of the immediate benefits of using a power meter is that it provides you with data that are unaffected by external variables such as wind, hills, heat, humidity, and diet. Power responds differently than heart rate and makes the heart rate monitor a more valuable tool. In addition, a power meter provides an instantaneous check of performance. Power meters express performance in watts: The greater your wattage, the more power you are generating and the faster you will travel for a given set of external conditions.

There are several areas in which power-based training can be an effective supplement to heart rate–based systems (all commercially available power meters incorporate a heart rate function). Power-based training is most effective in these areas:

- Early in a workout or a race, athletes tend to underestimate how hard they are working. A well-rested athlete will be able to produce significant wattage and/or lactate levels without immediately elevating his or her heart rate. A power meter is quite useful for regulating early ride intensity and quickly showing the impact of power spikes or surges.

- When used in conjunction with a heart rate monitor, a power meter is extremely useful for steady-state training. At the start of a long race or workout, an athlete can have confidence that, despite a lower heart rate, he or she is working at the correct intensity. Previously, coaches could only advise their athletes to "go easy" or "hold back" at the start of a race or training session. With a power meter, a specific power range can be determined in advance.

- In general, the time lag between effort and cardiac response is somewhere between 20 sec. and 2 min., depending on how early or late in the workout that heart rate is being monitored. This lag in cardiac response means that for short-duration efforts (intervals, in particular), heart rate is a poor indicator of actual work being done.

- Although nearly every athlete can produce a heart rate profile that rises while climbing, it takes practice to produce an even power profile over a climb. Typically, a "power novice" will generate his or her highest power output in the first 20–40 sec. of a climb. Following the peak output, power declines (as heart rate and blood lactate levels climb). This athlete may be under the impression that a higher heart rate implies increasing power output. A power meter will quickly show whether this is the case and will help the athlete learn to climb more efficiently.

- Regular use of a power meter enables an athlete to quickly realize when he or she is accumulating excessive fatigue within a training block. When an athlete is tired, it quickly shows in the power numbers. A lower-than-usual power–to–heart rate ratio and a higher perceived effort for a given level of power are clear indicators that an athlete should consider additional rest.

TABLE 7.2 HEART RATE AND CRITICAL POWER ZONES

HEART RATE ZONE	CRITICAL POWER ZONE	EFFORT DESCRIPTION
5c	CP0.2–CP1	Maximum effort
5b	CP6	Very hard or VO₂max
5a	CP30	Hard to very hard
4	CP60	Functional threshold
3	CP90	Mod-hard
2	CP180–CP240	Steady
1	Half of CP12	Easy

Power-based training, like any system, has its limitations. Power is most effective when used in conjunction with the full range of training variables available to an athlete (principally heart rate, pace, RPE, and cadence). In general, the shorter the workout or race duration and the fitter the athlete, the greater the role that "feel," or perception of effort, plays for an athlete. However, as you will find, fairly high-wattage figures can initially feel easy to a highly motivated and rested athlete.

The techniques presented in the following sections are a summary of what we use in our training as well as in the training programs for the athletes we coach who have access to power meters. For a more complete explanation of this topic, refer to the recommended readings at the end of this book. You are highly encouraged to review a copy of Joe Friel's "Training with Power Guide," available online at the Power-Tap Web site, and *Training and Racing with a Power Meter* (Allen and Coggan).

Table 7.2 is a rough guideline of the relationship between heart rate and critical power. As you will quickly discover, heart rate intensity zones do not track directly with critical power. This discrepancy is due to the variation in muscular endurance seen in the spectrum of athletes, from elite to novice. Also included in the table is a qualitative pace description of each zone.

■ *Power Zones*

Power training zones are based on functional threshold power (FTP), which is the power you can maintain for an hour—your CP60. There are several ways of determining your FTP. Perhaps the simplest is to do a 30-min. time trial workout alone. You are probably wondering why a 30-min. test tells you what your CP60 is. The reason is the difference in motivation between a 60-min. time trial race with competitors and your reputation on the line and riding by yourself with no one else seeing the results. We'll always go harder in a race and feel more sorry for ourselves in a workout. So the 30-min. solo effort winds up being about the same effort as a 60-min. race effort and serves as a good predictor of your FTP. Should you do a stand-alone 40K time trial race (not part of a triathlon), the average power from that event may refine your FTP if your time was close to 1 hour.

To set up your power zones simply use Table 7.3 along with a calculator and your known FTP.

Table 7.4 provides a more qualitative description of a range of aerobic training zones relative to CP30. Because of the challenges involved in relating power to heart rate, the values given in the table do not specifically match the heart rate estimations in the tables in Appendix A.

TABLE 7.3 POWER ZONES

POWER ZONE	AS PERCENTAGE OF FTP	HEART RATE ZONE (APPROX.)	RPE
7	>150	5c	Maximal
6	121–150	5b	Very hard or VO$_2$max
5	106–120	5a	Hard to very hard
4	91–105	4	Functional threshold
3	76–90	3	Mod-hard
2	56–75	2	Steady
1	<56	1	Easy

TABLE 7.4 AEROBIC TRAINING ZONES TO CP30

ZONE DESCRIPTION	PERCENTAGE OF CP30	PACE DESCRIPTION
Threshold	100	Hard to very hard
Cruise intervals	90–100	Hard
Sprint-distance triathlon	90–95	Hard
Olympic-distance triathlon	85–90	Hard
Half-Ironman-distance triathlon	80–87	Mod-hard to hard
Intensive endurance (long ride)	73–80	Steady to mod-hard
Base endurance (long ride)	67–73	Easy to steady
Easy training	<67	Easy

■ *Power-Based Training*

Although there is little on this issue in the scientific literature, the limited research available appears to indicate that when aerobic endurance improves, there is reduced heart rate drift relative to constant outputs of power and speed. Of course, the reverse of this is that when heart rate is held steady during extensive endurance training, output may be expected to drift downward.

Power Zones and Power Testing

These are the most common questions raised by athletes concerning power zones and power testing.

Why use a 30-min. time trial? The power methodology presented has been designed to be consistent with the training system outlined in this book. As your most frequent cycling test is a 30-min. time trial, your average power for this test is the starting point for discussing power zones. Although taxing, the test duration is short enough to be repeated every four to eight weeks to track your progress.

When should you test? Power testing is best done toward the end of a recovery week and more than forty-eight hours after a strength training or BT session. Athletes should prepare themselves by doing a thorough warm-up prior to testing.

What is a CP30 value? The average power generated across any time period is referred to as an athlete's "critical power" (CP). So the 30-min. average-power test would yield a 30-min. critical power, or CP30, value. Like any best average test, critical power testing is most accurate when you are able to hold the average power with as small a variation as possible. If you blow up midtest, then the results will likely be inaccurate. For this reason, we recommend that you build into your tests and

start a little easier than your anticipated best effort. Remember that you'll have a long career to improve your CP numbers!

How does power change over CP duration? A good rule of thumb is that average power decreases by 5 percent as duration doubles. So an athlete with a CP30 of 200 would be expected to have a CP60 of 190 (95 percent of CP30). The further you get from a test value, and the more anaerobic a test becomes, the less accurate this estimation becomes. For example, your CP60 would be a poor predictor of your CP6.

Are any other CP figures useful for the long-course athlete? Our experience to date shows CP30 is the most useful data point for long-course athletes. CP30 is a reasonable estimation of threshold power and easy to test. However, athletes will benefit from developing an understanding of their individual power profiles across a range of durations, intensities, and terrains.

For elite and strong cyclists, the CP12 value is a reasonable measurement of anaerobic endurance and can provide useful information for racing shorter distances. However, anaerobic endurance is rarely a performance limiter for long-course racing, so this test is more important for a short-course athlete.

This parallel relationship between input (heart rate) and output (power) is referred to as "coupling." When heart rate and power are no longer tracking in parallel, their relationship is said to have "decoupled." Excessive decoupling indicates a lack of aerobic endurance fitness.

Joe designed a function within software called WKO+® with this purpose in mind (available at www.TrainingPeaks.com and compatible with all power meters). It can help you to determine your degree of aerobic endurance conditioning by charting both power and heart rate and by measuring your level of decoupling. Once you achieve an excellent level of aerobic fitness, which translates into Ironman-distance race readiness, your workout heart rate and power graphs on WKO+ will be almost parallel.

Figures 7.1 and 7.2 illustrate this concept. In both figures, only the aerobic threshold main set is shown; the warm-ups and cool-downs have been omitted. The riders in each case were riding for about two hours while holding heart rates steady. The graphs reveal what happened to their power outputs.

Figure 7.1 shows a ride with heart rate and power coupled—meaning there was less than 5 percent decoupling over the course of the main set of the ride. Notice how the two graphs are

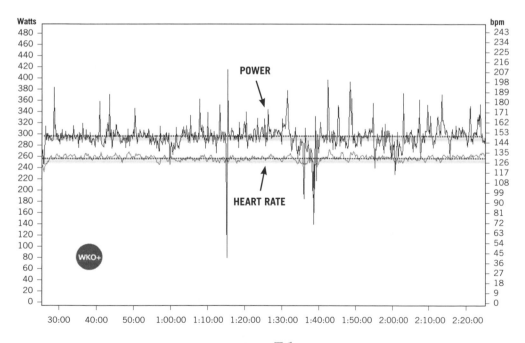

FIGURE *7.1*
HEART RATE AND POWER DECOUPLED 3%

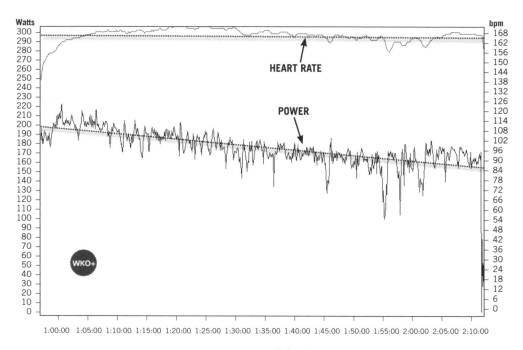

FIGURE *7.2*

HEART RATE AND POWER DECOUPLED 22%

almost perfectly parallel. This athlete was riding at about 73 percent of FTP. His aerobic fitness for 2 hours is excellent. In Figure 7.2, heart rate and power are decoupling right from the start, indicating that the rider's aerobic fitness was not adequate for the intensity of the ride. She was riding at 75 percent of FTP. Notice how the heart rate and power graphs are never parallel. The decoupling was 22 percent, which is extremely high. This athlete needs to lower the power and heart rate until they remain coupled for the entire 2 hours. Attempting to race at this intensity would almost certainly result in underperformance.

If you don't have WKO+ software, you can use the software that came with your power meter to manually determine your decoupling. The following is a description of how to make this determination.

The aerobic threshold portion of the workout is split into halves. For each half, the average power is divided by the average heart rate to establish two ratios. The ratios are then compared by subtracting the first-half ratio from the second-half ratio and dividing the remainder by the first-half ratio. This produces a power–to–heart rate ratio percentage of change from the first half to the second half of the workout. That percentage of change is your rate of decoupling.

The following list is an example of how power–to–heart rate ratio percentage of change is calculated.

1. Determine power–to–heart rate ratio for first half of ride.

    Power average: 180 watts

    Heart rate average: 135 bpm

    First-half power–to–heart rate ratio: 1.33 (180 ÷ 135)

2. Determine power–to–heart rate ratio for second half of ride.

    Power average: 178 watts

    Heart rate average: 139 bpm

    Second-half power–to–heart rate ratio: 1.28 (178 ÷ 139)

3. Subtract the ratio for the first half of the ride from the ratio of the second half of the ride: 0.05 (1.33 − 1.28).

4. Divide the remainder by the first-half ratio: 0.038 (0.05 ÷ 1.33). The decoupling rate is 3.8 percent.

Aerobically fit endurance athletes experience a decoupling rate of less than 5 percent when riding in their upper Zone 2. So one of your goals when working on race power is to keep decoupling to a minimum—less than 5 percent. When decoupling happens during a long ride in Zone 2 is just as important as how much decoupling occurs. In other words, it's possible for coupling to be present for the early portion of an aerobic threshold workout, followed by excessive decoupling in the latter portion. That variation may be acceptable when training for short-course races. Athletes who race in relatively short endurance events such as sprint- and Olympic-distance triathlons don't need as much aerobic endurance as long-course athletes. The importance placed on your aerobic threshold workouts remaining coupled is, to some extent, a function of your preferred race distance.

How long should optimal decoupling last relative to your race duration? Ironman-distance athletes must be able to stay coupled for 4 hours with steady effort in Zone 2. This workout may be done weekly, with the exception of rest weeks, for the last twelve weeks before the race. The last workout should be no closer to the event than three weeks.

The format is simple. Just include the Zone 2 coupling portion within your long ride. Warm up for 20–30 min. and then, on a relatively flat course, ride in the upper half of your Zone 2. The first of these Zone 2 portions of the long ride should be about an hour. Over the course of the next several weeks, increase the Zone 2 duration until you reach four hours. Whenever you discover

Using a Power Meter on a Hilly Course

In a hilly, long-course race, your focus must be on "smoothing" the course. The power on uphills must be restricted by gearing down and keeping your power output below your functional threshold power (FTP) (or even lower on longer climbs). The typical newcomer to Ironman-distance racing pushes far too hard on hills, especially early in the race, and pays the price later as high fatigue sets in.

- For short climbs of up to 5 min. duration, athletes should consider an effort ceiling of 90–100 percent of FTP.
- For longer climbs, consider an effort ceiling of 80–90 percent of FTP.
- For all climbs, it is very important to "save some watts" for cresting the apex of the climb. Novices tend to have their highest watts at the base of a climb. The intelligent athlete will have his or her highest watts over the top of a climb and accelerate down the backside. Experienced power users know that higher lactate levels can be cleared during the descent and after the rider has returned to cruising speed.
- On the downhill side, stop pedaling and coast in the aero position when your pedaling cadence becomes so high that you begin to breathe more heavily. If in doubt, coast the downhills so long as your speed is well above your average for the race.

that decoupling greater than 5 percent is occurring, you either need to repeat that duration until heart rate and power remain coupled or reduce the power and heart rate of subsequent rides.

Note that there are two ways to do an aerobic threshold coupling workout. You can ride or run while keeping heart rate steady to see what happens to power or speed. Alternatively, you can ride or run at a fixed power or speed and see what happens to heart rate. Try both to see which is more comfortable for you.

As well as being a result of poor aerobic endurance, decoupling may occur because of a failure to take in fluids at a rate that prevents excessive dehydration during a workout. Also associated with decoupling is environmental heat stress, which can cause heart rate to rise or power and speed to fall. One would expect the rate of decoupling to decrease as heat adaptation takes place. We know of no research on this matter, but Joe has seen it in athletes he coaches who live in hot places such as Phoenix, Arizona. Decoupling may also be expected to increase if you go to a high-elevation location such as Boulder, Colorado. Just as with heat, expect your decoupling rate to improve as you adapt to the higher elevation.

■ *Power-based Racing*

The Ironman-distance bike leg should be a steady effort raced at about your aerobic threshold. Getting this right is critical because in the first 30 min. or so, the effort, if paced correctly, will seem very easy. But if you started out too aggressively—which is common when you are rested, highly motivated, and surrounded by competitors and supportive crowds—the effort is likely to cause premature fatigue. If this happens, you will slow down dramatically late in the ride, your gut may "shut down," and you may wind up walking much if not all of the marathon. So it's critical that you get the intensity right immediately and maintain it over the entire 112 miles.

That level of effort could be defined and monitored using a heart rate monitor, but this technology presents some complicating factors on race day. Heart rate is slow to respond, so early in the race it may be difficult to know how hard you are working. If you had coffee before the race, your heart rate may be unusually high. The excitement of race morning and the start can set off a "fight or flight" response with hormones, causing your heart to beat faster. All of these factors mean the data you are getting from your heart rate monitor are suspect on race day, and you really can't count on the data being accurate until you're well into the race. It may be too late by then to undo the damage from starting too fast.

This is where a power meter is most effective. Power is unaffected by emotions, hormones, and nutrition. And it is immediately accurate—there is no delay in getting meaningful information about how hard you are going. The challenge in using a power meter is knowing what your power should be for the entire ride. Since it is raced at about aerobic threshold, we know that it will be somewhere around Power Zone 2 (again see Table 7.3). But 56–75 percent of FTP makes for a rather broad range of possibilities. For some, the upper end of this range will be too hard, and for others the lower end will be too easy.

HIGHLY TRAINED elite athletes may be able to sustain levels up to 5 percent above these Zone 2 guidelines.

E ELITE

NOVICE ATHLETES should consider racing at, or below, the bottom end of Zone 2.

N NOVICE

The best way to establish what your race power should be is by doing race-simulation workouts (like those shown earlier in this chapter). These rides have three major purposes. The first is to determine what your power should be in the race by comparing heart rate and power in long rides. The second is to build your race fitness on the bike gradually over the course of several weeks. The third is to dial in your nutrition relative to your intensity on the bike. One reason so many athletes experience stomach problems is that they don't properly match the types and amounts of fuel they take in with their race intensity. If you ride slowly enough—really slowly—you can eat anything you want. You can wolf down a hamburger and french fries. As the intensity of the ride goes up, your options for refueling go down. At the very highest effort levels, digesting even water is a problem.

■ *Power-based Race Planning*

The preceding guidelines are merely a starting point for helping develop your own race strategy, a strategy that should be field-tested well in advance of race day.

Athletes of all abilities will benefit greatly from not only training with a power meter but also racing with it. Knowing what your power should be and paying close attention to it during the race will prevent many common long-course racing mistakes. With post-race analysis, you will also learn a lot about what is needed in your training to perform better in future races.

Because an Ironman-distance race exacts a severe penalty for early pacing mistakes, you should start each race conservatively and build your power through the second half of the race. Walking even a single mile of the marathon can negate a lot of hard work on the bike!

CHAPTER 8

TRAINING FOR THE RUN

O f the three sports in triathlon, running is the most stressful on the body. It is also the sport that appears to cause the majority of injuries in both novice and experienced athletes. For this reason, you should approach run training with caution.

You have to be willing to let the race come back to you.

—LORI BOWDEN,
TWO-TIME IRONMAN WORLD CHAMPION

There is nothing "fast" about running well in an Ironman-distance triathlon; even the fastest competitors are running below their open marathon fitness level. Consistent volume over time correlates much more closely to success than fast 5K run times. We recommend that you build your run volume gradually by focusing primarily on your workout frequency.

STAGES OF RUNNING DEVELOPMENT

There are four stages in the life cycle of the development of a runner. These stages can also provide ideas for structuring your season if you are an experienced runner.

There are many ways to successfully train for running, and you should remain sensitive to the signals you receive from your body. With running in particular, your body typically gives numerous early warnings in advance of an injury occurring. Knowing when to back off is a valuable skill, whether you are a novice or an elite runner.

Adaptation

When you are making changes to your running form, your average pace may decrease. Endure the adaptation phase, as improved running economy is one of the easiest ways to improve your run speed. Genetics will set the upper limit on your aerobic gains; dedication and attention to detail will set the limits on your running form.

Superior technical form can enable an athlete to race beyond his or her inbuilt aerobic limitations.

Running well in an Ironman-distance race requires superior economy, exceptional durability, and excellent early pace control. Performance at functional threshold and VO_2max is a poor predictor of ultradistance race performance.

■ *Stage 1: Learning to Run*

The primary goal in this stage of training is to strengthen connective tissues and prepare your body for the stresses of the longer sessions in Stage 2. This process is enhanced by strength training, particularly if you are a novice, a cyclist, or, more importantly, a swimmer.

A secondary goal of this stage (and an important focus for all athletes) is technical improvement. Though the overall intensity of this stage is low, you will be able to maintain your quickness, enhance economy, and improve form through using speed drills such as strides, one-leg drills, high-cadence running, and technique exercises, all of which are described later in this chapter.

All runs should be done in heart rate Zones 1 and 2. If you are a novice, you may feel that this pace is too slow to produce any benefit. However, this stage of running development is essential for a long, healthy, and successful running career—and it is the *only* way to build a successful triathlon running career.

Frequency is essential; you should plan three to five runs per week. Each run should last 20–45 min. At least one of these runs is a short transition run following a bike ride, generally 15–30 min. The purpose of this transition run is to teach your body to quickly move from cycling to running. This combination of cycling and running is also known as a "brick," "combination," or "transition" (in International Triathlon Union terminology, the latter term now refers to the skills training required for effective transitions) workout. You do not need to run long or fast (that may come later). What you need to do is run until your muscles successfully transition from cycling to running.

If you are looking to speed your adaptation, you can supplement run training with hiking or backpacking and trekking, all of which are excellent ways to build endurance and complement run training. In many ways, an Ironman-distance marathon run has more in common with a long hike than with a true marathon.

The length of time that you spend in Stage 1 is highly variable, ranging from six months (if you are a fit cyclist or lean swimmer) to several years (if you are a novice and/or overweight). If you are new to running, you should spend a minimum of six months in this stage of development.

■ *Stage 2: Building Endurance*

The goal of Stage 2 is to build the endurance necessary to complete (rather than compete in) the run portion of your event.

Once your running base has been established, you can safely extend the duration of your longest run each week. The duration of your long run should increase no more than 5–15 min. each week in your training cycle. Your long run should be significantly reduced (25–50 percent) during recovery weeks.

When you are seeking to build endurance, the duration of your workout is more important than the overall intensity. Whenever you are extending your "endurance envelope," intensity should be kept down and your focus should be on maintaining your best form for the entire workout. Long runs provide an excellent opportunity to program/drill/habituate strong running technique into the neuromuscular system. These programs are what will appear when you are under stress in a race situation.

Once your long run has been built up to between 90 and 150 min., you should consider extending the duration of your second-longest run. Typically, if you are slow to recover or have running as a key limiter, you will find greater benefits in two moderate runs than in one megarun. The principal reason is recovery. The marginal benefit of a run longer than 2.5 hours is outweighed by the extended recovery period that is required and the heightened risk of overuse injury.

When you are able to comfortably run for the desired duration, intensity can be steadily increased. The most effective way of increasing intensity is to do it gradually through a workout. For example, a 2-hour run could start in heart rate Zone 1 and slowly build so that it finishes at the top of heart rate Zone 2. In general, when building base endurance it is best to avoid heart rate Zone 3 and above.

Though the main focus of this stage is to build run endurance, you should continue to work on your transition running and balance the long, slow distance work with one or two weekly strides and skills sessions. These sessions should be alactic in nature, meaning that they involve short periods of high-speed running rather than sustained high-intensity training.

You should not train beyond Stage 2 until you have been running for at least two years. You will benefit from building your endurance base for up to five years before starting focused muscular endurance work. The body adapts slowly, and the deeper the base you create, the harder you can work when the time is right.

■ Stage 3: Building Muscular Endurance

Once you have invested the time required to build up your endurance to complete the run, you will begin training to compete in the run. Do not progress to this stage until your run split is consistent with training performance. Athletes who underperform in running should focus on swimming endurance, cycling muscular endurance, and overall race pacing.

Long-course running is based on strength and muscular endurance because it follows a long cycling effort. Functional threshold speed is not a requirement for success, but superior muscular endurance is essential. Specific workouts to improve muscular endurance for cycling were included in the previous chapter, many of which provided a brick option. Here are some general ideas to incorporate into your muscular endurance run training.

Triathlons. Run or ride following a short, intense race. For novices, this could be a sprint-distance race, and for more experienced athletes, up to an Olympic-distance race. For example, after a sprint duathlon, you would ride 2–3 hours at a low to moderate intensity (heart rate Zone 1 or 2). Athletes using this strategy should watch their race frequency. Even a series of "easy" races can prove physically and mentally draining for any athlete.

Hills. Gently rolling courses provide natural fartlek training because intensity increases on the climbs and drops on the descents. (*Fartlek* is a Swedish term meaning "speed play" that refers to continuous training involving changes of pace.) Hill running, like hill cycling, builds your sport-specific strength. Endurance runs on rolling terrain are very useful for building race-specific strength, but you should be conscientious about your volume and how you balance hill work with your other training. You will need to allow ample recovery time from these challenging sessions. Hills are particularly useful for athletes who are seeking to boost running economy while training their aerobic system.

You should remember that hills are useful only to the extent that good form and a reasonable intensity can be held while climbing. A moderate grade is enough to promote the economy and strength benefits of hill running.

Tempo running.   These intervals will push your heart rate to Zone 3. Here are some ideas for tempo sessions:

- Work in up to three intervals of 5–20 min. duration in the middle of an endurance run.
- Insert a tempo finish to a transition or endurance run. The intensity should build to the top of heart rate Zone 3 by the finish. Elite runners should extend the duration of the tempo finish to be between 45 and 75 min. by the end of the Build period.
- A specific tempo run: Following warm-up, build to tempo pace and hold for 20–90 min.

Road races.   Up to 10 km for novices, 10 miles for experienced age groupers, and half-marathons for elite athletes. Short races enable you to place a higher level of aerobic stress on your system without compromising recovery times.

It is worth remembering that longer and harder are not necessarily better with this type of training. Combining appropriate recovery with focused sessions that gradually stretch your limits is more effective than training to the edge of fatigue or injury. Nearly all triathletes will achieve best results by focusing the majority of their training load on their bike sessions.

Trail running.   Best in the Prep and Base periods, trail running is excellent for building complete leg strength as well as improving agility. Trail running is less appropriate in the Build period because training should simulate race conditions. See the "Crosstraining: Hiking" sidebar for more on trail running.

Crosstraining: Hiking

For those with running as their greatest limiter, the early Base period is an excellent time for longer, low-intensity walking and running. These sessions provide the opportunity to

- Improve running economy
- Strengthen running-specific connective tissues
- Build base endurance

The most important thing to remember is that these sessions should be done at an easy pace and designed to gradually stretch your endurance. Trail running also provides an opportunity to improve your running economy. Trails, specifically inclines, give you the

continued >

< Crosstraining: Hiking, continued

opportunity to shorten your stride and increase cadence while building greater leg strength.

TRAIL TIPS

Form: Whether running uphill or downhill, maintain proper running form. Particular attention should be paid to the alignment of the foot and knee.

Technical improvement: Longer, low-intensity sessions are an ideal time to remove running flaws. There is a low level of training stress, leaving you free to focus on your personal limiters, such as cadence, arm carriage, pelvic and hip stability, foot strike, and body alignment.

Hydration: As the Base period generally occurs in the cooler months of the year, hydration needs are reduced. However, it is still important to maintain adequate hydration, particularly in long sessions. Products such as the FuelBelt are an excellent way to carry fluids on the trail.

Nutrition: Long, low-intensity sessions are an excellent way to promote fat burning if you are looking to improve your body composition. You should always bring plenty of food when hitting the trails. However, most will be able to get away with 100–300 calories per hour, depending on the duration of the hike.

Duration: You will get an appropriate workout from a hike lasting 2–6 hours. When trail running, a session of 1–4 hours is appropriate, depending on the severity of the terrain. As a general rule, go long rather than fast.

Terrain: Soft surface and rolling terrain with a variety of climbs lasting between 10 and 30 min. provide an opportunity to build "whole-leg" strength. A wide variety of grades will use the full range of running muscles. On steeper terrain, you should remember to keep your heart rate and exertion under control; even elite runners will walk hills.

Downhill running: Even when using a short, rapid stride, downhill running is quite stressful. You may benefit from inserting walking breaks of 2–10 min. into each 10- to 20-min. period of downhill running. When running downhill, focus on a relaxed body and maintaining a high, comfortable cadence. It is best to avoid striding out, as this can overload the leg muscles and soft tissues of the joints. Use extreme caution with downhill running if you are a novice runner.

Running with packs: Avoid running with a pack on your back, as it can overload the knees and lead to injury.

Considerations when weight lifting: Hiking and trail running are complementary to the early phases of your strength program. However, because of the risk of overloading the lower body, longer run sessions should not be undertaken when you are in a heavy strength training phase.

Clothing: Cycling clothing can be quite useful on the trail. A long-sleeved bike jersey will provide pockets for trail maps, food, and other supplies. In order to prevent the contents from bouncing or spilling onto the trail, pull a set of tights up and over the pockets. A hat and a thin windbreaker are excellent items to bring on any excursions in the cooler months.

Partners: Hiking is a great time to bring along the kids or a nontriathlon partner. A heavy pack can be a great equalizer for even the strongest athlete.

Even when you are focusing on building muscular endurance, it is essential to maintain your running endurance. Many strong runners find that good results can be achieved by a combination of cycling and tempo run training.

In planning their seasons, experienced runners can use half-marathons and 10K races for building intensive aerobic endurance. Half-marathons in the spring season are particularly useful because pace and heart rate data provide an excellent indicator of running fitness. Half-marathon efforts measure running fitness without major muscular damage or long recovery periods.

Two final things to remember are:

- Avoid high-intensity running when strength training is at a high intensity.
- When building muscular endurance for long-distance triathlon, keep the overall intensity well below functional threshold for the quickest recovery. High-intensity running is for only the strongest athletes, and the marginal benefit is not worth the injury and recovery considerations for most athletes. Until your run splits are in the top 10 percent of your age group, muscular endurance work is the safest way to build triathlon run speed.

> **RUNNERS WITH ENDURANCE AS A KEY LIMITER** should remember that cycling endurance and muscular endurance are more important than speed for long-distance triathlon. Although many athletes enjoy running fast, it is rarely the best strategy for long-course triathlon success. You should ensure that your run training does not compromise the quality of your bike training.
>
> **NOVICE**

■ *Stage 4: Building Superior Threshold Speed, Elites*

What follows is the final stage of a runner's development. This kind of training is appropriate only for athletes with all of the following characteristics:

- You have been running without injury for at least the past twelve months.
- You have successfully completed twelve months of muscular endurance training.
- You recover well from your key sessions and do not have endurance (bike or run) as a key limiter.
- You consistently place in the top 10 percent of your age group at international-level races.

The first step is to determine your VO_2max pace using the test provided in Appendix B. This test will identify your sustained speed (SS) pace, which will dictate your speed in anaerobic endurance workouts, like those detailed at the end of the chapter. Typically, this kind of training will start in the late Base period and extend to the beginning or middle of the Build period.

There are many ways to build running speed, and the protocol that follows is an effective one for certain athletes. You should take the guidelines and workouts throughout this book and interpret them in the context of your specific goals and limiters. What follows is a summary of the key points for anaerobic endurance training.

Here are some important points to remember with this kind of training:

Once per week. As a long-distance triathlete, you need to do only one of these sessions every seven to ten days. Increased frequency will result in lower-quality sessions in the rest of your training week.

Moderate volume leads to the best results. Studies have shown that 10–15 min. of this type of work once a week is sufficient to achieve results, with improving threshold speed as well as economy. Early sessions should be done at 4–10 sec. per 400 m slower than your SS pace. You should gradually increase the speed and the workload.

Focus on technique. You will find that when you focus on form and relax, the pace will be challenging but comfortable. If you are experiencing trouble hitting target pacing, then either your splits are too challenging, you need additional recovery, or you are starting each interval too quickly.

Timing. As mentioned earlier, this type of training should be started eight to fifteen weeks before your first A-priority race of the year. Each block should last no more than six weeks.

Pacing. If you are a strong runner, then you will be able to run these sessions at faster than SS pace. Research shows that running at a faster pace is not necessary and will only prolong recovery times. Stick to your VO_2max pace (see Appendix B); you will get the same benefit and recover more quickly.

Warm-up and cool-down. Hard BT sessions are best done later in the day following a deep warm-up. In addition to an extensive warm-up of 35–40 min., you may benefit from 20–30 min. of easy cycling prior to arriving at the track. Here is an example of a warm-up:

- Run 800 m easy.
- Run 1,600–3,000 m with a mix of easy, steady, and running drills.
- Run eight strides with walk-back recovery. Strides are best done barefoot on grass. Do thirty left-foot strikes, run at 800 m race pace, focus on perfect form, about 19 sec. per repetition (95 rpm cadence). Walk-back is essential to drop heart rate.
- Run 800 m easy, with builds to test effort.
- Fully recover for 3–5 min.

Core conditioning work and running skills can be incorporated into the warm-up to more effectively use your time. Following the main set, a proper cool-down, including light stretching, will help promote recovery. You should also plan your nutrition needs in advance of this session.

Testing. If you plan to do more than four weeks of anaerobic endurance training, then you should repeat the VO_2max test every four to six weeks (see Appendix B). It bears repeating that if you are new to running or injury-prone, then the risks of this training far outweigh the benefits.

After four to six weeks of this intense training, you should begin to focus more on threshold and subthreshold running; this involves extending the interval duration and lowering the intensity and pace of the sessions (see the sample workouts at the end of this chapter).

RUNNING TECHNIQUE

There is no athlete in triathlon who doesn't want to figure out how to improve his or her running speed. One of the most common statements we hear from highly motivated athletes is "I have to run faster." Too many athletes believe that the quickest way to run faster is to run more and run harder. In fact, most athletes are already running close to, or more than, the run volume required for success. The purpose of this section is to give you some ideas on how to run smarter and how to get the most speed out of a given level of aerobic fitness.

What is good running form? In our experience, it is

1. *Smooth:* The athlete looks comfortable; the head, shoulders, and hips are stable and travel in a consistent horizontal plane. In other words, there is very little vertical movement of the head, hips, and shoulders.

2. *Balanced:* The athlete's legs, hips, and arms all contribute to forward (as opposed to lateral) movement. Viewed from behind, the athlete has no lateral movement and the pelvis remains stable.

3. *Relaxed:* The athlete's shoulders, jaw, and arms are relaxed. The only tension in the body is specific muscle tension required for running. All nonrunning muscles are relaxed. Breathing is rhythmic and calm.

Many athletes who are seeking to improve their running form start with a focus on their feet, in particular their foot strike. Although heel striking is a sign of poor economy, it is a symptom rather than a cause of poor form. Athletes often eliminate a heel strike by pointing their toes at the moment of impact. The heel strike disappears, but the overall stride is no more economical. In fact, this modification can lead to a wide range of overuse injuries, as the muscles and tendons of the lower leg must decelerate the runner with each impact.

So where to start? The most effective approach is to seek a combination of correct body alignment and cadence. These two factors account for the majority of economy gains that you can attain. Speed comes from the correct manipulation of body alignment and cadence. Stride length is the result, not the source, of speed.

■ *Body Alignment*

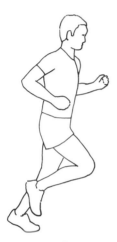

Body alignment is often referred to as an athlete's "pose" or "stance." The proper configuration is for the shoulder, hip, and ankle joints to all be aligned (Figure 8.1). For ease of explanation, let's call this alignment the "Stance Line."

Once a correct stance is achieved, forward motion is generated by moving the top of the Stance Line forward of the center of balance so that the athlete is, effectively, falling. Cadence is then used to efficiently transform gravity's downward pull into forward motion. Watch any child run and you will quickly see this principle in action. You will also see what happens when the child's cadence is unable to keep up with the body's inclination. The child falls down!

Athletes unaccustomed to this stance will find that the position feels very "vertical"; this is a good cue for proper alignment. A technique for maintaining good body alignment is to focus on running tall, with the chin slightly down. With experimentation you will find that you need very little tilt of the Stance Line. In fact, at all speeds up to a 7:00-per-mile pace, the correct stance is very close to vertical.

FIGURE *8.1*

When making the transition from cycling to running, many triathletes find that their hip flexors tighten and their stance is compromised. Here are four things to watch for when running off the bike:

Excessive trunk lean. Athletes with this issue often have good leg turnover but, in order to achieve the required lean, bend at the waist and put their hips behind their Stance Line (Figure 8.2). An athlete can correct this problem by focusing on keeping the shoulders back, head up, and/or pelvis open.

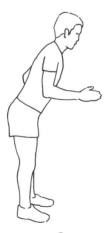

Tight shoulders. This problem is common when athletes seek to increase their speed. Tension enters the body, and the athlete finds that he or she is

FIGURE *8.2*

shrugging (Figure 8.3). Focusing on relaxed shoulders is more economical and also increases lung capacity.

Head imbalance. Allowing the chin to drop toward the chest or to be excessively elevated will also cause the athlete to be out of balance (see Figures 8.4 and 8.5). Viewed from the side, a runner with efficient form will have his or her neck in alignment with the spine, with no excessive curvature either forward or backward.

Wide elbows and open arm carriage. Coming off the bike, athletes often run in a very open manner, with arms extended and elbows out to the sides of the body (Figure 8.6). This reduces economy because energy is spent stabilizing the upper body. An easy correction is to lift the hands, orient the thumb over a soft fist, and relax the shoulders.

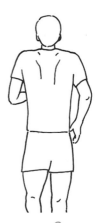

FIGURE *8.3*

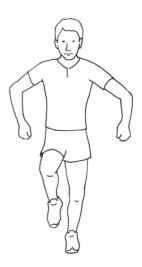

FIGURE *8.6*

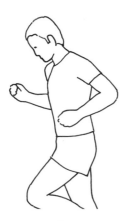

FIGURE *8.4*

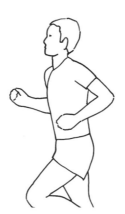

FIGURE *8.5*

 Cadence

Watch any good runner within a group of novices, and you will quickly note that he or she almost always has faster leg turnover. Leg turnover in itself is not necessarily economical because it is important for the foot strike to occur at the base of the Stance Line. Foot strike in front of the base of the Stance Line requires the athlete to support the body as it moves over and beyond the point of impact.

When most novice runners seek to increase their cadence, they find that their heart rate increases materially. If this happens to you, shorten your stride until you are able to run at the desired intensity. You will likely feel that you are running with "baby steps," and that is probably the best sign that you have it right. Indeed, athletes running at up to a 5:20-per-mile pace with good form will continue to feel as if they are running with short strides.

As a general rule, most runners should seek a minimum cadence of 85 cycles per minute for their long, slow distance pace and 90 cycles per minute for 10K race pace and faster. Depending on your speed, 5–10 cycles per minute quicker is even better. If you are currently running with a cadence significantly lower (for example, more than 5 cycles per minute) than these targets, you should seek to gradually lift your cadence over a series of six to eighteen months. Rapid changes in cadence place undue stress on the body.

FORM DRILLS

It is essential that you understand the objective of each drill as it relates to your personal technical limiters. Simply doing drills will not improve running economy, but specific drills will help you learn movement patterns and enhance your overall technical awareness.

In addition to strides, the following sequence is recommended to help guide you through the correct movement pattern for your legs. When most of us were "taught" to run (something we already knew how to do as children), we were instructed to raise our knees high. The trouble with running with high knees is that athletes tend to draw the heel forward when lifting the knee, which results in a foot strike in front of the Stance Line.

Rather than focusing on knee lift, focus on heel lift. Heel lift occurs when the heel is drawn up along the Stance Line. But wait! The elite runners whom you have seen always have their trailing heel well behind their Stance Line. However, this is a result of their forward velocity, and the correct firing pattern is to draw the heel up the Stance Line. The easiest way to start learning this firing pattern is to use the mirror drill.

MIRROR DRILL. Stand sideways in front of a full-length mirror and draw your left heel up your right inseam, allowing your toes to hang down (Figure 8.7). You may find that your heel tends to pull forward or backward. You want your heel to track straight up your inseam (note that your inseam is along your Stance Line when you are standing still). When learning the mirror drill, start with a slow movement, one leg at a time. Keep your foot relaxed as you lift your heel. Once you have mastered the movement pattern, hold your upper body in your run-

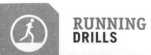

**RUNNING
DRILLS**

ning stance. Continue with this drill until you are able to perform rapid heel lifts with perfect tracking and form.

MARCHING DRILL. The next progression is the marching drill. With a full-length mirror at your side for feedback, alternate heel lifts (see Figure 8.7). Start slowly, and gradually speed your transitions from leg to leg. When you feel comfortable with your form, take this drill outside and slowly move forward while combining perfect heel lift with slow forward motion and proper arm carriage. Remember that the goal of this drill is to teach your legs the correct movement pattern. The speed of forward motion does not matter. Indeed, many athletes will find that they make very little forward progress at all.

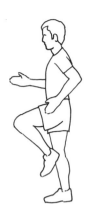

FIGURE *8.7*

TOE DRILL. When you feel that you have mastered the marching drill, you can progress to the toe drill. In the toe drill, you complete each heel lift by moving onto the toe of the supporting leg (Figures 8.8a and 8.8b). This drill enhances your proprioceptive skills and increases pelvic stability. It should be done with slow to moderate pacing, as the benefits are balance and strength related.

SKIP DRILL. The final step in the drill progression is to add a skip to the toe drill. This is called the skip drill. As you move onto your toe, insert a slight forward skip. The skip drill enables you to increase your cadence and train the rapid firing of the muscles required to generate heel lift. When it is done correctly, the head, shoulders, and hips are stable with minimal vertical lift.

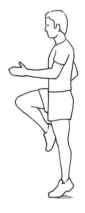

FIGURE *8.8a*

The toe and skip drills are complementary and can be included in your warm-up or inserted into the middle of the walk-back recovery used during strides.

ACTIVE RUNNING DRILLS

These drills can be used as part of a warm-up for an SS session and as part of a running strength/core conditioning session. Some of these drills require a fair degree of coordination. If you are doing the drills only one or two times per week, give your muscles plenty of time to "learn" correct technique. It is normal for some of the drills to feel a little awkward at first.

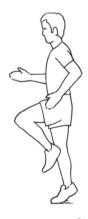

FIGURE *8.8b*

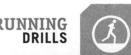

RUNNING DRILLS

With economy training, it's best to do short workouts frequently rather than long ones infrequently. Once the nervous system begins to tire or you experience difficulty maintaining focus on technique, no further improvements will take place. For the same reason, these workouts are best early in a session. Don't do them when fatigued.

Though these drills can be done anywhere, doing them on a soft surface is highly recommended. Note that the explosive drills are stressful on the body. Start slowly with a small number of repetitions. Typically, we recommend a selection of drills four to six times for 20–80 m. In between the drills, jog easily or walk. Because these drills are either technique or strength oriented, there is no need for concern about average heart rates.

■ *Strides*

Strides are our preferred drill for improving run economy. Put simply, strides are short bursts of fast running with perfect form. Strides are an excellent way to improve running technique and should be incorporated year-round.

Protocol. Do strides at least once a week. A single set per session is sufficient, with six to eight intervals per set.

Recovery. Recover by walking back to the starting point. Remember that this is a skills session, not an aerobic training session. Therefore, the recovery interval is intentionally long to ensure that you maintain perfect form throughout the session.

Timing. Novice athletes should undertake strides at the start of a run session or as a stand-alone workout. In the early season, athletes may find it time-effective to include strides in advance of a cycling skills session, also known as a skills reverse brick (see "Skills Reverse Brick" sidebar for a session example; also refer to Appendix D for brick options). Athletes with strong running technique may wish to do strides at the end of a run workout. All athletes will benefit from using strides as part of their race and run test warm-ups.

Pacing. Strides should be done at between 800 m and 1-mile race pace. Strides should not be done all-out. Many athletes find it beneficial to start easy and increase speed through each interval as well as across a set of strides. Quite often, you will find that tired legs will come alive during a set of Strides that starts easy and builds through the set.

Distance. Each stride should last for 30 left-foot strikes, a total of 60 foot strikes. You will find it easiest to count the foot strikes on one side.

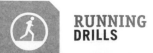

RUNNING DRILLS

Skills Reverse Brick

Doing a traditional brick means that you would be fatigued for the strides. For those of you who want to improve your running form and economy, it is essential that you be fresh and relaxed when doing strides.

Run 10–15 min. at an easy pace to warm up, then do six to eight strides with walk-backs; focus on cadence and run easy to steady for the rest of the workout.

TRANSITION

Bike 10–15 min. easy: Low-cadence riders focus on a slightly higher cadence, then begin speed drills—dominant leg, single leg (if on trainer), and/or spin-ups. Continue to focus on cadence and ride easy to steady pace for the rest of the workout.

TIPS FOR RUNNING STRIDES

1. Relax, particularly your shoulders, upper back, and jaw.
2. Concentrate; know what aspects of your form you are trying to improve.
3. Remember that the walk-back is essential. Take your time with the recovery. This is a skills session. The rest of your week is for adding endurance.
4. Do your strides with bare feet wherever safe to do so.

Cadence. Aim to complete each stride in about 19 sec.; this implies an overall cadence of 95 cycles per minute. Athletes can enhance leg speed by doing downhill strides as well as running with the wind.

Equipment. Strides are best done barefoot on grass. When weather or safety conditions do not permit bare feet, very light shoes can be used. Barefoot strides increase the natural feedback that occurs when an athlete is heel striking. Much of this valuable feedback is lost with a highly cushioned shoe. Check the area first to make sure it is free of glass, thorns, or anything else that may cut. Don't run barefoot if there are breaks in the skin on your feet.

Downhill Strides

After a warm-up, run down a very slight grade for 20 sec. at about the pace you would run a 400 m race. In other words, the pace is well short of a sprint but is fairly quick. Run six to eight of these strides, relaxing during each. Walk back after each stride, taking about 90 sec. to do so. Walking is important for the success of this workout—don't run the recoveries.

RUNNING
DRILLS

Uphill Strides

Hills and stairs can also be used to enhance heel lift. Athletes can use short-duration stair and hill repeats (on long recoveries) to help increase proper heel lift. When using hills and stairs for technical improvement, interval duration should be short and recovery periods long. The best stairs for this kind of work are the "half stairs" found in most stadium bleachers. Remember that the goal is to train your ability to rapidly lift your heel up your Stance Line. Run six to eight strides, as before, and walk back after each.

■ *Plyometrics and Run-Specific Strength*

In a weekly session, spend 10–20 min. working on power with plyometric exercises. Just as with uphill running, this type of exercise has been shown to improve economy in runners. This form of training is best done during the Base period. Be careful with plyometrics because the risk of injury with certain types of exercises is great.

SIDEWAYS RUNNING. Step to your right with your right foot and then bring your left foot up to your right without crossing over it. Continue this movement—you will be almost bouncing. Repeat drill in the reverse direction.

SIDEWAYS CROSSOVERS. The same as sideways running, only this time you cross over and rotate your hips (but not your shoulders) as the left leg moves in front of and then behind the right leg. Think fast feet on this one. It's best to start slowly and then build up the speed.

BACKWARD RUNNING. Hold normal running form and jog easily backward. Speed can be increased over time. You can also do quick accelerations to forward running from the backward running.

HANDS-ON-HEAD RUNNING. Alternate between normal running and hands-on-head running. If you have any lateral movement in your normal running gait, then it will become more pronounced. This is a good drill for promoting running stability.

FRONT BENCH DRILL. Face a bench and place your left leg on the bench. Draw the right heel quickly up toward your butt (Figure 8.9). The goal is a quick movement up and a minimization of ground contact time. Hold arms in regular running position. Start with 10 repetitions with each leg and build gradually toward 30. Once you hit 30 repetitions, drop back down to 20 and add another set. The purpose of this drill is to train the ability of the leg to fire quickly and lift the heel up the Stance Line. This is an explosive drill and should be done only by strong and experienced athletes.

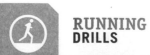

RUNNING DRILLS

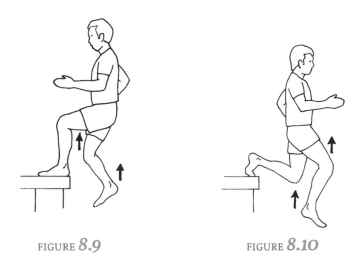

FIGURE *8.9*   FIGURE *8.10*

REAR BENCH DRILL. Facing away from the bench, place your left leg up on the bench behind you (knee bent, toe resting on the bench), draw your right heel up toward your butt, and hold your arms in normal running position (Figure 8.10). You may find that you need to do a little jump with your right leg to get it off the ground. The resting leg does not contribute anything to this drill (aside from balance). Aim for a quick action with minimal ground contact time. Start with 10 repetitions with each leg and build gradually toward 30. Once you hit 30 repetitions, drop back down to 20 and add another set. Like the front bench drill, this is an explosive drill that should be done only by strong and experienced athletes.

KNEE LIFT. Come up onto the ball of your left foot while raising your right knee. Grab your right knee and lift up while maintaining proud form (Figure 8.11). If you have trouble with balance, keep your supporting foot flat on the ground. Speed is not important on this one.

QUICK FEET. For this quickness drill, take baby steps and work on a very, very fast leg action. Arms and feet move very quickly. There should be little in the way of knee action; movement is on and off the balls of the feet. Forward speed is not important, as the goal is to quickly fire the legs so that the heel travels up the Stance Line.

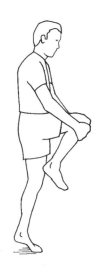

FIGURE *8.11*

RUNNING DRILLS

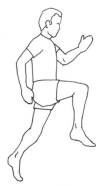

FIGURE *8.12*

BOUNDING. Running tall, extend the push-off phase and bound. Relax the shoulders and use your arms as part of the drive phase (Figure 8.12). This is a plyometric drill designed to build run-specific strength; it can be incorporated into warm-ups, hill repeats, and endurance running sessions.

LOPING RUN. From a crouched position, bound forward with a side-to-side component (Figure 8.13a). Your feet should strike the ground about 5 feet apart (Figure 8.13b). Rather than driving forward, the body is driven side to side. In the previous drill, you push straight ahead; in this drill, your arms swing from side to side.

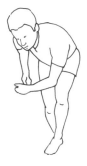

FIGURE *8.13a*

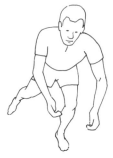

FIGURE *8.13b*

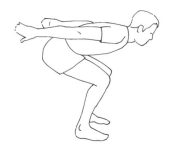

FIGURE *8.14*

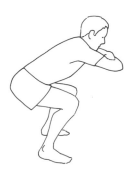

FIGURE *8.15*

TWO-LEGGED JUMPS. This is a great drill to load the legs before doing an interval, or just as a drill on its own. Swing the arms forward when jumping. Start from a low position. Absorb the impact by bending the knees quickly on landing (Figure 8.14). The legs act like springs, coiling down on impact and springing forward when jumping. It is important that the legs, rather than the knees, and hips absorb the impact.

LOW WALKING. Get into a crouch with your thighs parallel to the ground and arms folded across your chest (Figure 8.15). Walk around in this position, or stay still and (ever so slightly) oscillate up and down. Maintain until the quads start to burn, then maintain some more.

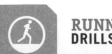

RUNNING DRILLS

KEY TRAINING SESSIONS

▪ *Run/Walk Protocol*

If running is a limiter for you, a run/walk protocol is likely to deliver the improved running endurance you need to finish your Ironman race strong. Coach Bobby McGee has helped many elite triathletes to become more successful runners using this technique.

Determining where to start with the run/walk method depends on your current level of fitness and volume of run conditioning. McGee recommends that athletes follow these guidelines:

- Use run/walk for all runs longer than 30 min.
- Use walking for the rest interval for all workouts involving running above heart rate Zone 3.
- Use the method for all longer bricks—those with a total duration over 2.5 hours and/or a running component greater than 30 min.

The basic recommended pattern is 10 min. of running and 1 min. of walking. However, the run portion can fall anywhere between 5 and 15 min., and the walk portion can be from 15 sec. to 1 min. The exact mix can be varied based on your abilities and training level.

> **ADVANTAGES TO RUN/WALK TRAINING (AND RACING)**
> - Increased volume (per workout, per week, per phase)
> - Reduced recovery time
> - Improved mental preparation for training and racing
> - Improved speed in most cases
> - Improved lipid metabolism
> - Increased functional leg strength

RUN/WALK ENDURANCE WORKOUT

Goal: Build volume quickly and safely
Note: If you are currently running fewer than four times per week and looking to build volume, variations on this workout will help you build endurance and distance.

MAIN SET

Break run into following intervals:
6- to 10-min. run, 1-min. walk
Coach's tip: Add 10–15% to all runs weekly. For a 10% increase, the run-to-walk ratio should be closer to 10:1. For a 15% increase, the run-to-walk ratio is closer to 6:1.

N   **NOVICE**

RUN/WALK VOLUME AND PACE WORKOUT

Goal: Increase both volume in long runs and pace in higher-intensity workouts
Note: This approach is most effective for advanced runners.

MAIN SET

10-min. run, 1-min. walk
Build incrementally

I/E   INTERMEDIATE/ELITE

You may consider breaking runs into intervals as long as 30 min. However, often you will find that with blocks longer than 15 min., you have a hard time starting the run again. In some cases this problem can be rectified by ensuring that the walk-stride rate stays high (shorter steps and high cadence). Use a brisk walk and remember that the purpose is to cover ground rather than thinking, "Ah, rest!"

Also ensure that your arm carriage remains in running mode while you are walking. Allowing the arms to drop slows the stride rate and increases the stride length. This in turn leads to "switching off" or "derecruits," with the lengthened levers placing the pelvis and hamstrings under increased stress.

These guidelines will help you to stay prepared for running and to easily start the next section with renewed vigor.

Considerations for long runs. The purpose of long runs is to develop endurance and train the body's ability to metabolize lipids as a fuel source. McGee points out that a coach (or athlete) can objectively measure increases in vascular capacity in long runs by observing the athlete's decoupling rates (the point when pace slows while heart rate remains constant). The basic idea is to be able to increase your long-run pace while maintaining predetermined subthreshold heart rates. A run/walk approach is by far the easiest method to improve this component of running endurance. McGee has found that most athletes achieve the best results by keeping the ratio at 10:1 (run/walk). As you improve, reduce the walk segment by 5–10 sec. until you reach a minimum walk period of 15 sec.

Considerations for racing. The run/walk method may be used effectively during racing as well as training. Sub-2:30 open marathons have been achieved by runners using a run/walk technique. If you are going to race this way, then you should train this way.

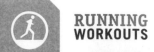

■ *Workouts for Intermediate and Elite Runners*

ANAEROBIC ENDURANCE WORKOUTS

Goal: Increase VO_2max, increase threshold pace, and improve running economy
Note: See the sample warm-up described in Appendix B for an appropriate warm-up routine. SS pace is determined in VO_2max test (Appendix B).

WORKOUT 1	
10–15 x 1 min.	30 sec. at SS pace, 30 sec. at 50% SS pace

WORKOUT 2	
10–15 x 400 m	200 m at SS pace, 200 m at 50% SS pace

WORKOUT 3
Note: Interval time is 3 min., or such length as gives approximately a 1:1 work-to-rest ratio.

3, 6, or 9 x 400 m descending	Interval 1 at SS pace + 4 sec. Interval 2 at SS pace + 2 sec. Interval 3 at SS pace

Repeat based on desired number of sets.

WORKOUT 4

3–5 x 1,000 m at SS pace
Recovery 1:1 work-to-rest ratio

I/E   **INTERMEDIATE/ELITE**

THRESHOLD/SUBTHRESHOLD WORKOUTS

Goal: Improve threshold and subthreshold running
Note: See the sample warm-up described in Appendix B for an appropriate warm-up routine. SS pace is determined in VO_2max test (Appendix B).

WORKOUT 1
Note: If your goal is to run a 3:10 Ironman-distance marathon (7:15 average pace), 5:45 is the mile pace for these 800s, so run 2:52 for both the 800 and the 400 RI.

6–12 x 800 m at fresh marathon goal pace less 90 sec. per mile
(400 m RI on the same total 800 m split)

WORKOUT 2

6- to 12-min. repeats at goal race pace less 30–45 sec. per mile
Easy jogging recovery (recovery 4:1 or 3:1 work-to-rest ratio)

WORKOUT 3

3–5 x 2,000 m at 10K race pace
400 m easy jogging recovery between each interval

I/E   **INTERMEDIATE/ELITE**

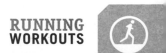

RUNNING WORKOUTS

OTHER CONSIDERATIONS

Keep these factors in mind when training for the run.

The role of nutrition. Probably the single greatest thing that most age-group athletes can do in order to improve their run performance is to improve their nutrition strategy. Ideas on this topic are included in Chapter 10.

The role of economy. There aren't many sources of "free speed" in sport, but running economy is an easy way to maximize performance from an existing aerobic base. To promote economy, you should incorporate strides into your weekly program. In addition, pay particular attention to your running form toward the end of long runs or when you are running off the bike. Reviewing video footage of running performance when fatigued can offer valuable insights into areas for improvement.

Running tired. Many coaches and athletes believe that it is beneficial to learn how to "run tired," so they schedule long runs for the day following long rides. This training does benefit a few, but it is accompanied by a greatly increased risk of injury and illness. For this reason, you will see both safer and more rapid results by starting your key running BT workouts as fresh as possible. If running is a limiter for you, then this approach is even more important. The benefits of training fresh are higher-quality sessions and more rapid recovery times.

Marathon running for age-group athletes. Many Ironman-distance triathletes are tempted to improve their running by competing in early-season marathons. However, because of the training time lost to the taper and subsequent race recovery, this strategy is a poor one for most triathletes. If your key limiter is running endurance, focus on your nutrition and long endurance sessions. If your key limiter is running muscular endurance, you can often achieve a substantial improvement by targeting an early-season half-marathon and using an appropriate mix of sustained speed and muscular endurance sessions.

"Recovery" runs. Given the stresses associated with running (at any speed), running workouts should rarely be used for active-recovery sessions. Recovery workouts are best done on the bike, in the pool, or in another nonimpact activity, such as yoga.

Intensity. High-intensity running is powerful training. If you have a history of injuries or biomechanical problems, it is best to remember that a marginal gain in running speed will not matter if you are injured or miss key BT workouts. Once endurance is built, cycling muscular endurance should be the number-one focus for all endurance athletes.

3-hour runs. Some athletes like to include 3-hour, or longer, runs in their training program. You should exercise caution in using runs of this duration, as recovery times are normally 48–72 hours. There are rapidly diminishing returns in running longer than 2.5 hours. The reason is the risk of extended recovery required after the session, as well as the risk of injury. Therefore, such sessions can have an adverse impact on cycling and swimming BT workouts. It is far better to do a 2-hour run and be able to get back on your training program after a single recovery day. Consistent training is the most important aspect of preparing for an ultraendurance event. Long endurance sessions are best done on the bike or as a combination workout.

Running is a very important part of Ironman-distance racing. However, a quick review of any set of race results will show that raw speed is not a requirement for race success. What is required is a multiyear apprenticeship that safely builds endurance and mileage as the body adapts to constant training. If you seek shortcuts, then injury is a likely result. Persistence, consistency, and patience are the essential attributes of success.

Beyond the Basics

PART III

CHAPTER 9

STRENGTH TRAINING

Given the endurance focus of triathlon, many athletes wonder if they stand to benefit from strength training. Even among leading coaches, there is a wide range of views on the benefits of traditional strength training. Of the three sports in triathlon, cycling appears to receive the greatest boost from strength training. However, running and swimming will also benefit from the gains associated with a properly constructed strength program.

> *Training is the act of breaking down muscle tissue. . . . The body builds strength during the recovery phase. Skip that and you deny your body the opportunity to get stronger.*
>
> —BRENDAN BRAZIER,
> IRONMAN COACH AND ATHLETE

For some athletes, a minimal commitment to strength training will be more than adequate. Men, particularly those under 30, have the ability to hold their strength through the season. For these athletes, it can make sense to strength train a few months a year or avoid lifting altogether. Building general endurance rather than spending time in the gym will also better serve many time-constrained athletes.

Given their physiology, women and masters athletes have much to gain from year-round strength training. Because these athletes are prone to lose strength over time, a maintenance program of at least one session per week is recommended even when sport-specific intensity is high. Aging athletes find the greatest benefit from strength training in maintaining the performance level that they already have achieved.

Athletes who are seeking to improve cycling performance will see benefits from increasing their lower-body strength. Traditional strength training can provide a suitable platform upon which the athlete can launch the higher-intensity work associated with the late Base and Build periods.

Athletes who are prone to injuries will benefit from including a strength regimen in their Prep and Base periods. Once biomechanical and equipment causes are ruled out, many aches and pains (particularly in the knee and back) are actually caused by either structural weaknesses or muscular imbalance—problems that may be addressed by a properly designed strength training program.

STRUCTURING YOUR PLAN

Before starting any training plan, it is worth spending a little time deciding on your goals. The first step of this process is to consider which of your key triathlon limiters can be specifically addressed through the strength program.

Many athletes have muscular imbalances that favor the front of their bodies—that is, the chest muscles, biceps, abdominals, and quadriceps dominate the muscles of the back, triceps, glutes, and hamstrings. The major posterior muscle groups are very important in triathlon, and most triathletes will benefit from incorporating exercises to strengthen these muscles.

Your strength plan should include a solid focus on core muscles, as well as hip flexors, once or twice per week. A strong core is key to racing the Ironman distance comfortably, as it keeps the pelvis in a neutral position on the run, keeps the legs and hips up while swimming, and enables you to generate more force on the bike. A strong lower back also means a more comfortable aero position on the bike. The advantages of strong hip flexors are numerous. The main hip flexor (the iliopsoas) is not only the primary mover to get good knee lift and drive you forward; it is also the major trunk stabilizer, keeping your lower spine stable when running and cycling.

After you define the goals of your strength training, you need to decide on the duration of the strength plan. In general, you should start strength training four weeks after your last A-priority race and switch to strength maintenance no less than seven weeks before your first A-priority race of the upcoming season. These guidelines give most athletes four to six months for focused strength training. Table 9.1 shows guidelines for strength training periodization.

Each phase is assumed to last four weeks (note that the Anatomical Adaptation [AA] phase consists of three subphases). Owing to scheduling constraints, some athletes may have to reduce some of the phases to three weeks' duration. This reduction makes sense when you want an early-season race to fall at the end of a recovery week.

You should start each block at the top end of the repetition range. As the block progresses, weight can be gradually increased and repetitions reduced, except in strength maintenance (SM). In the AA phase, it is very important to avoid repetition failure.

TABLE 9.1 STRENGTH TRAINING PERIODIZATION

	ANATOMICAL ADAPTATION 1	ANATOMICAL ADAPTATION 2	ANATOMICAL ADAPTATION 3	MAXIMUM STRENGTH	STRENGTH MAINTENANCE
Goal	Muscles and connective tissues are conditioned to regular strength training	Build a muscular base with increasing intensity	Specifically prepare body for the rigors of the MS phase	Increase maximum strength for all lifts	Maintain strength; sport-specific and functional strength training dominates
Exercises	Wide range of whole-body exercises	Wide range of lower-body and core exercises; upper-body exercises become more focused	Specific range of upper- and lower-body exercises, continued range of core exercises	Specific range of lower- and upper-body exercises, continued range of core exercises	Limited number of exercises, selected in light of athlete's limiters
Intensity	Low intensity, never to strain or failure	Moderate intensity, some strain on final repetitions of last set, never to failure	Moderately high intensity, final reps of both sets require focus, never to failure	High intensity, final reps of last 2 sets require heavy focus; spotter might be required on final rep of final set	Low to moderate, inversely related to the intensity of sport-specific and functional training
Sets	1–2 sets	2 sets	2 sets	4 sets	2 sets (including warm-up set)
Reps	25 reps	15–20 reps	12–15 reps	6–10 reps	6–10 reps (after warm-up)
Rest interval	30–45 sec.	30–45 sec.	60–90 sec.	2–3 min.	30–60 sec.

The repetition and intensity protocol for core exercises is different from the guidelines for other exercises. You should start with a core session that lasts for 5 min. and builds to a session of 15–20 min. duration.

In all exercises, emphasize perfect technique and relaxed breathing. The absolute amount of weight lifted is of limited importance. Focus your energies on gradual, consistent improvement. The greatest increases in strength will happen during the AA3 and maximum strength (MS) phases. Give your body adequate time to prepare for the increased stress associated with these phases of the program. Rushing the body's natural speed of adaptation can lead to injury.

If you are uncomfortable with the intensity of the MS phase, you should consider skipping the MS phase and moving directly to the SM phase.

Assuming that each phase lasts four weeks, it will take four blocks to move through to SM. Many athletes assume that additional benefits will result from extending the MS phase. However, we recommend that the MS phase last for a maximum of four weeks. Athletes will show superior gains from moving to sport-specific strength work rather than repeating the MS phase. Those living in a climate conducive to year-round training will find sport-specific work, particularly for cycling and running, much more valuable than gym-based muscular endurance work.

WEIGHT TRAINING EXERCISES

▪ *Timing*

For all AA and MS sessions, it is best if strength training is the first workout of the day in order to get the full benefit from your session. If this timing is not possible, you should try to get as much rest as possible between your morning aerobic session and your evening strength session.

In the AA1 phase, the intensity is low enough for some athletes to include some light aerobic work before lifting. However, in AA2 and beyond, it is best for the strength work to come first. In the AA3 and MS phases, the goal is to increase maximal strength, so it is essential that you be fresh.

Many athletes wonder about the risk of injury in doing aerobic training after lifting. The risk varies tremendously by athlete as well as by the intensity of the lifting. You should be cautious about scheduling any activity after intense strength training; running in particular should be avoided. Keep all sessions light in the 24–48 hours after strength training. Athletes in the SM phase have more scheduling flexibility.

Table 9.2 shows strength targets. Stronger athletes should never exceed these weight targets. Rather than increasing weight beyond these points, you should increase the number of repetitions. Specifically, stronger athletes should bear in mind that squatting more than 185 pounds is likely unnecessary. The safest place to overload your legs is the leg press (sled).

TABLE 9.2 **STRENGTH TARGETS**	
Squat	1.3–1.7 x BW
Leg press (sled)	2.5–2.9 x BW
Step up	0.7–0.9 x BW
Seated row	0.5–0.8 x BW
Standing, bent-arm lat pull	0.3–0.5 x BW

◼ *General Tips*

Change is the key to making progress. The body adapts to the training stress, and by varying that stress, you are able to achieve constant adaptation, and thus progress.

Heavy weights will affect the quality of sport-specific sessions. For this reason, it is best to complete the MS phase no later than the middle of the Base period. During that time of the year, you are training in endurance and technique. Therefore, the strength gains outweigh the negative impact on the sport-specific work.

Start out easy, as muscles adapt more quickly than connective tissue. Many athletes have seriously injured themselves by rushing the natural pace of their bodies. This is a powerful argument for avoiding all supplements that are designed to speed muscular adaptation, regardless of ethical reasons.

Be especially conservative with increasing intensity until you are six to eight weeks into your program (twelve weeks for novices). Relax about the amount that is being lifted, and remember your program goals. Often novices will find themselves becoming numbers-driven. The safest and most effective approach is to establish excellent technique, prepare the connective tissues, and then increase intensity. Training with consistency and patience will ensure the best results. You will get significant gains in the first eight weeks of any strength program because of the "recruitment" of your muscles. Initially, the training teaches your body to use the muscles it already has. By the time you have tapped much of these gains, your muscles will also be stronger from the training.

Four weeks of MS lifting is plenty for triathletes. The goal of this strength program is to build sport-specific strength. Once the majority of the gains have been made, it is time to switch to sport-specific work. We recommend that these lifts be done in the order they are listed.

For AA1, we recommend a wide range of full-body exercises. For AA2 and beyond, we recommend the following exercises, and in the order they are listed. MS exercises are in bold; athletes who are short on time should focus on these.

- **Squats and/or leg press** (always do a light set to warm up)
- **Lat pulldowns** (to front)
- **Knee extension**
- **Hamstring curl**
- **Straight-arm pulldowns**
- **Core**
- **Calf raise**
- **Seated row**
- Dips (use dip machine)
- Triceps extension

Ten to 15 min. of light aerobic activity should always precede strength training. As a cooldown, many athletes enjoy a brief swim or cycle. Stretching should follow.

With all lifts, start lighter than the weight you think you need. Avoid the natural urge to rush. Focus on repetition quality because good form yields the most benefits. However, good form means that you will not be able to use as much weight. You will be well served by leaving your ego in the locker room and remembering that you want to impress only yourself on race day.

After lifting is the ideal time for an extended full-body stretch and to improve flexibility. Gyms are warm, dry environments where you can focus on your limiters. You should also stretch briefly after each set to help maintain range of motion and ensure an adequate recovery after each set. You will find a progression of stretches at the end of this chapter.

THE SQUAT IS ONE OF THE MOST DANGEROUS OPTIONS for the novice athlete, and great care is necessary to protect the back and knees; therefore, the leg press is recommended. For both squats and leg press, correct technique is essential to avoid injury or muscular imbalances.

N NOVICE

Squat

Goal: Improve force delivery to the pedal in cycling

Rotate your feet 5–10 degrees outward, as this position promotes the correct firing of the muscles. Keep the squat bar moving vertically, without any forward or backward movement (Figure 9.1a). Your pelvis should rotate forward and down as you lower the weight. Never descend past 90 degrees

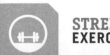

STRENGTH
EXERCISES

(Figure 9.1b), but 100–110 degrees is fine for the strength gains required for triathlon. Control the speed of each repetition, and never "bounce" off the bottom. Breathing should be controlled and deep; exhale in a controlled fashion when extending.

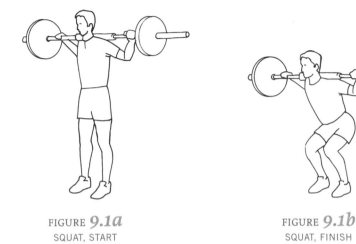

FIGURE **9.1a**
SQUAT, START

FIGURE **9.1b**
SQUAT, FINISH

Leg Press

Goal: Improve force delivery to the pedal in cycling

Keep your back perfectly flat against the backrest (Figure 9.2a). As with squats, never descend past 90 degrees, and do not push on your knees on the extension (Figure 9.2b). Your breathing should be controlled and deep; exhale in a controlled fashion when extending. Many athletes find single-leg work to be effective—if you use this technique, ensure that guards/braces are placed to prevent injury.

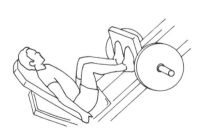

FIGURE **9.2a**
LEG PRESS, START

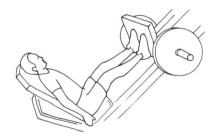

FIGURE **9.2b**
LEG PRESS, FINISH

**STRENGTH
EXERCISES**

Knee Extension

Goal: Improve the balance between the lateral and medial quadriceps

Begin with your knee slightly bent (Figure 9.3a), and extend it to be fully straight. Restrict your movement within the range of 120–180 degrees (Figure 9.3b). Focus on the final 20–30 degrees, where you should achieve maximum extension. A 90-degree or greater range of motion has been shown to irritate the patella tendon.

> A COMMON PHENOMENON IN CYCLISTS IS KNEE TROUBLE, typically as a result of the quadriceps not firing properly. The best way to correct this problem is to focus on the final 15 degrees of the knee extension exercise, maintaining a solid contraction of the inner quadriceps. You can actually do further damage if you fail to do the full extension, so reduce the weight if you begin to lose proper form.

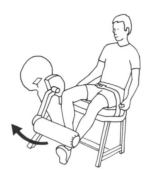

FIGURE **9.3a**
KNEE EXTENSION, START

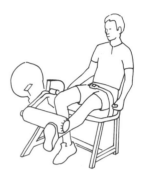

FIGURE **9.3b**
KNEE EXTENSION, FINISH

Hamstring Curl

Goal: Improve the strength ratio between the quadriceps and hamstrings

This exercise is best done one leg at a time. With a controlled movement, pull your heels to your buttocks (Figures 9.4a and 9.4b). Keep your core stable and your repetition speed slow. Rocking the hips and using a rapid lift speed can cause injury.

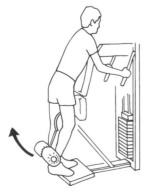

FIGURE **9.4a**
HAMSTRING CURL, START

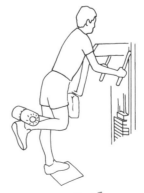

FIGURE **9.4b**
HAMSTRING CURL, FINISH

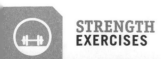

STRENGTH EXERCISES

Calf Raise

Goal: Improve force delivery to the pedal for cycling and improve running strength

Keep your feet aligned (Figure 9.5a) (you may turn your heels slightly inward). Your legs, hips, back, and shoulders should be aligned at all times as you lift (Figure 9.5b) and lower.

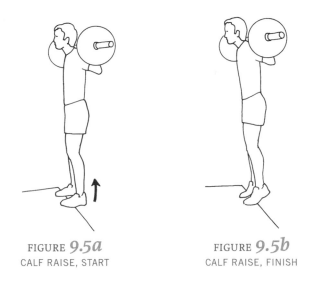

FIGURE **9.5a**
CALF RAISE, START

FIGURE **9.5b**
CALF RAISE, FINISH

Seated Row

Goal: Strengthen your core and lower back

Your back should be vertically aligned. Grasp the bar so that your thumbs are pointing up (Figure 9.6a). Your chest should remain out in a "proud" position, your elbows should be drawn backward and positioned close to your body, and your back should not rock (Figure 9.6b). Reduce the weight if you find yourself rocking.

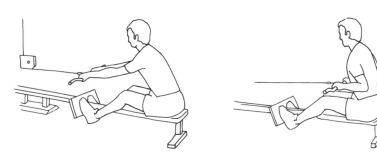

FIGURE **9.6a**
SEATED ROW, START

FIGURE **9.6b**
SEATED ROW, FINISH

**STRENGTH
EXERCISES**

Lat Pulldown

Goal: Stabilize the shoulders

Keeping your shoulder blades pulled down (Figure 9.7a), pull the bar to a "proud" chest (Figure 9.7b). You should always pull to the chest, not the shoulder blades (as illustrated on some gym equipment) and maintain controlled movement for both the pulldown and return phases of the lift.

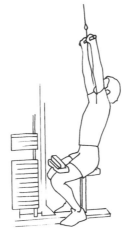

FIGURE **9.7a**
LAT PULLDOWN, START

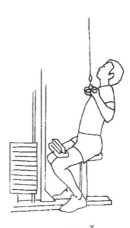

FIGURE **9.7b**
LAT PULLDOWN, FINISH

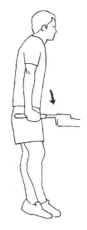

FIGURE **9.8a**
TRICEPS DIP, START

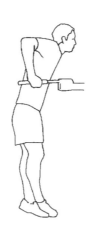

FIGURE **9.8b**
TRICEPS DIP, FINISH

Triceps Dip

Goal: Improve finish of the swim stroke

Your elbows should be kept close to the body at all times. Position your hands at slightly wider than shoulder width (Figure 9.8a). Superdeep or superwide dips should be avoided, as they are not required for the targeted strength gains. A 90-degree angle is the most you need to improve swim-specific strength (Figure 9.8b).

STRENGTH EXERCISES

Triceps Extension

Goal: Improve finish of the swim stroke

Keep your elbows locked for this exercise. Pause at full
extension (Figure 9.9b) and keep tension on your triceps
at the top of the cycle (Figure 9.9a). You may choose to
alternate between rope extensions and bar extensions
(both attachments are available in most gyms).

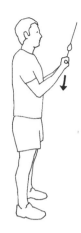 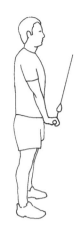

FIGURE *9.9a*
TRICEPS EXTENSION, START

FIGURE *9.9b*
TRICEPS EXTENSION, FINISH

Standing Straight-Arm Pulldown

Goal: Improve force for swimming

This exercise simulates the catch and pull of swim stroke. As in swimming, you should focus
on maintaining a high elbow. Maintain correct swimming form in both directions—pull down
(Figures 9.10a and 9.10b) and return to start. Many athletes will achieve a higher-quality exercise
by using stretch cords. Exercises using stretch cords are discussed in more detail in Chapter 6.

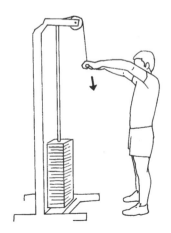 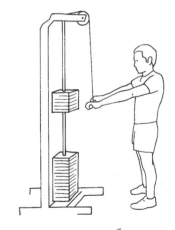

FIGURE *9.10a*
STANDING STRAIGHT-ARM PULLDOWN, START

FIGURE *9.10b*
STANDING STRAIGHT-ARM PULLDOWN, FINISH

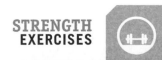

**STRENGTH
EXERCISES**

COMMON CONCERNS

Many athletes worry that weight training will result in bulking up. For the vast majority, it is extremely difficult to add muscle mass. For triathletes, endurance training makes it even tougher. Although some athletes will add some muscle mass during the winter, it tends to "burn away" in the spring once the longer endurance sessions begin.

Some athletes respond very quickly to weight training; if this is the case for you, then you should keep the MS phase specifically focused on the areas that you are seeking to improve. For example, if you carry a lot of upper-body muscle, you will likely find that focusing primarily on the lower body and core region makes the most sense.

Another common concern is that strength training will reduce quickness and agility. An easy way to address this issue is to maintain speed-skills sessions in all sports. However, slowing down is normal in the MS phase. In fact, if you don't slow down, you may not be working hard enough (assuming you have the appropriate strength and technique base for pushing MS). You will also find that your hill-climbing ability and power generation decline. This is normal, and your power will return once you ease off the weights.

A reduction in range of motion can also be a concern. The 10- to 20-min. period after strength training is an ideal time to undertake a full-body stretching program.

CORE STRENGTH EXERCISES

Correct technique is essential to working the core. You should maintain a slow repetition speed and incorporate a wide variety of the exercises described here. The vast majority of athletes have greater strength in their upper abdominal region, and if you have the same imbalance, you should focus on the lower abdominals, obliques, lower back, and glutes. Your training objective should be slow, high-quality repetitions that utilize a wide range of motion.

If you already have a strong core, meaning you have been doing fifty or more crunches in a traditional manner, it is time to shake things up a little. The following exercises will help you put together an advanced core workout—the perfect solution to a core routine that is becoming too easy. Aside from incline twisting sit-ups, these exercises require no equipment. Remember to exercise caution when beginning a new routine.

SUPERMAN. Your body is in push-up position, except your elbows are together directly under your shoulders. Your elbows and forearms are on the ground at a 90-degree angle from your shoulder, and your elbows are about 6 inches apart as if you are praying (Figure 9.11). Keep

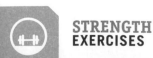

STRENGTH
EXERCISES

Core Exercise Tips

- Be very careful with new exercises. They are a different form of muscular contraction from crunches and traditional sit-ups. You can easily strain yourself for days if you overdo it.
- Remember to breathe!
- Use slow, controlled movements in all core exercises.
- If possible, do these exercises at a track where you can run easy (and tall) for 100 m

between sets. If you are at the gym, stand and do some torso stretching in between sets. Don't rush these exercises because they are tough.

- Go easy when you start. This point can't be emphasized too much. You don't want to be "crunched" for four days afterward.
- Quality over quantity.

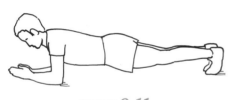

FIGURE **9.11**

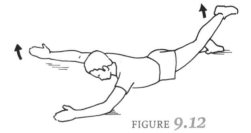

FIGURE **9.12**

your shoulder blades together (no curve in shoulders). Keep your hips a little higher than in a push-up and your back perfectly straight, on your toes with legs straight.

Hold for 15 sec., then move your elbows forward 2 inches and hold for 15 sec., then move your elbows forward another 2 inches and hold for 15 sec. Your hips may be falling now; keep them up—no bow in the back. Keep extending until you really feel it. If you aren't shaking after 45 sec., the technique needs modification (if body is straight, then make sure hips aren't too low). Flip over and do twenty slow crunches, then repeat the Superman. You will feel this one in your back and abs.

REAR SUPERMAN. Lie flat on your belly with arms and legs extended. Lift your right arm (thumb pointing up) and left leg (Figure 9.12). Tighten your glutes hard, crunch, and hold for 10–15 sec. Lift your left arm (thumb up) and right leg. Alternate four to six times on each side, keeping tension in the glutes, both thumbs pointing up, with no rotation of the core.

STRENGTH EXERCISES

PIKE. Place your hands together on the ground, keeping your arms straight and directly under your shoulders (Figure 9.13a). Make a triangle. The points of the triangle are your hands, shoulders, and feet. On your toes, keep your body perfectly straight. Slowly open upward by rotating your torso outward (Figure 9.13b). Keep both arms straight (one will be coming off the ground). Continue to rotate until you have gone 90 degrees and you are in a "cross" position, arms fully extended, one still on the ground (Figure 9.13c). Hold, return, rotate in the other direction, and repeat as desired. Keep the movement slow.

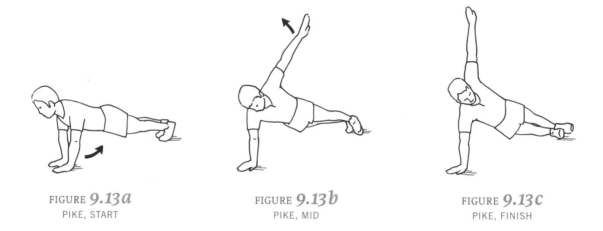

FIGURE **9.13a**
PIKE, START

FIGURE **9.13b**
PIKE, MID

FIGURE **9.13c**
PIKE, FINISH

OBLIQUES. Your neck remains neutral, with no "pull" on the head. The lift comes solely from your obliques (Figures 9.14a and 9.14b).

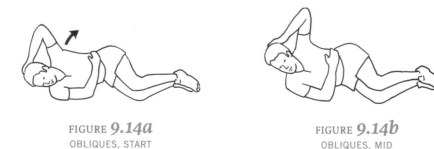

FIGURE **9.14a**
OBLIQUES, START

FIGURE **9.14b**
OBLIQUES, MID

**STRENGTH
EXERCISES**

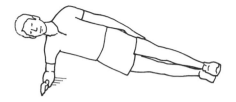

FIGURE *9.15a*
ADVANCED OBLIQUES, START

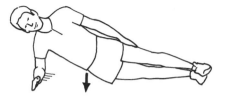

FIGURE *9.15b*
ADVANCED OBLIQUES, MID

ADVANCED OBLIQUES. Lie on your side and support your upper body with your elbow. Keep your higher arm flat against your side. Your body is straight, with chest and hips perpendicular to the ground. Lift your hips so your waist is 8–12 inches off the ground (Figure 9.15a), and hold for 10 sec. Lower slowly for a 5-sec. count (Figure 9.15b), then lift back to ready position. Five repetitions on each side are suggested for beginners. Work up to ten reps.

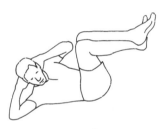

FIGURE *9.16a*

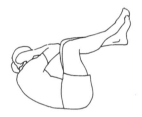

FIGURE *9.16b*

LOWER ABDOMINAL/OBLIQUE COMBO. Lying on your back with your knees bent, perform a twisting crunch, and touch your left elbow to your right knee (Figure 9.16a). Alternate sides, checking that the outside of your elbow touches the outside of your knee (Figure 9.16b).

■ *Swiss Ball Core Strength Exercises*

Before beginning these exercises, open your hips and stretch your back by lying backward over the ball. Work through the exercises in a "bottom-up" order. The last thing you raise is your head. Begin with exercises requiring balance. Upper abdominal exercises like the Swiss Ball crunches should be done last, as these are generally the strongest core muscles for most athletes. We recommend these be done in the order listed.

> **SWISS BALL CORE STRENGTH COMES FROM**
> * Remembering the goal is the work, not the reps.
> * Moving slowly and staying in control.
> * Breathing fully and smoothly.

STRENGTH EXERCISES

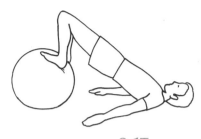

FIGURE **9.17**

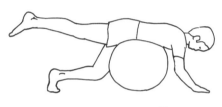

FIGURE **9.18**

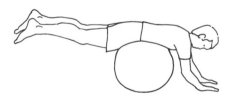

FIGURE **9.19**

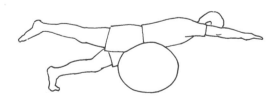

FIGURE **9.20**

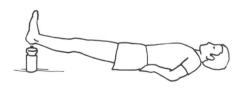

FIGURE **9.21**

SWISS BALL BRIDGE. Lie on your back with arms extended at your sides. Place your feet on the ball about shoulder width apart, and lift your hips so your torso is straight. Bend your knees so your lower legs are perpendicular to the ground (Figure 9.17). Hold for 1–3 sec., relax, and repeat.

ALTERNATING LEG LIFT. Lie on your belly over the ball and roll so that your arms are resting on the ground. Lift and extend one leg at a time. Move slowly and smoothly through the full range of motion (Figure 9.18).

DUAL-LEG LIFT. Same focus and movement as the alternating leg lift, only this time lift and extend both legs (Figure 9.19). Hold for 10 sec. You will feel this in your back and abs.

TRADITIONAL BACK EXTENSION. Lie on your belly over the ball with your right leg extended behind and your right arm extended forward (Figure 9.20). Move slowly and smoothly through the full range of motion, a side at a time. Increase the degree of difficulty by crossing your arms on your chest.

OVER AND AROUND. Lie on your back on the floor, with a water bottle at your feet. Keeping the small of your back pressed against the ground and your legs extended, lift your legs up and over the bottle (Figure 9.21). Repeat side to side. This exercise targets your lower abdominals.

**STRENGTH
EXERCISES**

IN AND UP. Lie on your back with legs extended. The first movement is to lift your legs just off the ground and pull your heels back to your buttocks (Figure 9.22), then extend back to the starting position. The second movement is to lift your legs straight up and perpendicular to the ground. Keep movement speed slow and controlled, so you feel the exertion in your lower abs.

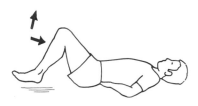

FIGURE *9.22*

SWISS BALL OBLIQUE CRUNCH. Lie on your side across the ball with your inside leg bent against the ball and your outside leg extended. Place your upper hand on the ball and rest your head on your bottom hand. Laterally lower and raise your torso slowly, keeping your hips and shoulders aligned (Figure 9.23).

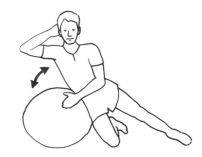

FIGURE *9.23*

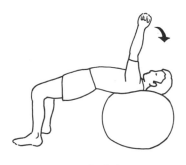

FIGURE *9.24a*

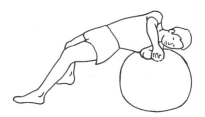

FIGURE *9.24b*

RUSSIAN TWIST. Lie on your back with the ball under your shoulders. Move your feet about shoulder width apart and lift your hips up so your body is parallel to the ground (Figure 9.24a). Extend your arms and roll back and forth, twisting at the abdomen (Figure 9.24b). The key to this oblique exercise is to roll the *ball*, not the body.

SWISS BALL CRUNCH. Lie with the small of your back against the ball and feet shoulder width apart. Place your hands across your chest or at your temples. Slowly crunch, lifting your shoulders and upper back off the ball (Figure 9.25).

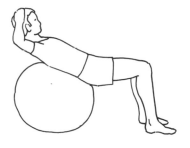

FIGURE *9.25*

STRENGTH EXERCISES

■ *Medicine Ball Core Strength Exercises*

Key points to remember when exercising with a medicine ball are: Start with a light ball (you can always switch to a heavier ball later), learn the movement pattern *before* you add speed, and add resistance only after speed has been added.

CHOP TO ANKLE, KNEE, AND WAIST. To the ankle, start with the ball held overhead and off to one side (Figure 9.26a). Chop down and across to the opposite-side ankle (Figure 9.26b). Be sure to bend, flexing at the ankle, knee, and hip. Stand up fully and reach as high as possible after each repetition. Repeat five times each side. To the knee, start with the ball overhead and off to one side, then chop down to the opposite-side knee (Figure 9.26c). Repeat ten times for each side. To the waist, start with the ball overhead and off to one side, then chop down to the opposite-side hip (Figure 9.26d). Repeat ten times for each side. Always bend at the ankles, knees, and hips when performing this exercise.

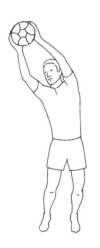

FIGURE **9.26*a***
CHOP, START

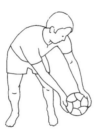

FIGURE **9.26*b***
CHOP, FINISH

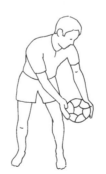

FIGURE **9.26*c***
CHOP TO KNEE

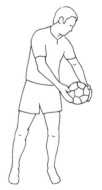

FIGURE **9.26*d***
CHOP TO WAIST

LUNGE. Start with the medicine ball held at your side (Figure 9.27a). Move the ball across the front of your body as you lunge forward in a controlled manner. The ball will end up outside the lunging leg (Figure 9.27b). Return the ball to the starting position as you return to the "ready" position. For an advanced exercise, use the same starting position. Swing the ball as if you are chopping wood. The ball will travel in an arc from over your head (Figure 9.27c) to the same finishing position (Figure 9.27d). Return the ball to the "ready" position by swinging it back. Lunges should always be done in a controlled manner. Maintain alignment between your third toe, knee, and ankle. Ensure that your leading knee stays behind your leading toes when lunging.

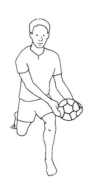 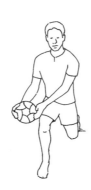 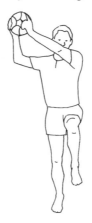 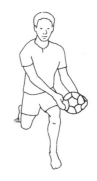

FIGURE **9.27a**
LUNGE, START

FIGURE **9.27b**
LUNGE, FINISH

FIGURE **9.27c**
ADVANCED LUNGE, START

FIGURE **9.27d**
ADVANCED LUNGE, FINISH

TWISTING "THROW." Start with the ball between your knees with your butt down, as if you are doing a squat (Figure 9.28a). As you extend upward, twist your body as if you were throwing the ball over one shoulder (Figure 9.28b). Move in a controlled manner and perform ten repetitions each side. This exercise places a dynamic load on the back, so use caution when learning it.

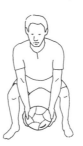 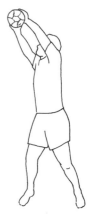

FIGURE **9.28a**
TWISTING THROW, START

FIGURE **9.28b**
TWISTING THROW, FINISH

STRENGTH EXERCISES

HIP-DRIVE EXERCISES

As with core exercises, the key for improving hip flexors is 100 percent correct technique and stable core support. Here are three levels of exercise to strengthen your hip flexors (iliopsoas). Ensure good posture and body position when doing these exercises. If all your muscle groups are stable around the hips, then you will get the most out of the exercises, recover more quickly, and achieve better stability.

For all these exercises, you will need a 2 m piece of bungee cord, or you can use stretch cords. Most gyms will have a good selection of stretch cords. Begin with a light-resistance cord and move to heavier resistance as you get stronger.

After a session of hip flexor work, it is important to loosen up with an easy jog or high-cadence (90 rpm) easy cycle and a good stretching of your hip muscles.

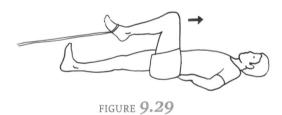

FIGURE **9.29**

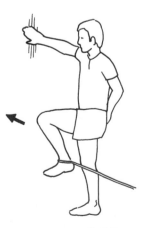

FIGURE **9.30**

BASE-LEG DRIVE. Attach the bungee cord around the bottom of a solid table leg. Lie on your back far enough out from the table so there is some resistance on the cord around your foot (Figure 9.29). Place your hands under your lower back. Bring your knee to your chest with a fast, controlled movement. Slowly lower your leg back to the floor on a 5-sec. count. On the backward movement, make sure that your back is flat and the pressure remains on your hands. You can have your non-bungee leg slightly bent to make this easier. Repeat until fatigued—fifteen to thirty repetitions—or until you lose the ability to control your lower spine.

STANDING HIP DRIVE. Stand with your right hand against the wall, and place your left hand behind your back so you can touch your right buttock muscle. Before beginning the movement, squeeze your buttocks together. Stand tall in an upright position and drive your left knee forward (Figure 9.30). Ensure that

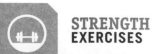

STRENGTH EXERCISES

your upper body remains stable and your right buttock muscle is tight. There should be no lateral movement. Slowly lower the leg back to the starting position. Repeat until fatigued—twenty to thirty repetitions.

DYNAMIC HIP DRIVE. Start free-standing with the bungee cord in the same position as in the standing hip drive (Figure 9.31). The purpose of this exercise is to mimic the movement pattern of uphill running. After you drive your knee forward, hold your body position at the top of the movement for a moment. This requires the constant activation of not only your hip flexors but also the buttock, calf, and abdominal muscles. Drive your knee forward using a running-style motion with your arms. Just before the top of the movement, come up onto your toes and extend your hip. This requires good stability and strength, and you will initially be unstable. Repeat until fatigued—thirty to forty repetitions.

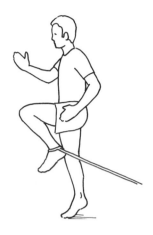

FIGURE *9.31*

FLEXIBILITY

If you want to have a long and successful career, a commitment to a structured flexibility program such as yoga is essential. The benefits include recovery, strength, and economy. One to two hours per week is the minimum amount of time required to see results. A little flexibility training each day goes a long way toward reducing injury risk and increasing economy.

If possible, try to find an instructor who is familiar with multisport or endurance athletes. Discuss what you are trying to achieve and have him or her develop a personal program for you involving a fusion of various styles. When you are tired, stick to mainly floor work. As you learn and become more flexible, begin adding more traditional poses; however, be sure that you are ready for the progression. A few exercises in isolation might not be best for most people.

For working athletes, we recommend a flexibility program rather than a full-on yoga regimen. One session a week is okay, but you should supplement with at least two solo sessions of a minimum of 20 min. These sessions should focus on employing the stretching techniques that cover the parts of your body where you hold tension. The hip flexibility routine at the end of this chapter is a good example of an effective program.

TIPS FOR YOGA
- Start slowly.
- Learn the fundamentals.
- Take your time.
- Maintain a smooth, relaxed breathing pattern.
- Focus on the seated postures first.
- Never force a pose.
- Most importantly, focus on frequency.

FLEXIBILITY EXERCISES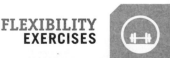

Your yoga should focus on restorative poses. Avoid strenuous poses. Standing poses can be quite tiring for many people and interfere with recovery. Do a lot of floor work, and keep it mellow.

Many athletes tend to drop yoga sessions unless they schedule them. The first thing they drop is stretching. However, experience has shown that this is a big, big mistake. Stretching has one of the largest rates of return (per hour invested) of all training activities for an athlete with pretty reasonable flexibility. An inflexible athlete would have an even greater rate of return.

■ Sample Flexibility Program for the Hips

Because most athletes store stress and tension in their hips, here's a flexibility routine that works as a progression and is best done in the order listed, completing the routine for one side of the body before working the other side. (Please note that the figures show a mix of left- and right-side stretching.) Stretch only as far as you can comfortably breathe, and remember that quality of stretch is more important than range of stretch.

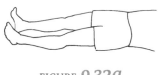

FIGURE **9.32*a***

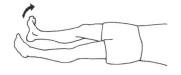

FIGURE **9.32*b***

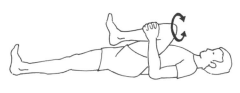

FIGURE **9.33**

1. To prepare for the sequence, lie on your back and slowly roll one leg at a time from side to side (Figures 9.32a and 9.32b). When rolling, your hips remain stable and your foot moves from 3 to 9 o'clock. Repeat eight times on both legs.

2. Bend one knee and clasp your hands together over your knee, pulling it back toward your chest (Figure 9.33). Hold and relax eight times. To reduce the intensity of the stretch, slightly bend your other leg. As your flexibility increases, your goal is to keep your nonstretching leg straight, your foot flexed upward, and your knee on the ground.

3. Still holding your knee, slowly rotate your leg in small semicircles, working in both directions and with a variety of circle sizes.

4. Place a belt or band under (or slightly behind) the ball of your foot. Keeping both legs straight, gently lift your leg toward your head. Stretch only as far as is comfortable. In most cases, your knee should remain locked, and you should have the sensa-

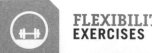

FLEXIBILITY
EXERCISES

tion that you are extending through both legs. If you are unable to achieve a 45-degree angle, then bend the leg that is against the ground—you should always keep the stretching leg fully extended (Figure 9.34).

5. Place your ankle across the opposite knee and gently push your bent leg away (Figure 9.35). Push and relax eight times.

6. Place your ankle across your knee (as above) and clasp your hands behind your thigh. Pull your knee straight back to your chest (Figure 9.36). To increase the stretch, clasp your hands on your shin just below your knee.

7. Place a belt or band around your foot, bend your leg, and pull your knee down toward the ground. Your lower leg should remain perpendicular to the ground (Figure 9.37). To increase the stretch, grab your foot with your hand.

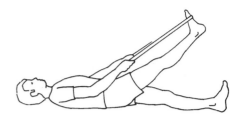

FIGURE **9.34**

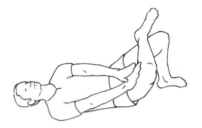

FIGURE **9.35**

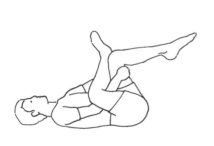

FIGURE **9.36**

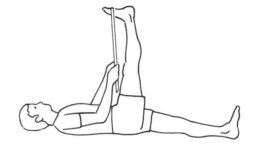

FIGURE **9.37**

8. Draw your leg up toward your chest, supporting your knee with the arm on the same side, and use your opposite arm to guide your leg across your body line (Figure 9.38). Then draw your knee up and slightly across your body line. The opposite leg will remain outstretched and still. You can increase your range of motion in this stretch by making semicircles with the knee, moving your working leg back and forth across your body.

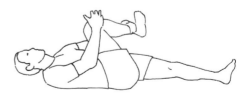

FIGURE **9.38**

FLEXIBILITY EXERCISES

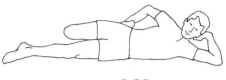

FIGURE *9.39*

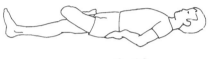

FIGURE *9.40*

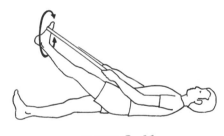

FIGURE *9.41*

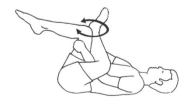

FIGURE *9.42*

9. Lie on your side with your bottom arm extended to support your head. Your pelvis should be forward, and one knee should be on top of the other. Clasp your top ankle with your hand and bend your knee, pressing your heel toward your buttocks (Figure 9.39). Be careful not to overextend your knee. Stop if you feel any pain.

10. On your back in a half-lotus position, lift and press down your bent knee (Figure 9.40). When you are lifting your bent knee, use your lower abdominal muscles to press the small of your back against the ground. You will find that the movement assists with the opening of this stretch. You are likely to need a belt to support the ankle of your bent leg. Complete fifteen to thirty cycles.

11. On your back, place a belt or band under the ball of your foot and repeat the straight-leg hamstring stretch. This time, slowly make circles with your straightened leg, alternating small to big to small in both directions (Figure 9.41).

12. Cross your ankle over your knee again. This time make circles (Figure 9.42) with your knee (instead of drawing it straight back). This stretch should give you feedback as to whether you have been successful in opening your hips a little more.

Be patient with your body. Most athletes find that it takes six to eight weeks before they notice a material range-of-movement improvement. The routine outlined here, if done three times per week as part of a program, will enable you to achieve a better aero position in twelve to sixteen weeks.

CONCLUSION

Apart from the benefits to endurance athletics, we believe that everyone benefits from lifelong strength training. The information contained in this chapter is our best advice for how you can incorporate strength work into an active, healthy life.

FLEXIBILITY EXERCISES

CHAPTER 10

NUTRITION:
THE FOURTH DISCIPLINE

Nutrition can be the toughest part of the performance equation. It requires a total dedication
to eating only the best foods at the right times. You
need to learn the right balance based on your genetics, body size, and training load.

*Human successes, like human failures, are
composed of one action at a time and
achieved by one person at a time.*
—PATTY H. SAMPSON

There is no magical formula for identifying your optimal diet. This chapter will give you the
guidelines for good nutrition as you train, but you must discover what mix of foods works best
for you. If you have never experimented with your preferred mix, don't assume you have found it
already. You may be surprised at what happens when changes are made at the training table. Once
you find a nutrition strategy that gives you plenty of energy and leaves your weight stable, you are
there. At that stage, you can slightly trim your energy intake for a slow, safe weight loss. If you cut
your caloric intake too drastically, you will compromise your recovery and your immune-system
function. A diet that is light on calories, particularly protein, can cause you to lose valuable lean
muscle mass. The ideal weight-loss formula will vary from athlete to athlete.

THE OPTIMAL DIET FOR AN ATHLETE

Based on our personal experience, our research, and the experience of the athletes that we
coach, the optimal diet for endurance training incorporates the principles contained in *The*

Paleo Diet for Athletes by Loren Cordain, PhD, and Joe Friel. The concepts of the paleo diet are quite simple:

- Eat lots of fruits and vegetables.
- Eat lean protein with every meal.
- Eat high-glycemic-index carbohydrates during and after training for recovery.
- Avoid eating foods that contain saturated and hydrogenated fats.
- Eat moderate amounts of good fats.

If you are like most people, transitioning to the paleo diet entails eating more fruits and veggies and knocking cheese, butter, cream, and fast food out of your diet. It is also important to cut out starchy foods. Traditional Western diets can cause people to become "starch addicted." If this is the case, you will experience a withdrawal period (from the blood-sugar spikes that typify a high-starch, high-sugar diet). The length of the transition period varies, but normally it will last two to four weeks.

You will need to adjust your diet with increased training or intensity. Otherwise, the paleo diet seems less relevant given the nature of long-course training. Long, intense training sessions will require you to eat more and eat often. For example, elite athletes training twenty-five to thirty hours per week and doing multiple sessions every day can find that they need to eat constantly. Typical age-group athletes will find that higher-glycemic-index carbohydrates are required after their longest sessions but not so much after short, intense sessions. If your recovery starts to suffer or energy levels dip, then you might not be refueling quickly enough. It is essential to eat high-GI carbohydrates (with protein) immediately after every training session or race lasting 90–180 min. or longer. More experienced athletes will have greater fat-burning

Glycemic Index

The glycemic index (GI) ranks carbohydrate-containing foods according to their immediate effect on blood-sugar levels. High-GI foods elicit a fast blood-glucose response, and low-GI foods elicit a slow, sustained response. Therefore, you will want to consume low-GI foods before training and competition and throughout most of your day. Medium- and high-GI foods will help speed recovery during and after your training. Total carbohydrate intake, combined with a high GI, is the most important factor in speeding recovery.

ability and therefore less need to use high-GI carbohydrates. Table 10.1 identifies the GI of common foods to help you make better choices for improved performance and recovery.

Intense training has been shown to depress the immune system. This is why so many athletes find themselves sick in the ten to fourteen days after their toughest training periods. To avoid placing undue stress on your body, you need to master both the timing and type of carbohydrate you eat. With smart timing of carbohydrates, you can maintain a stable blood-sugar level, which has proven to reduce stress on the immune system. Many athletes make the mistake of depending on highly processed carbohydrates following intense training (for example, bars). This practice increases the stress on the body because such foods lack the nutrients essential for recovery.

TABLE 10.1 GLYCEMIC INDEX (GI) OF SELECTED FOODS

LOW GI (<50)		MEDIUM GI (50–79)		HIGH GI (≥80)	
Grain-based foods					
27	Rice bran	51	Vermicelli	80	Muesli
38	Pasta, spaghetti, protein enriched	58	Rice, parboiled	81	Wild rice, Saskatchewan
45	Barley (pearl)	60	All-bran cereal	82	Semolina bread
45	Spaghetti, white, boiled 5 min.	61	Spaghetti, brown, boiled 15 min.	87	Oatmeal
46	Fettuccine	63	Wheat kernels	89	Rye bread, whole-meal
48	Rye	65	Bulgur	93	Couscous
		68	Rye or pumpernickel bread	95	Rye crispbread
		68	Oat-bran bread	95	Barley-flour bread
		69	Multigrain bread	95	Gnocchi
		74	Buckwheat	96	Muesli
		75	Bulgur bread	100	Whole-meal wheat bread
		79	Brown rice	103	Millet
Dairy products/substitutes					
43	Soy milk	52	Yogurt		
46	Skim milk				
Simple sugars					
31	Fructose	65	Lactose	92	Sucrose
				138	Glucose
				152	Maltose

continued >

TABLE 10.1 CONTINUED

LOW GI (<50)		MEDIUM GI (50–79)		HIGH GI (≥80)	
Vegetables					
12	Bengal gram dal	50	Green peas, dried	80	Potato, new, boiled
20	Soybeans	50	Lima beans	80	Sweet corn
32	Dried peas	54	Brown beans	88	Beet
37	Red lentils	55	Pinto beans	99	Rutabaga
43	Black beans	57	Haricot (navy) beans	100	Potato, mashed
45	Kidney beans, dried	59	Black-eyed beans	107	Pumpkin
46	Black-eyed peas	60	Baked beans (canned)	108	Broad beans (fava)
46	Butter beans	65	Green peas, frozen	117	Cooked carrots
46	Baby lima beans	65	Romano beans	118	Potato, instant
47	Rye kernels	68	Green peas	128	Potato, russet, baked
49	Chickpeas (garbanzo beans)	70	Potato, sweet	139	Cooked parsnips
		74	Yam		
		74	Kidney beans (canned)		
Fruits					
10	Nopal (prickly pear)	53	Apple	80	Mango
32	Cherries	55	Plum	84	Banana
34	Plum	58	Pear	91	Raisins
36	Grapefruit	59	Apple juice	91	Apricots, canned
40	Peach	60	Fresh peach	93	Cantaloupe
44	Apricot	63	Orange	94	Pineapple
49	Strawberries	63	Pears, canned	103	Watermelon
		66	Pineapple juice		
		66	Grapes		
		69	Grapefruit juice		
		74	Orange juice		
		74	Peaches, canned		
		75	Kiwi		
		79	Fruit cocktail		

If you frequently get sick after hard BT workouts, you should look at increasing your carbohydrate intake for the three to seventy-two hours after exercise. However, be careful that this increase does not cut into your protein intake. Low protein contributes to frequent illness, loss of muscle mass, and lethargy.

Many athletes who eat a high-fiber diet can find it difficult to get enough calories, as the fiber and grains leave them feeling full. This is a good point for people who are chronically skinny to consider; a huge fruit intake could be counterproductive for an athlete who has trouble maintaining lean body mass.

The optimal diet for peak performance varies based on the athlete.

REALIZING YOUR IDEAL BODY COMPOSITION

Before you begin training, you need to evaluate your body composition. Given the fact that you are training for an Ironman-distance triathlon, the chances are good that you have a relatively healthy body composition because of your dedication to fitness. Still, many of us who work out regularly and eat healthy may still carry some extra weight. Would you race stronger and minimize the strain on your body if you weighed 10 pounds less? Do you struggle to maintain your weight when training intensities and durations pick up? Are you frequently battling illness or injury?

The following five steps will help you reach your ideal body composition. Even if you are satisfied with your current body composition, you can use these tips to help reinforce your healthy lifestyle. You will notice that we are not giving you a means of calculating your daily intake of calories, protein, carbohydrates, or fat. It is more important that you have the information you need to make smarter choices, ultimately changing poor eating habits and focusing on the nutritional quality of your diet.

> **A WORD OF CAUTION:** Make changes gradually, and allow at least three weeks for your body to adapt to a new diet before passing judgment on how you feel and your performance in training. It usually takes two weeks of adaptation before seeing any results. During the adaptation period, you may feel strange and train poorly. For this reason, changes in diet are best done early in the season—not in the last few weeks before an important race.
>
> Age is another concern in making dietary changes. As you age, changes may occur in body chemistry that require further shifts in diet. Recent research has shown that aging athletes need a considerable amount of vegetables and fruits in their diets to maintain calcium and nitrogen balances.

■ *Step 1: Understand Your Food Choices*

It is important to understand your motivation in making the food choices that you do. You may identify with some of the points below as they describe your relationship with food.

Food as signal. Thinking back over the years, the times when you made the poor food selections may have been the times when you were under the greatest levels of stress. Stress can come from a variety of sources: training, relationships, children, work, finances, a partner's alignment with your life goals, and others. When these sources of stress are reduced, your food choices will improve. Poor eating habits may merely be a symptom of bigger issues in your life that need to be addressed.

Food as nourishment. There may be times when you feel a sense of guilt at meals. It is almost as if food has become an enemy that is preventing you from achieving your ideal self. This feeling is dangerous because it sets up a negative cycle. Food is essential for your survival, period. When you view food as a source of strength, it is far easier to establish a virtuous cycle in which your nutritional choices move you toward your ideal self. By acknowledging a flawed view of food, it will become easier to see food for what it really is: a source of energy and pleasure.

Food as self. There may be periods in your life when you believe that you are a "good" person when you eat well and a "bad" person when you make poor food choices. In order to establish a healthy relationship with food, you should avoid defining yourself by your food choices. Once a choice has been made, it is in the past. All you can do is focus on the next opportunity and realize that you are the same person regardless of your food choices. This point is important, particularly in conjunction with an understanding of why we are drawn to certain types of food. For example, have you ever wondered why we like fatty or sugary foods? It's because they taste good and make us feel good (at least they create that illusion). It's not because we're losers!

Every athlete faces stress in his or her work, personal, and family life. The first step toward effective nutrition is taking full responsibility for your own food choices. Only you have total control over what you eat—it isn't determined by your coworkers, your family, or your personal background.

With a few medical exceptions, the way you look today is dictated by a huge number of tiny decisions that you make on a daily basis. What you will look like six months from now is based on the decisions you start making now. In order to change, we need to take responsibility for ourselves. This is a classic conflict between short-term pleasure and long-term gain. When you see an elite athlete, you are looking at the result of tens of thousands of little decisions that he or she has made over many years.

Before getting into a discussion of useful techniques, you should ask yourself how much you are willing to commit and how important improvement is to you. There are no shortcuts, and good nutrition is a lifestyle decision. As in any endeavor, the results are dictated by your commitment and dedication.

■ Step 2: Know What You Eat

You can get started by keeping a food log for an entire week. Record what you are eating, not how much, and make an honest assessment of your current eating habits. Make sure you include everything you eat, not just the major meals. This will help you become aware of mindless eating—the occasional handful of candy at the office or the bowl of cereal after dinner. Remember, you're not judging yourself, but you need to know your nutrition patterns.

When you are keeping your log, be honest. Anyone can "eat right" for seven days. There is no point in fooling yourself, your coach, or your nutritionist. In order to make changes, you need to have a realistic assessment of where you are.

Armed with the log, you are now in a great position to analyze your diet objectively.

■ Step 3: Recognize Energy-Dense Foods

Energy-dense foods are those that are high in calories relative to their size or volume. Some examples are cheese, whole milk, butter, french fries, burgers, sweets, energy bars, and soft drinks. These types of foods can put a lot of calories in you at times when you don't need them.

There is a time and a place for many energy-dense foods. However, when you are trying to shed fat, you need to know what you are eating. In general, athletes who are seeking to improve their body composition should limit their intake of energy-dense foods and increase their intake of nutrient-dense foods, such as fruits, vegetables, fish, poultry, and lean cuts of other meat. Highlight the energy-dense foods in your log.

■ Step 4: Choose Nutrient-Dense Foods

The next step is to swap half of your energy-dense choices for nutrient-dense choices. Why only half? We have limited willpower, and we should apply it sparingly. We are trying to change habits that have been formed over years—and, quite often, generations. This is powerful programming that needs to be adjusted. Although quitting "cold turkey" works for some people, more often they return to their old eating habits after shedding pounds.

Your ultimate goal is to develop a healthy, long-term lifestyle that will bring out your ideal self. Make this long-term change in a manner that maintains your quality of life.

It sounds so easy—write a log, swap half your food, and presto, you'll be transformed into your perfect self. Seems hard to believe. But what we are talking about is a long-term transformation. It could take up to six months before you notice a major transformation (although your friends will notice before that). Our bodies change very slowly, and you will need to have patience. However, if you make the changes, the results will come. There are many success stories from athletes who have followed this advice.

■ *Step 5: Embrace Long-Term Change*

The following steps will help make your new regimen a lasting change.

Housecleaning. Clean out all the foods that are inconsistent with achieving your ideal self. It is much easier to make excellent food choices when they are all around you. Keep plenty of fresh fruit in your office, home, car, and training sites. This makes it a lot easier for you to stick with your plan.

Treats. Think about some of your favorite foods. During or after your long sessions, treat yourself to moderate amounts of these foods. Focus on eating them slowly and consuming nutrient-dense foods with them (this helps moderate intake).

Acceptance. Constantly remind yourself that your goal is to bring out your ideal self. Visualize the person within that you are helping to strengthen and bring forward. This philosophy is useful for making positive choices in all aspects of your life. It changes your mindset from "denying yourself a candy bar" to "feeding your ideal self a peach."

Serving. Serve your meals in the kitchen rather than having large plates of food on the table. Like many people, you are likely to continue to eat well past being hungry if there is food in front of you. When trying to improve your body composition, try the following suggestions:

- Use smaller plates and bowls.
- Eat as much as you want, but wait 5 to 10 min. between servings.
- Make a conscious decision to eat slightly more slowly than usual.
- Increase your intake of foods that are high in fiber but relatively low in calories.

Patterns and habits. Each of us has our own particular patterns and habits that either result in poor food selections or lead us toward poor choices. Pay attention to when and why you are engaging in self-sabotage. Show yourself some compassion, and see if you can understand the motivation behind the feelings or situations that lead you down familiar paths.

Perhaps you have a habit of going out for pizza and beer a few times each week. By changing that pattern to stir-fry at your place, you might be able to achieve better food choices and see your friends at the same time. Sometimes a simple change is all it takes.

Scales. Weighing is counterproductive for many athletes trying to improve their body composition. Why is that? Scales encourage a short-term focus, whereas nutrition is a long-term strategy. Tracking your daily weight will show artificial highs and lows (quite often based on nothing more than your hydration levels). Wake up 2 pounds lighter, and you are happy all day. Find out that you are up 3 pounds, and the world had better watch out!

Scales give inaccurate feedback. What we weigh says very little about our ability as an athlete (or our worth as a person, for that matter). Although there are a number of sports in which it is beneficial to have a high power-to-weight ratio, many athletes lose power faster than they lose weight.

Athletes who focus excessively on weight tend to underhydrate and skimp on recovery nutrition because they want to "save" the weight they just lost. In reality, fat has been burned, and food and water are necessary to replenish glycogen, rebuild muscles, and restore hydration levels—all essential in order to be able to train and burn more fat. Proper nutrition is an essential part of this virtuous circle.

Finally, and most important of all, it's not about how much you weigh. It is about how you look, how you feel, how you recover, and how you perform. A scale tells you nothing about these things (although your mind might trick you into thinking it does!).

Spend some time considering your relationship with your scale. Is it affirming your ideal self or helping the part of your mind that beats you up? You may be better off pitching it into your housecleaning box.

Go natural. Probably the easiest thing to remember is to maximize your intake of fresh fruits, fresh vegetables, fish, poultry, and lean cuts of other meat. Focus on achieving a balanced, natural diet, and you are well on your way to good health.

Cooking. Many athletes have limited time in their lives, and finding time to cook can be difficult. We all have the same amount of time. The only difference is how we use it. In order to save time, make extra quantities when you cook "healthy." That way you have leftovers for the days when you are busy.

Fat. Very low-fat diets involve a lot of stress on your system, as there is a high degree of "background hunger" associated with avoiding fats. A more moderate approach to fats works best. Include small amounts of "good" fat in your diet. Sources of good fat include olive oil, canola oil, raw nuts and seeds, and avocados in small amounts as well as substantial amounts of organic, free-range, lean meat and coldwater fish (see "Sources of Good Fat" sidebar).

Starches. When choosing rice, pasta, breads, and other foods with a large amount of starch, look for foods that have been subject to minimal processing. Avoid boxed cereals, white breads, white pasta, and white rice in

SOURCES OF GOOD FAT
- Albacore tuna
- Almonds
- Avocados
- Cashews
- Cod-liver oil
- Flax meal
- Flaxseed oil
- Macadamia nuts
- Mackerel
- Olive oil
- Olives
- Pecans
- Salmon
- Sardines
- Trout
- Walnuts

favor of whole-grain breads, unsweetened grain-based cereals, whole-wheat pasta, and other whole grains. Limit your consumption of starchy foods to after training, and combine them with nutrient-dense foods.

Fuel for performance. Given our habits and conditioning, we often misinterpret appropriate hunger for cravings. When you start giving yourself balanced nutrition, you will discover that you feel better and many of your cravings disappear. They will still appear from time to time, but you can better deal with them through the other strategies given earlier in this chapter.

When you put these tips into action, you will realize that you don't need all the poor food choices that you thought would make you happy. By caring for your ideal self, you will find that it will become increasingly easy to make choices that support your long-term goals.

You can do it! Achieving your body composition goals is the result of a conscious decision to start a journey toward your ideal self. Make a decision today, and take it hour by hour. There will be hurdles to overcome, but the rewards are worth the dedication required. Always remember that you get a fresh start every morning and can take it one meal at a time.

Show compassion to yourself, make gradual changes, and build the habits that strengthen your ideal self. Soon you will see that it's been there all the time.

Tips for Changing Your Diet

- Make small and gradual changes—this is the only way to ensure long-term success.
- Try to reduce saturated and partially hydrogenated (trans) fats—cheese, crackers, snack foods, etc.
- Ensure that you get enough protein. Tuna and other fish are good sources, as are meats from free-range cattle and poultry. It is important, particularly for female athletes, to eat protein with every meal.
- Don't watch your calories, but do watch your "bad" fats (saturated and hydrogenated). Also be aware of your omega-6 polyunsaturated intake (mostly vegetable oils and snack foods) because these fats, though beneficial in some ways, may increase your risk of inflammation. If you eat plenty of fruits, veggies, lean protein, and "good" fats such as monounsaturated and omega-3 polyunsaturated (olive, flaxseed, and canola oils; nut butters; and fish oils), you will be fine.
- Eat more fruits and veggies. Whole fruits are superior to juices because the fiber keeps them lower on the GI scale.

EATING TO PREVENT MUSCLE LOSS

Popeye was right: Eating spinach can make you stronger and more muscular, especially if you're over 50 years of age. This is because as we grow older, we lose muscle mass. Although this loss is slowed somewhat by weight lifting and vigorous aerobic exercise, it still happens. Athletes in their 60s typically demonstrate considerably less muscle than they had in their 40s.

Now research by T. Remer and F. Manz has shown why. Nitrogen, which is an essential component of muscle protein, is given up by the body at a faster rate than it can be taken in as we get older. This effect is due to a gradual change in kidney function that comes with aging, producing an acidic state in the blood. Essentially, we are peeing off our muscles as we pass the half-century mark in life.

With a net loss of nitrogen, new muscle cannot be formed. This acidic state of the blood also explains why calcium is lost with aging, resulting in osteoporosis for many, especially women, with advanced age.

The key to reducing, or even avoiding, this situation is to lower the blood's acid level by increasing its alkalinity. There are studies demonstrating that taking a supplement of potassium bicarbonate increases the blood's alkaline level by balancing nitrogen in the body. However, potassium bicarbonate is not currently available as an over-the-counter supplement, and there are no long-term studies of its effects on health. There is some evidence that it contributes to irregular electrocardiogram readings.

The natural way of achieving the same result is eating foods that increase the blood's alkalinity—fruits and vegetables. Fats and oils have a neutral effect on blood acid. All other foods, including grains, meats, nuts, beans, dairy, fish, and eggs, increase the blood's acidity. If your diet is high in these foods but low in fruits and vegetables, you can expect to lose muscle mass and bone calcium as you age.

Remer and Manz's study ranks foods in terms of their effect on blood acidity and alkalinity. For example, the food that has the most acidic effect, therefore contributing to a loss of nitrogen and ultimately muscle, is parmesan cheese. The food that has the greatest alkaline effect, thus reducing nitrogen and muscle loss, is raisins. Among vegetables, spinach is the most alkaline food. So, you see? Popeye was right.

Table 10.2 ranks common foods by their effect on alkalinity and acidity as demonstrated by Remer and Manz's study (which has since been confirmed by several follow-up studies). The higher a food's positive acidic ranking, the more likely it is to contribute to a loss of muscle

TABLE 10.2 **ACIDIC VERSUS ALKALINE FOODS**	
ACID FOODS (+)	
Grains	
Brown rice	+12.5
Rolled oats	+10.7
Whole-wheat bread	+8.2
Spaghetti	+7.3
Corn flakes	+6.0
White rice	+4.6
Dairy	
Parmesan cheese	+34.2
Processed cheese	+28.7
Hard cheese	+19.2
Cottage cheese	+8.7
Whole milk	+0.7
Legumes	
Peanuts	+8.3
Meats, fish, eggs	
Trout	+10.8
Turkey	+9.9
Chicken	+8.7
Eggs	+8.1
Beef	+7.8
ALKALINE FOODS (–)	
Fruits	
Raisins	–21.0
Black currants	–6.5
Bananas	–5.5
Apricots	–4.8
Vegetables	
Spinach	–14.0
Celery	–5.2
Carrots	–4.9
Lettuce	–2.5

mass and bone-mineral levels. The more negative the food's alkaline ranking, the more beneficial the effect on these measures.

PERIODIZATION

An optimal diet to enhance training, racing, and recovery involves not only eating moderate amounts of the macronutrients —including carbohydrates, protein, fat, and water—but also varying the mix of these foods throughout the year. In other words, diet should cycle just as training cycles within a periodization plan. Protein serves as the anchor for the diet and stays relatively constant throughout the year as fat and carbohydrates rise and fall.

In our experience, it all comes down to three key choices you can make for better health and performance.

- Eliminate processed foods from your diet.
- Obtain the majority of your energy needs from whole fruits, fresh vegetables, and lean protein.
- Limit your use of starchy and sugary foods to during and after your longest or most intense sessions.

These nutritional guidelines will have a significant impact on your body composition and give you a good nutritional foundation for your triathlon training.

If the "Key Three" are applied against perhaps 80 percent of everything you eat, while including good fats, then you will not have to be concerned with ratios or counting calories. You'll also recover better and race faster.

In the Base period, when training volume is relatively high and intensity is low, eating a diet rich in "good" fats is beneficial to improving your ability to burn fat for fuel while conserving glycogen stores—a physiological goal of training at this time of the season. Such fats include monounsaturated oils with some polyunsaturated oils. Avoid saturated and partially hydrogenated fats.

Simply emphasizing these foods, along with plenty of lean protein, fruits, and vegetables, puts you on the right track for this time of year.

Good snacks in the Base period, and year-round, are nuts and seeds. If you find that you need additional energy, then dried fruit may be mixed with the nuts in the Build period to boost your carbohydrate intake. Go light on snack foods and remember the "Key Three."

In the Build period, when the intensity of training increases as you prepare for the first A-priority race of the season, the fat-carbohydrate balance should shift toward carbohydrate. But be careful—this doesn't mean you should pig out on starch and sugar. Treat these (highly processed carbs such as bread, packaged cold cereals, sports bars, and "fat-free" snack foods) strictly as recovery foods because they are nutrient-poor. As discussed in the next section, they may be eaten in considerable quantities immediately after a hard or long workout to restore glycogen levels but should otherwise be avoided. Consider them as "junk" food, along with sports nutrition products. Get your carbohydrates primarily from fruits and nonstarchy vegetables. The density of vitamin and mineral micronutrients in these foods far exceeds that of the starches and simple sugars. You'll recover faster, control weight, and be healthier.

Throughout the season, keep your intake of lean protein high by including such foods in every meal. The best sources of such foods are free-range cattle, chicken, turkey, and eggs. Try to avoid products from animals that are feedlot-raised. Their body compositions are not suitable for good health—either theirs or ours.

NUTRITION FOR TRAINING AND RECOVERY

Food is important to aid and speed your recovery. It is very important to immediately reload the carbohydrates lost during long or intense workouts. Carbohydrates are necessary to replace spent glycogen, a primary fuel source in exercise. Protein is needed to rebuild muscle and other protein-based tissues. Fat, especially monounsaturated, maintains the immune system and other vital physiological systems. Also important are the micronutrients, such as vitamins and minerals, found in high-quality foods. You should eat a wide variety of foods in a condition as close to their natural state as possible while minimizing sugar and highly processed products. Appropriate amounts of water are required to prevent recovery-delaying dehydration. If any of these factors are neglected, the time to full recovery is pushed back several hours or even days.

When training for long-course triathlon, the greatest challenge is recovery. Long workouts done twice a day can push the body to its limits. To achieve the level of fitness you're seeking, consider recovery to be at least as important as workouts. Exercise and recovery are the yin and yang of training. Without a balanced approach you'll be going through the motions, but you really won't be "training."

The starting point is to accept that your workouts are the central events of each day and that the types of foods you eat are determined by when those workouts take place (see Table 10.3). For serious athletes, that's a fairly easy notion because they generally have a "training is life; everything else is just the details" way of seeing the world.

Each workout has feeding times linked with it called "stages." Here's how it works.

■ *Stage 1: Before the Workout*

The goal of this stage is to have adequate carbohydrate stored in order to get you through the workout. This is especially important for early-morning workouts. Eating 200 to 400 calories primarily from a moderate-GI, carbohydrate-rich food two hours before the workout would be perfect, but that often isn't possible. Few are willing to get up at 3 a.m. just to eat before a 5 a.m. masters swim session. In this case, take a bottle of your favorite sports drink or a couple of gel packets with 12 ounces of water to the workout. Ten minutes before the warm-up begins, start taking in your "breakfast." It isn't quite as good as eating a real breakfast two hours before, but it's far better than training on a low fuel tank.

■ *Stage 2: During the Workout*

Now you need to take in carbohydrate, mostly in the form of liquids from a high-GI source. The best choice is your favorite sports drink. You could also use gels chased immediately with lots of water. The longer the workout, the more important carbohydrate is. For a workout lasting an hour or less, water is all you need, assuming you filled the tank in Stage 1. As the workout gets longer, the amount of carbohydrate you take in per hour also increases. This could be as little as 120 calories or as much as 500 calories per hour, depending not only on workout length but also on body size, workout intensity, and your experience. It's a good idea for the liquid fuel source to include sodium. The research is less than overwhelming on other ingredients, including potassium, magnesium, and protein. Include them if you want to.

TABLE 10.3 TIMING YOUR NUTRITION

WHEN	GOALS	WHAT TO EAT	HOW MUCH TO EAT	NOTES
Before workout	Replenish carbohydrate stores to fuel workout.	Moderate-GI, carbohydrate-rich foods	200–400 calories 2 hours before workout or 100–200 calories up to 10 min. before workout	Before early-morning sessions, a bottle of sports beverage can suffice.
During workout	Keep body fueled for duration of the workout.	High-GI foods, mostly in liquid form. For longer workouts, include sodium or more solid sports nutrition products.	120–500 calories per hour, depending on workout length and intensity and personal needs	This stage can be skipped for workouts lasting less than 1 hour.
Immediately following workout	Replace the carbohydrates burned.	Carbohydrate-rich foods with some protein	3–4 calories per pound of body weight	This is the period when your body is best able to take in and store carbohydrates.
Following workout (for as long as the workout lasted)	Continue to replenish carbohydrate stores for recovery; focus on nutrition.	Medium- and high-GI carbohydrates with some protein	Eat until satisfied. After long workouts, you will probably want to eat a meal in this phase.	This is a good time to eat starches.
Between workouts	Focus on long-term nutrition.	Return to the "Key Three" food guidelines. Eat low-GI carbohydrates, lean proteins, and natural foods high in nutrients.	Varies with individual needs	If you are doing multiple workouts per day, you may not reach Stage 5 until after your last workout

■ *Stage 3: Immediately After the Workout*

This and the next stage are the key times in the day for taking in carbohydrate. When athletes say that eating in stages doesn't work for them, it is invariably due to not taking in enough fuel in Stages 3 and 4.

Your purpose now is to replace the carbohydrate you used up during the workout. In the first 30 min. or so after a workout, your body is several hundred times more sensitive to carbohydrate than at any other time of the day. The longer you wait to refuel, the less likely you are to completely refill the gas tank. Take in 3 to 4 calories per pound of body weight, mostly from carbohydrate, in this stage.

You can buy a commercial product, though they tend to be pricey. Or you can make your own by blending about 16 ounces of fruit juice with a banana; 3 to 5 tablespoons of glucose (such as Carbo-Pro), depending on body size; 2 to 3 tablespoons of protein powder, especially from egg or whey sources; and 2 or 3 pinches of salt. Drinking this in the 30-min. window is critical for recovery. It should be your highest priority after a hard workout. If the workout lasted less than an hour and was low-intensity, omit this stage.

■ *Stage 4: As Long as the Workout Lasted*

For the next several minutes, or as long as the preceding workout lasted, continue to focus your diet on carbohydrate, especially from moderate- to high-GI sources, along with some protein. You'll be ready to eat a meal at some time in Stage 4 if the workout was long. Now is the time to eat starches such as pasta, bread, bagels, rice, corn, and other foods rich in glucose to maintain the recovery process. Ideal foods to eat at this time are potatoes, sweet potatoes, bananas, and raisins. Eat until satisfied.

■ *Stage 5: Until the Next Workout*

Now you're at work, back in class, spending time with the family, doing yard work, or whatever it is you do when not training or racing on a given day of the week. Although this part of your day may look ordinary to the rest of the world, it really isn't. You're still focused on nutrition for long-term recovery.

This is the time when many athletes get sloppy with their diets. The most common mistake is continuing to eat a diet that is low in nutrient value and high in starch and sugar, as was common in Stages 3 and 4. Such foods are relatively poor in vitamins and minerals. Again, the most nutrient-dense foods are vegetables, fruits, and lean protein from animal sources, especially seafood. Snack on nuts, seeds, and berries. All of these foods are rich in vitamins, minerals, and other trace elements necessary for health, growth, and recovery.

Avoid foods that come in packages, including those with labels that say "healthy." They aren't. If your great-great-grandmother couldn't have eaten it, then it is best avoided. That includes foods invented by sports nutrition scientists. Just eat *real* food in Stage 5.

If you are doing two or three workouts in a day, you may not get to Stage 5 until late in the day, and Stage 4 may replace Stage 1 with closely spaced workouts.

SPORTS NUTRITION PRODUCTS

In the past four decades there has been a revolution in sports nutrition supplements. It started in the 1970s with a sports drink developed at the University of Florida—Gatorade. There are now more products on the market than can be sampled in a four-hour workout.

The field has expanded well beyond just drinks consumed during exercise. Now there are carbohydrate-loading drinks, recovery drinks, sports bars, energy gels, and more. To help clear the confusion, here is a quick primer in sports nutrition products.

■ *Sports Drinks*

There is no shortage of sports drinks on the market. Every year new ones with slightly different recipes enter the fray. What all these drinks have in common are carbohydrate content and the inclusion of sodium. Both have been found to speed fluid's movement from the stomach into the small intestine, where it can be absorbed.

Sports drinks should be used during exercise lasting an hour or more. Generally, an athlete should take in 16 to 32 ounces (480 to 960 milliliters [ml]) per hour, depending on race duration, body size, known rate of fluid loss, and heat. A few big gulps every hour have been shown to work better than frequent small sips. Cool liquids are also more effective than warm drinks.

Carbohydrate-loading and meal-replacement drinks appeared in the early 1980s as carbohydrate loading came into general practice before long events such as marathons, and companies began marketing drinks that would help loading with less bulk than solid foods such as pasta. Such products are sometimes used on the last day before an event lasting 90 min. or more. They help the body store more carbohydrates, thus pushing fatigue farther away from the start line. They are typically easy for the nervous athlete to digest. Besides carbohydrates, they usually contain some fat and protein to mimic a meal. Some athletes have started using them during events lasting longer than four hours, such as Ironman triathlons, since it's difficult to get in enough calories otherwise. Care must be taken in doing this because loading drinks containing more than 3 grams of fat per serving could delay absorption and lead to dehydration. High protein concentrations can also lead to slow digestion and a foamy sensation in the gut during an Ironman-distance race. What you primarily need during a race is carbohydrate. Be cautious of any other additives.

■ Recovery Drinks

There is a lot of crossover between loading and recovery drinks. The common element of products intended to speed recovery following long or intense exercise is protein along with carbohydrate.

A small amount of the fuel used during exhausting exercise comes from protein. While small, it is not insignificant. If it is not replaced soon afterward, there may be a loss of muscle mass and a delay in recovery. These drinks should be used immediately following exercise in Stage 3 recovery for best results.

■ Sports Bars

In the mid-1980s, PowerBar launched a new category into the sports nutrition market—sports bars. Although they look much like a candy bar, the primary ingredient is usually carbohydrate, and all contain some fat and protein. Most have fewer than 3 grams of fat, although some have twice that amount.

Bars may be used in low-intensity exercise lasting longer than about 90 min.—three to four hours or longer is probably more appropriate. The major limiter for these products is their absorption rate. You must drink 8 to 16 ounces of fluid with every bar eaten, yet it still may take 30 min. or more for the fuel to get to your working muscles. In an Ironman-distance race, bars should be viewed as an occasional break from all the liquid sources of fuel, not as the primary fuel source.

■ Gels

In the early 1990s, energy gels appeared on the market. These are gooey liquids that come in ketchup-sized pouches to be torn open so the contents can be sucked out. Their main attraction is the convenience of a small package with a high-energy yield—about 100 calories per packet. Essentially what you are doing when using a gel is mixing a sports drink in your stomach rather than in a bottle.

During exercise lasting an hour or more, take one every 30 min., drinking 8 to 10 ounces (240 to 300 ml) of fluid with each. During four-hour or longer events, consume a packet every 15 min., especially later in the contest.

Drink enough water when using sports bars and gels. If you don't, your gut will pull fluid from the blood to help in the digestive process, which causes dehydration.

■ *Chewable Gels*

A relatively new entry in the category of sports nutrition, chewable gels are like the gummy-bear candies that kids, and some adult athletes, snack on. They are basically gels with most of the fluid removed, leaving small chunks of what is mostly carbohydrate. Just as with gels, you must make sure to take in plenty of fluid when using these. Like bars, they should be viewed as something you use during a race as a break from sports drinks and not as a primary source of fuel. Compared with sports drinks, they are slow to digest and can cause stomach problems in a race.

SUPPLEMENTS

Supplements should be supplemental to an overall nutritional program that is consistent with the advice provided in this chapter. It is not possible to overcome weak nutritional choices with powders and potions. Supplements are, however, effective in compensating for a deficiency that has been identified in partnership with your medical adviser. What follows are our thoughts on the most popular supplements being used today.

The nutritional supplement market is virtually unregulated, so athletes should be aware that taking supplements carries a risk of cross-contamination from banned and prohibited substances. For this reason, many athletes subject to drug testing have decided to move away from all forms of nutritional supplementation. The most difficult aspect of assessing the value of any nutritional supplement, dietary strategy, recovery technique, or training tool is that we have so much going on in our lives that it is tough to single out one aspect.

Quite often many of us are looking for a magic pill, session, or piece of equipment that will offer breakthrough success. Athletes should be very skeptical of any supplement appearing to offer huge benefits.

One thing for sure is that most working athletes would go faster if they managed to get an extra hour of sleep every night. Sleep is a natural performance enhancer, and a lack of it is probably the single greatest challenge facing most working athletes.

Following is a review of some of the most common supplements. This is not an exhaustive review of all the supplements on the market. We have evaluated those supplements that we believe are beneficial as well as certain others that are widely used by athletes.

■ *Antioxidants, Iron, and Calcium*

Medical treatments and lifestyle practices that slow the aging process are often beneficial to athletic performance. A good example is antioxidants. They have been shown to prevent the damage that advances the aging of cells and help to ward off such diseases as cancer and heart disease.

Antioxidants are part of an elaborate defense system the body employs to check cellular damage caused by free radicals—highly reactive atoms formed when oxygen interacts with certain molecules. The damage that free radicals cause to cellular components such as DNA or the cell membrane may be equated with what happens when rust forms on metal.

If you do only one thing in the way of supplements, antioxidants should be it. Take daily 400 to 800 IU of vitamin E (d-alpha tocopherols, not dL-alpha), 1 gram of vitamin C, and 2 to 5 grams of fish oil high in omega-3 DHA and EPA. When choosing vitamin E, d-alpha (a natural source) is superior to dL-alpha (a synthetic source), as it is more readily absorbed by the body. Although flaxseed oil is a source of omega-3 oils, studies have shown that fish oils are better absorbed by the body.

Omega-3 fats are powerful antioxidants, antiaging aids, and cancer fighters. They also help the athlete reduce inflammations that are common when training stress is high. Omega-3s bind to free radicals (waste from exercise) and help remove them from the body. They reduce bad serum cholesterol and are precursors to sex hormones that lead to normal body function and faster recovery. They also support the immune system, as do vitamins C and E.

Some athletes may need to supplement their diet with iron, but you should never take iron supplements except under the specific guidance of a physician. Unmonitored supplementation of iron can be very dangerous to your health.

Many athletes wonder about the need to supplement calcium to keep their bones strong. Generally, calcium supplementation is not necessary when you are eating according to the guidelines expressed in this chapter. Eating alkaline foods (vegetables and fruits) in abundance will also maintain bone strength. After all, our ancestors for the better part of four and a half million years did not eat dairy and did not suffer from osteoporosis. Finally, the large amount of weight-bearing exercise done by triathletes makes a sound positive contribution to overall bone health. Keep in mind that swimming and cycling are not weight-bearing sports, but running and strength training are.

Increased fitness from regular exercise also means greater resistance to free-radical damage. Although regular and consistent exercise is effective for boosting the body's natural resistance to free-radical breakdown, "weekend warriors" create significant stresses on their bodies. Infrequent and excessive exercise overwhelms the body with free radicals and is too inconsistent to promote our natural defense system. This is one reason why sedentary people are urged to keep their periodic episodes of exercise brief and at low intensity.

The human body contains several enzymes that prevent or reduce the severity of this damage by interacting with free radicals to render them harmless. This is the body's natural antioxidant system. There are also certain nutrients found in food that bolster this defense system. The principal dietary antioxidants are vitamins E and C. It has been well established that a deficiency of these vitamins greatly reduces endurance capacity. Other nutrients, especially beta-carotene, and to a lesser extent selenium and coenzyme Q10, have also been shown to be effective at combining with free radicals.

Vitamin E (d-alpha tocopherol) is present in nuts, seeds, vegetable oils, fish-liver oils, and wheat germ. Vitamin C (ascorbic acid) is found in citrus fruits and juices, sweet peppers, raw cabbage, berries, kiwifruit, cantaloupe, and green leafy vegetables. Such foods as carrots, sweet potatoes, spinach, cantaloupe, broccoli, dark green leafy vegetables, and orange vegetables and fruits are rich in beta-carotene, which is a precursor of vitamin A.

Some studies have shown that supplementing the diet with antioxidants well in excess of the recommended daily allowance (RDA) reduces free-radical damage in athletes. Although we recommend eating a diet rich in antioxidants, it is difficult to consume enough food to achieve the levels used in some of these studies, especially for vitamin E. Although it is somewhat controversial, supplementation is recommended for serious athletes.

The RDA for vitamin E is 15 IU for men and 12 IU for women. This amount may be well below what is necessary for serious endurance athletes. Recent studies have successfully supplemented with amounts as high as 200 to 800 IU daily. The RDA for vitamin C is 60 milligrams (mg), but once again, dosages as high as 250 to 1,000 mg per day have typically been used by athletes. With a diet very high in plant foods, the lower end of this vitamin C dosage may be attained without supplementation.

Antioxidants are generally believed to play no direct role in performance enhancement. In other words, you won't be faster because of taking vitamin E and C supplements. On the other hand, at least one study, as reported by O. Anderson in *Running Research News*, has shown a direct relationship between performance at high elevation and vitamin E supplementation.

So, should you supplement your diet with antioxidants? Although not overwhelming, the evidence at this time seems to indicate that there is good reason to do so. However, this advice applies only if you are not on certain medications such as blood thinners or pain relievers; if you are, vitamin E supplementation may cause complications. If you are on any medications at all, check with your physician before supplementing.

■ *Caffeine*

Many athletes use caffeine to "boost" their race day performance or to get a "jump" before a BT workout. Several studies over the past fifty years have shown that it delays fatigue during endurance exercise and enhances high-intensity activities such as interval training. Other studies found that when used during endurance exercise, caffeine improved performance. We should point out that there have been studies that showed no benefit for endurance performance from caffeine intake. Others have shown that eating a high-carbohydrate meal along with caffeine prevents an endurance benefit. But on the whole, the research seems to support caffeine as an ergogenic aid.

If you aren't used to caffeine, it is best to start with a single cup of coffee. Caffeine works best in low to moderate doses and at high levels is detrimental to performance. If you start to shake, you'll know you have gone too far. There are, however, side effects from the use of caffeine.

- It is easy to become habituated to the response. Some research indicates less of a beneficial effect in habitual drinkers.
- You will sleep better if you have had no caffeine during the day. Many athletes experience disrupted sleep patterns from caffeine. Given the recovery benefits of sleep, caffeine use is likely counterproductive for these athletes.
- Stomach upset is common. Experiment with dosages during race-simulation training and B- and C-priority races. Use less caffeine in an A-priority race because of the additional stresses associated with a race situation.

■ *Creatine*

Some athletes supplement with creatine to aid recovery and enhance strength. It has been shown to improve performance when doing very short intervals such as fast, 50 m repeats in the pool. However, this substance is useful only for people who have power (not muscular endurance) as a limiter, and it is not recommended for endurance athletes. For endurance athletes, there is still quite a bit to be learned about this ergogenic aid, and there is likely to be a downside. Probably the greatest risk that you face in using any strength-oriented supplement is inadvertent doping owing to poor quality control by the manufacturer. In recent years there have been a number of studies that have shown a lack of purity in dietary supplements generally.

■ *L-Glutamine and Branch-Chain Amino Acids*

One study has shown that taking 8 grams of the amino acid glutamine immediately after stressful exercise improved the capacity to recover by improving the glucose absorption rate. Such research is still in the preliminary stages.

This amino acid was once considered "nonessential." It is now thought of as "conditionally essential." There is evidence that under traumatic conditions (heavy periods of training, stage racing, or bodily injury), the body is unable to produce enough glutamine. Glutamine is essential to muscle growth, has positive effects on the immune system, and may improve insulin metabolism. It has the ability to preserve skeletal muscle mass in times of stress, which is one of the reasons it is added to IV bags for hospital patients.

Should you decide to supplement with L-glutamine, consider starting conservatively, with 2 grams per day.

Branch-chain amino acids (BCAAs) may also enhance recovery during heavy periods of training. All of the amino acids can be found in meats, and a nutritional analysis will provide information about adequate protein. However, if it is unclear whether the quantity of amino acids in your diet is sufficient, then consuming 35 mg of BCAA for each pound of body weight each day during periods of high stress may be beneficial.

In the case of both BCAAs and L-glutamine, supplement half the dose after training or racing with a recovery drink and the other half with a snack before bed. Food slows the absorption rate and helps the body utilize more of the supplement. If you decide to use any supplements, record the dose taken, the time, and other particulars in your training diary. Also comment on whether you believe the supplementation helps compared with past seasons of heavy racing or training. We do not recommend taking these supplements daily, year-round. Whereas the typical athlete's diet, one that is high in grains and starches, will challenge and deplete your glutamine stores, you will get plenty of glutamine and BCAAs if you eat a paleo diet with plenty of lean meat, fish, and seafood.

■ *Sodium*

Those at the greatest risk for electrolyte problems are the thirteen-hour-plus Ironman-distance athletes because their pace is slow enough that they can drink large quantities of fluid all day. Combine that rate of consumption with a high sweat rate, and you risk seriously disrupting your electrolyte balance.

For longer, hot races, the use of salt/electrolyte tablets has proven successful. A common rate of sodium loss is in the range of 1.8 grams (not mg) to 3.5 grams of sodium per liter of sweat. The low figure is for a fit, acclimatized athlete, and the high figure is for an unfit, nonacclimatized athlete.

The average person has about 80 grams of sodium in his or her body and consumes 5 to 20 grams of sodium per day. As you can see, you have to sweat an awful lot to end up salt depleted. However, the issue is more complicated because sodium balance affects your ability to move fluid from the stomach to the bloodstream. For this reason, many athletes view sodium supplementation as a source of insurance while racing. They may not need the additional electrolytes, but they feel better taking them.

Many middle-of-the-pack and back-of-the-pack athletes overhydrate, thus diluting the sodium content of their blood. Two ways to avoid this result are to drink less or supplement. Supplementation is the safer choice in an Ironman-distance race.

Once again, you should experiment during training in order to recognize what works for you. If you have hypertension or are on a low-sodium diet, then consult your physician before starting any sodium supplementation. Indeed, as we mentioned earlier, you should discuss any potential supplementation with your physician.

CONCLUSION

Aside from training wisely, the most important things most working athletes can do to improve their performance are to get an extra hour of sleep every night and improve their nutrition. If you have difficulty reaching your ideal body composition, or your performance or recovery is lagging, we recommend that you commit to a few sessions with a good sports nutritionist. The ideal consultant will be familiar with the demands of long-course triathlon. The benefits of an effective nutritional strategy flow into all areas of training and will greatly improve the quality of your life.

CHAPTER 11

TRAINING THE MIND

Never give up, for that is just the place and time that the tide will turn.

—HARRIET BEECHER STOWE

he mind is a powerful ally, but it can also be a formidable adversary. The techniques in this chapter are designed to help you achieve an effective mindset to maximize your race performance. Everyone can improve performance through the application of these concepts. Why? Because it's all in your head!

Before getting into this chapter, we recommend that you take some quality time to answer these three questions:

1. What are your long-term goals in the sport of triathlon as well as the other important areas of your life (work, family, community, friends, and other interests)?
2. What is your level of commitment to achieving your triathlon goals?
3. What price are you willing to pay in order to achieve your goals?

Be as honest as possible in making this assessment. One of the most effective ways to develop these goals is to sit down and write for 15 min. each morning. Write down whatever comes to mind, resist the urge to judge, and save everything. After seven to twenty-eight days of these sessions, go back through your notes and highlight items that repeat. Then create a short list of overall goals. You can find out more about this technique in a book by Julia Cameron called *The Artist's Way* (see "References and Recommended Reading").

These three questions are a natural place to begin working on your mental training. When you consider your triathlon goals alongside your other long-term goals, your athletic success is only one component of a fulfilling life. The size of this component varies from person to person. As for commitment, the subconscious mind is highly attuned and will quickly see through anything other than true commitment. You should strive for total commitment to whatever level of dedication you believe is appropriate.

Finally, in order to maximize the benefits from implementing the techniques discussed in this chapter, your mind needs to be in a state of harmony. Both harmony and success are achieved when your life goals are working in concert with each other.

BE YOUR GOALS

Probably the quickest method for achieving any goal is to "be" that goal. This means that you should aim to replicate as many things as possible that are consistent with your goals. For example, if your goal is to be the very best, then you could do the following:

Eat like a champion. Dedicate yourself to following a suitable nutrition strategy.

Train like a champion. Focus on high-quality BT workouts. Training hard is often the easiest task for a highly motivated athlete.

Recover like a champion. Know when to back off, and ensure that you get adequate levels of sleep each night. An inability to listen to the body's signals has been the downfall of many athletes. Champions are sensitive to all aspects of their health and know that rest is their ally.

Behave like a champion. Strong ethics are essential. If you follow a well-developed set of ethics, you will find it much easier to achieve harmony. Always remember that success does not imply arrogance.

Be a champion. Walk like a champion, talk like a champion, stand like a champion—in as many areas as possible, let your conduct be consistent with your goals.

Many athletes have a fear of truly committing to their goals. It is important to remember that seeking excellence is never something that should cause you embarrassment. When you are on a path of excellence that is in balance with other aspects of your life goals, success is close at hand.

Many athletes feel that they have to hide their successes, often out of a fear of the response of others. You may even find friends, peers, and acquaintances belittling or undermining your athletic goals. In this situation, the time spent considering your goals is highly valuable. It is much harder for people to negatively affect us when we are working toward our goal in harmony. The most stinging comments are often reminders that we have strayed from our path.

CONTROL YOUR THOUGHTS

Almost every athlete would like to improve his or her mental conditioning. The difficulty most of us face is finding a formula for achieving success. What follows are some practical ideas for controlling your thoughts.

Edward Wilson presents some novel concepts about the mind, genes, free will, and thoughts in his book *Consilience* (see "References and Recommended Reading"). He believes that the mind is a powerful analog computer—a series of arrays that are constantly running various scenarios. The ability to generate and interpret successful scenarios is what determines intelligence and a person's adaptability within his or her environment.

One key implication of the "brain as array" model is that the scenarios we focus on and repeat most often are the ones that are most likely to become reality. Just as we train our neuromuscular pathways, so can we train our neurological pathways. Though it is difficult to control our thoughts (particularly if our brain is running a wide range of them at any given time), we can control a few things.

■ *Guide Your Written and Spoken Thoughts*

Control over the written word is probably the easiest type of control to exercise. Writing is a deliberate act, less subject to habitual patterns than other actions, and can be an effective way to help us guide our thoughts. Our diaries, e-mails, training logs, and other materials are areas where we can use the written word to help strengthen our desired thought patterns and outcomes. Speech requires a more advanced level of control. Words, particularly about the self, are very powerful guides to patterns. The first step to verbalizing our intentions is to say them out loud when we are alone. State the goal, desire, or intended outcome. Note the thoughts immediately after you've made your statement. Some people like to write these down and mark "OK" beside the notes. This practice can be a useful tool for uncovering your biases as well as clues to your current self-image. The purpose of the "OK" is to acknowledge the validity of any thought that you may have (a simple acknowledgment of self-acceptance).

■ *Address Your Fears*

If you can't write it or say it, then odds are that it will be quite difficult to do it. Many athletes have a fear that if they write down or speak their goals, they will be devastated if they don't achieve them. This is an irrational fear. There is really only one "failure" that cannot be overcome: death. Everything else is only as serious as you want to make it.

The act of writing and speaking your goals makes them real. It can also flush out issues around the goals. If you are having trouble making your goals concrete, you should examine the source of your trouble—the source of your fear.

If you feel nervous about making your goals concrete, or if you tend to have difficulty dealing with others' opinions, you are likely to be best served by keeping your goals to yourself or sharing them only with trusted advisers (such as your coach, physician, nutritionist, or another member of your athletic network).

Though a weak self-image is a common challenge, the opposite can also occur when an athlete is subject to goal inflation regarding targets that are too challenging. Goals should be challenging yet achievable. When an athlete continually falls short of his or her goals, either the goals are too challenging or the athlete's mental skills need sharpening. An example of the latter case is the athlete who excels in training only to underperform on race day.

■ *Improve Your Attention and Focus*

After you have gained experience with controlling written and spoken words, the next step is to work on your attention and focus. Consider how you spend most of your time—what are you actually thinking about (positive outcomes, negative outcomes, past injustices, future fears)? One way to track such thoughts is to keep a short diary that contains thoughts, feelings, and filters (the kinds of negative emotions that make us prone to misinterpret reality) along with notes summarizing what triggered them. By first understanding our existing patterns, filters, and triggers, it will be easier to move toward our desired outcomes. The results of this exercise are almost always surprising.

■ *Stick to Your Plan*

All of these exercises assume that you know where you want to go. Once you have a plan, take every opportunity to support this direction through words and actions that are consistent with it. When situations arise that are inconsistent with the plan, it is best to calmly move on toward your goals. Classic examples are sickness, injury, and concerns over current fitness levels. Sitting on the couch worrying about the results of a time trial or about the fitness lost during a recent illness will not move you toward your goals. Learning from your challenges and taking concrete actions will lead to achievement.

Creating Your Race Plan

DURING TRAINING

- Write a list of your reasons for doing the race.
- Write a list of your life priorities.
- Write a list of your goals for the race.
- Ensure that all of the above are in harmony.
- Ensure that your partner/family/work/friends support your goals.

RACE PREPARATION

- Issues list—two columns (issue, solution).
- Get solutions to issues from experienced athletes and coaches.
- Take action early to address outstanding issues.
- Write things down—identified issues are normally minor and easily addressed.
- Ensure that thought patterns support goals—spoken and written words should be in complete alignment with life and race goals.
- Use visualization techniques to reduce stress and improve probability of success.

RACE STRATEGY

- Create a written race strategy that covers pacing, hydration and nutrition, equipment lists, transitions, and contingency issues.
- During race week, review the race strategy daily.
- Race strategy should include as much detail as possible.
- Pace should be effort-based, not time-based. External factors can affect time goals (flats, etc.), but effort goals are independent and 100 percent controllable by you, the athlete.

RACE WEEK

- Beware of goal inflation—maintain perspective.
- Avoid that "one last" megasession.
- Rest and prepare mentally.
- If you make any mistakes, do "too little."
- Ensure that you have 30 to 60 min. quiet time each day.
- Remember that changes in sleep patterns are normal.

DURING THE RACE

- Focus on the present—maintain a task orientation.
- Leave the past behind.
- Take the race in pieces, little chunks.
- Move forward at all times.
- Manage the emotional cycles (hold back in the peaks, endure the valleys).
- If you find yourself obsessing or flip-flopping, it's a sign you need to refocus.
- Control the controllables—leave all externals alone.

KNOW WHAT YOU CAN CONTROL

What is the greatest obstacle that stands between you and the things you desire? Money? Education? Social status? Genetics? Time? Opportunity? None of the above! The greatest obstacle that you face is yourself, and more specifically, your doubting self. The doubting self is the little voice inside your head that says, "You can't," "You'd better not," and "You'll never make it."

As we just discussed, there are only two things under your direct control: your words and your actions. You may think these are easy to control, but you'll realize it's not the case when you actually listen to what people are saying at any race: "I'm so out of shape"; "I haven't done enough training"; "There's no way I'm going to finish." Some may say that these people are releasing pre-race tension. It may be more accurate to say that they are programming failure.

Mentally strong athletes understand that the body will follow where the mind leads, and they are careful where they lead their minds. By controlling your words and actions, you eventually become your goals. Your words and deeds become so habitual that your mind has no choice but to follow.

Successful athletes have the ability to focus on the areas that are under their control and let go of factors that are beyond it. In long-distance racing, there will be many factors on race day that are not under your control.

Understanding Control

OUT OF YOUR CONTROL	UNDER YOUR CONTROL
Weather	Preparation (race strategy, course knowledge, training)
Equipment problems (flats, unexpected mechanical issues)	Equipment (appropriate, serviceable)
Swim conditions (surf, temperature, currents, course accuracy)	Pacing
Bike conditions (wind, temperature, road debris, other riders, vehicles)	Technique (form, cadence, economy)
Run conditions (cloud cover, temperature, terrain, other runners)	Nutrition
Competition	Hydration
Aid stations (volunteers, supplies, location)	

Though every effort should be made to become as informed as possible, you would be wise to spend very little time focusing on these factors. Given the nature of long-distance triathlon, challenges will appear in every race.

It is the factors that you can control that lead to improved race performance. The weather, the possibility of equipment failure, and the level of competition around you are all best left alone because either they have no direct impact on you or they affect all of the other athletes too.

YOUR MIND AND RACING

It is common to have two conversations going on in your head as you roll toward your A-priority race.

Conversation 1 is your mind telling you that you are woefully unprepared and you will surely crash and burn. Hogwash! Remember this when you are at the track, in a pack, at the pool, naked in front of the mirror, or on the start line—anytime you need confidence, say to yourself, "My body did the training. I belong." We all need to boost our confidence!

Conversation 2 is your taper telling you that you can win your age group; qualify for Kona; knock one, two—heck, even three hours off your personal record; or crush the course record. Maybe you race farther back in the pack and catch yourself thinking about a daylight finish when two months earlier your goal was simply to cross the finish line with a smile. When this happens, think back to what your goals were when you signed up for the race. These are the goals that you have been working toward for the last three to nine months. These should be the goals around which you have built your season.

Both of these conversations are natural, and it is worth sitting down and having a rational discussion with yourself. It is important to focus on your original goals. If you have set them properly, you are now very close to achieving them. You have done the training, and all you need to do is stay calm and execute your plan.

During a race, you may find either of these conversations starting again. Your reaction to such a diversion often goes one of two ways, commonly referred to as "fixation" and "splitting." Fixation is an obsession with an element that is in the past or out of your control (other athletes, a flat tire, the weather). Splitting is when you start that internal conversation ("You can't do it"/"You can do it"). Both fixation and splitting are signals that you have become diverted from your focus. If you succumb to the diversion, then economy, decisions, and timing all deteriorate. By spotting the diversion early, you can refocus on task orientation.

Try this exercise before your next A-priority race to help clear your mind. Say, "I feel the best I've ever felt." Write down the first thought or feeling you get from this statement. Then write "OK" beside it and sign it. Continue writing down the resulting feelings or thoughts until your mind is empty.

If you are truly feeling the best that you have ever felt, your mind will be empty. The statement will be true and float in the air. The mind will feel no compulsion to prove a true statement. It is important to say the statement aloud and write down the mental response (if any). When there is doubt, accept and clear the doubt.

Other examples are:

"I love myself and truly enjoy my life."

"My body is strong and powerful."

"I am going to race the best that I have ever raced."

LEARNING TO PUSH

Many triathletes find it difficult to maintain a "fighting spirit" for an entire race. Quite often you may be disappointed that you cannot push for the full duration of a long-course event. The truth is that this is a very hard skill to master. It can take years of practice to be able to push on when the mind wants to ease off.

How do you learn to push? Start small and then build. Train the body and the mind to remain focused for a shorter period, and then expand your boundaries. One of the most useful aspects of short-course racing is that it trains you to endure high levels of intensity.

Indeed, the layout of a typical season is well suited to learning to push. The early season's focus on endurance, technique, and strength requires little in the way of intense mental focus. Early in the race season, you will have a series of C-priority races, some of which will be shorter in length. By midseason, you will be mixing shorter races with BT and race-simulation workouts. All of these sessions will help you build the skills necessary to race mentally strong.

Another factor you should remember is that every individual has a unique breaking point. For this reason, a conservative early pace can pay large dividends. One should never underesti-

> **IF YOU KEEP YOUR GOALS REASONABLE YET** challenging, your mind will be your friend throughout race day as you hit your targets and perform. Even if things don't work out, you'll know you are doing the best you can do. If you have the desire to be the best, you must be willing to serve an apprenticeship. It takes a very long time to become a master at any skill. Typically, those who are new to the sport place too much pressure on themselves to perform at a high level right away. By realizing that an apprenticeship is required and committing to paying your dues over the long term, you will enjoy the journey more and enable yourself to achieve a higher level of ultimate performance.

mate the psychological impact of being stronger than one's competitors late in the race. This is a concept of mental pacing as well as physical pacing.

Finally, remember that an Ironman-distance triathlon involves a lot more "waiting" than "pushing." Successful long-course athletes practice a combination of patience and fortitude.

FACING YOUR FEARS ON RACE DAY

All athletes experience pre-race jitters—the people who look calm at races are probably doing their best to "be" their goals! Here is a progression that works for many people when they find themselves face-to-face with fear.

> **AN EFFECTIVE TECHNIQUE FOR PREPARING TO RACE** is to use certain key words during training. Words such as *power*, *control*, *pace*, *endure*, *jump*, *push*, *calm*, and *breathe* can be used to invoke a certain state. Choose your own words and then incorporate them into key moments of your training. The words can become a preprogrammed performance cue that you can summon at the appropriate time in a race.

Acceptance. Accept the fact that you are nervous, or even scared. Accept yourself for being scared and know that it is both natural and a sign that you are ready for competition.

Channeling. After you have acknowledged your fear, focus on where it is taking root physically. For example, many people experience shortness of breath when they are scared. If you are one of these people, then some trunk and abdominal stretching combined with a short period of deep breathing will quickly make you feel better. By breaking fear's physical chain, you will be able to regain your focus. This technique of fear management can easily be built into any pre-race routine.

Perspective. There is nothing like context to help in dealing with the doubting self. Quite often this side of your personality will attempt to take over your mind when you are feeling stressed. At these times, it is useful to pause and remember that it's only a race! The worst-case scenario is that you learn something new about your current limits, which is hardly a disaster. An obvious exception to this rule would be if you find yourself in a situation where your personal safety is at risk (such as a swim in rough surf). In those situations, caution is the best course of action. There will always be another race.

Reflection. Take some time to identify the source of the fear. Quite often a solution presents itself as soon as the source is identified.

Naming. Once the source of the fear is identified and acknowledged, it can be quite effective to name the fear. An example of this might be a fear of racing in the wind. Perhaps you give the wind a name: Mr. Blowhard. In you pre-race visualization, you talk with Mr. Blowhard and

Common Risks, Fears, and Solutions

RISKS AND FEARS	SOLUTIONS AND KEY POINTS TO REMEMBER
Weather-related • Wind • Heat • Cold • Humidity • Choppy water	• Same weather conditions for everyone in the race. • Appropriate pace varies based on the conditions you are experiencing. Increased weather stress requires a reduction in target race effort. • Consider weather-simulation workouts to prepare your body and mind for likely conditions. • For cold races, determine your bike clothing choices before the race start, then stick to them. You will be warm when you leave the water in your wetsuit. You will also not be thinking straight. Take time to put on clothes. It is a long day, and you want to be as comfortable as possible.
Equipment-related • Flat tire • Unexpected mechanical problem • Goggles break • Bike wobbles at high speed	• There are some risks that we must accept when we participate in a triathlon. Unexpected bike issues can be mitigated but not eliminated. • Well in advance of competition, practice changing flat tires as well as operating CO_2 inflators (if you plan to use them). • Well in advance of competition, have your bike serviced and check your shoes, cleats, and tires to ensure that they are in good condition. • In your pre-race bag, pack spares for an unexpected flat tire on race morning as well as backup goggles. • If bicycle stability has been an issue for you, then do not use deep-dish rims, especially on your front wheel. Nothing slows you down like crashing, and fear isn't aero.
Nutrition-related • Flat energy • GI shutdown • Dropping personal nutrition • Loss of appetite • Dehydration	• The most important thing to remember about nutritional risks is to start your day as relaxed as possible. There is little time to be made, or lost, in the first two hours of the day. However, if your GI system shuts down, then you will have hours of discomfort that will prove costly. • Create some personal nutrition backup plans. If you use a product not available on the course, then place ample quantities in both special-needs bags and your second transition bag. If it will be a hot day, then remember that your product (if not in powder form) will likely be quite warm when you receive it. • Remember to stop for dropped nutrition. • In your race-simulation workouts, remember to hydrate and eat at goal race levels. • Remember that it is normal to lose your appetite. Shift toward liquid sources of calories as your day progresses. • If you suspect that you are low on calories/hydration, or if your mood suddenly deteriorates, then slow immediately and eat/drink.

RISKS AND FEARS	SOLUTIONS AND KEY POINTS TO REMEMBER
Pacing-related • Low energy • Inability to run the marathon • Maintaining proper effort in the swim • "Losing time" early in the day	• Remember that race day is similar to every other day in your life. You will face variations in mood and energy. You will also face unexpected challenges. Coping with these potential distractions is a key part of successful long-course racing. • Humans are not great at forecasting the future when faced with immediate stress (swim starts, early bike pacing). Focusing on relaxed breathing and superior technique is an effective way to stay centered in a hectic situation. • As an athlete, you are in total control of the pace that you select to use. If you make an error in the first seven hours of your day, then go "too easy." The first four hours of an Ironman-distance event should feel very comfortable. • While swimming, if you think that you are trying too hard, then you are. Back off, relax, and focus on your breathing. • It is not possible to "bank time" during an Ironman-distance race. Early errors in pacing will be repaid late in the day. Be most wary of surges in power/pace, as these are the most stressful to your digestion and energy reserves.
Performance-related • Underperformance • Disappointment • Failing to meet own expectations • Others' opinions • Pain and discomfort	• Until you are at complete peace with your race performances, never make public predictions about your potential performance in a race. • Have a private, written race plan and focus your effort on executing that plan to the best of your ability. • Focus on superior execution rather than relative performance. • Remember that we are so wrapped up in ourselves that we rarely remember the performances of others. • Remember your goals one, two, and five years ago—you may be creating stress with goal inflation that has nothing to do with the reason that you participate in sports. • Acknowledge that the race is a challenging undertaking—be honest about what you will face. There will be discomfort to manage. • The race will get difficult on its own timetable; with conservative pacing, you will have the mental reserves to cope when the day becomes challenging.

continued >

< Common Risks, Fears, and Solutions, continued

RISKS AND FEARS	SOLUTIONS AND KEY POINTS TO REMEMBER
Preparation-related • Can I go that far? • Am I prepared? • Have I done the right training? • Have I rested too much?	• A written training log provides a clear reminder of the preparation that you have done. • Well before race day, ensure that your race-simulation workouts have been completed. • Given that most athletes arrive at the start line tired, resist the urge to test your fitness in the final two weeks before a race. • If you are concerned about your endurance, then adjust early race pace downward to build a cushion into your day.
General • Where should I line up at the start? • Swimming with others • What if I have to go to the bathroom? • What if I get sick before the race? • What if I get injured before the race? • How will I handle the course terrain?	• In many races, there can be no "clear water," and you will be faced with a crowded swim leg. Practice close-quarters open-water swimming and include crowded swimming in your pre-race visualization techniques. • Wear comfortable clothing that you have tested in race-simulation workouts. Ensure that you can go to the bathroom easily with your race kit setup. • If you need to go to the bathroom, then stop. Being uncomfortable costs you time. • If you have a history of sickness or injury in the final weeks before an A-priority event, then reduce the training stress in your Build period. Athletes who are frequently sick or injured in their Peak period need to reduce training stress in their programs. • If you are concerned about course terrain, then perform race-simulation workouts in the terrain or conditions that worry you and choose races that play to your strengths, not fears.

explain that there is nothing he can do to disrupt your race. By making the fear tangible, you can address it with thought-specific visualization.

Listing. As with naming, there are many benefits to writing down fears because the action makes the issues clearer. Write a list of risks, fears, and concerns and rate them on a scale of 1 to 10. When under stress, the mind can blow things out of proportion, so it helps to decide the rank of situations in advance. Then make a two-column list: At the top of one column is "Risk/ Fear" and at the top of the other is "Solution." Use all the resources at your disposal (books, the Internet, experienced athletes, online forums, friends, coaches) to find a solution for every risk. There are some risks (most uncontrollable) for which the only solution is to accept it.

Humor. Another effective method for dealing with fears is to treat them with humor. When you are able to view your fears, flaws, and failings with compassion, they are much easier to bear. This does not imply a lessening in your resolve to improve; however, it does imply having patience with your imperfections.

Action. Ultimately, the only way to deal with any persistent fear is to face it down—to turn to it and say, "You are not going to beat me." It can take tremendous strength of spirit to truly face your fears, but the payback is enormous.

In combating fear, remember that the goal is not to remove all fear but to acknowledge the fear and achieve superior performance notwithstanding its presence. Fear makes us feel alive. It heightens our arousal and challenges us to be our best. Rather than overcoming all fear, learn to dance with your fears, all the while becoming stronger in both body and spirit.

STRATEGIES FOR SUCCESS

What constitutes a successful race for you? Is it your finishing time? Your age-group ranking or overall placement? Actually, it would serve you better to define a successful race as one in which you did your best throughout every leg and every transition. When we focus on doing our best at each moment during the race, a successful outcome is much more likely. This has been the secret to many athletes' best races—a sharp focus on the present. The past is gone, and the future will take care of itself. If you focus only on doing your best (right now), then every race, every training session, every moment can be a success.

■ *Breathing*

How do you build a strong focus? Try focusing on your breathing. Feel the air moving in and out of your lungs. When you are centered on your breath, it is more difficult for your mind to generate those thoughts you'd prefer to do without. You can use this technique on the bike and when running. In the water, think about the feel of the water moving against your body, particularly your forearms.

■ *Visualization*

A technique used by almost all elite athletes is visualization. Visualization can be used to increase the probability of positive outcomes, create comfort, reduce anxiety, and improve technical skills.

There are two main styles of visualization: Movie Screen and Video Camera. Movie Screen visualization is when you watch yourself perform as if you are outside your body. The goal is to run a movie of your desired outcome. Video Camera visualization is when you picture the scene from within yourself, as if you are looking out through the lens of a camera.

No matter which style you prefer, you should try to picture as many aspects of the scene as possible: what the setting looks like, the quality of the sunlight, the color of the water, and the people around you. The goal should be to create as realistic a scene as possible.

In the final two weeks before an A-priority race, spend 10 min. per day visualizing key aspects of the race and positive outcomes. Pay particular attention to reinforcing positive images regarding any area of concern. A good time for this type of visualization is when lying in bed.

Those who have the opportunity to train alongside technically proficient athletes should use such opportunities to create mental images of excellent form and economy. These images can be replayed during visualization sessions.

In addition to evening visualization, you can use the last 10 min. before you fall asleep to focus on one thing that was good about that day's workout. Play that one good thing over in your mind, and relive the experience as you fall asleep. This technique is particularly useful if you have confidence issues.

THE POWER OF BELIEF

All of the techniques in this chapter are designed to enhance your self-belief. Ultimately, the beliefs that you have in your preparations, your experience, and your race strategy are the key determinants of your mental strength on race day.

Long-course racing presents hurdles for every athlete on race day. The extent to which you prepare your mind will determine how well you do in navigating the challenges that will inevitably arise.

CHAPTER 12

CASE STUDIES

By now, even if you are new to Ironman training, you've learned a lot about how to structure your training and plan a season. Sometimes it can be helpful to consider how it all comes together. In this chapter we will take a closer look at the annual training plan of four triath-

Before you can get your race together, you need to get your life together.

—MARK ALLEN,
SIX-TIME IRONMAN WORLD CHAMPION

letes. In our experience, the three most common scenarios are the novice, the runner, and the experienced athlete. You can review the profile of each athlete, note their key limiters, and see how they detailed their goals and structured their Base, Build, and Peak training periods. The final case study presents an alternative to strict periodization that you might find effective if you are an athlete with limited time or simply in need of a more streamlined approach to your training.

In the annual training plans that follow, goals and tactics are outlined for each period, but we have not indicated the weekly training volumes. For best results in planning your workouts, we recommend that you build the entire training period at one time. Place your workouts in your weekly schedule by using this priority system:

- First note your races and nontraining commitments (travel, business, family obligations).
- Schedule the workouts that address your period goals—your breakthrough workouts.
- Block out appropriate recovery time (passive or active) following your breakthrough workouts.

- Add workouts to ensure appropriate frequency in each sport (workout frequency can vary between weeks and throughout the year).
- Note the session details for each of your scheduled workouts, refer back to your period goals, and ensure that your training focus is appropriate for the time of year.

If you are a novice or time-constrained athlete, then you should stop at this stage. Extra volume will merely reduce the quality of your training and slow your BT workout recovery.

If you think you can handle greater volume, then schedule additional sessions in line with your period goals and tactics. It is good for athletes at all levels to increase volume, but keep in mind that the important points are to start with less than you think you can handle and remember that quality, not quantity, of training will determine your ultimate success. Here are some tips for considering appropriate levels of weekly volume:

- In the Prep and early Base periods, keep the volume comfortable in all weeks.
- In the middle of the Base period, it is OK to have one "stretch," or challenging, week per period.
- In the late Base period, experienced athletes may be able to handle two stretch weeks per period.
- If scheduling a Build period is appropriate, then you should stretch by way of race-specific intensity rather than volume.
- If you are aiming for a late-season peak, ensure that you schedule a two-week midseason break from structured training.

If you make a scheduling mistake, err on the side of too little volume and too much base training.

Although none of these case studies is likely to describe you perfectly, you should be able to get a good idea of how to apply the concepts in this book to map out your own personal training plan.

THE NOVICE

Nick the Novice has been in the sport of triathlon for three years. He's done a few triathlons and at the end of last summer completed his first half-Ironman-distance race. His main goal for this coming season is to complete an end-of-season Ironman-distance race. Although he'd like to post a solid time, his overriding goal is to have a good experience. Nick works full-time and has two kids. Sunday is family day, and therefore he likes to limit his volume on that day.

In his half-Ironman-distance race, Nick swam 40 min.; his key swim limiter is technique. He's never swum more than 2,800 m in any workout and is concerned about his overall endurance. He has access to a masters squad, but the people in that group swim hard, and he has to struggle to keep up.

In preparing for his goal race last summer, Nick's longest ride was 4 hours. His bike split in the race was 3:25 on a moderately difficult course. He has access to all kinds of training terrain. Nick has a tough time on the hills and is concerned about some long climbs that are a feature of his goal race. Darkness and weather limit his weekday riding time in the winter.

Nick has never run a marathon and expects that he will use a run/walk strategy for his first Ironman-distance race. In a recent half-Ironman race, he used a run/walk strategy for a run split of 2:20. (Refer to the "Run/Walk Protocol" section in Chapter 8 for an explanation of this strategy.)

Nick's season will be structured around building his overall endurance to complete his goal race (Tables 12.1–12.4). His training will start with a frequency and technique focus, then move toward building endurance. He will target a late-spring half-Ironman-distance race and have a midseason break to ensure that he remains fresh through the summer. Heading into his goal race, he will cut back on his racing to better enable him to focus on (and recover from) his key endurance BTs. In order to build his confidence, two century rides and a long open-water swim have been scheduled.

TABLE 12.1 NOVICE NICK'S ANNUAL TRAINING PLAN AND TACTICS

		GOALS	TACTICS
PREP 1	**Strength** AA1 **Weeks to Race** 24–27	Reestablish structured training	Workout frequency
		Improve strength training technique	2 sessions with personal trainer to review program
		Improve technical skills	Solo technique-oriented swim sessions
PREP 2	**Strength** AA2 **Weeks to Race** 20–23	Improve swim balance	Solo technique-oriented swim sessions
		Extend overall endurance	3 of 4 Saturdays are long, low-intensity aerobic training
		Improve flexibility	Start yoga; continue twice weekly to end of Base 2
		Prepare body for longer runs	2 of 4 weeks have increased run frequency
PREP 3	**Strength** AA3 **Weeks to Race** 16–19	Increase strength	Lower reps and increase intensity in gym
		Improve swimming stroke mechanics	Start swim cords; continue twice weekly to end of Base 2
		Increase running endurance	2 of 4 weeks have 1 long and 1 moderately long run
		Half-marathon (B-priority)	
BASE 1	**Strength** MS **Weeks to Race** 12–15	Increase strength	Maximum strength training phase
		Improve swimming body position	Continue as per previous block
		Increase cycling endurance	Target 2 long rides; in poor weather, crosstrain
BASE 2	**Strength** SM **Weeks to Race** 8–11	Increase cycling endurance	Target 3 long rides; in poor weather, crosstrain
		Increase running endurance	3 of 4 weeks have long run; 1 weekend BT is all-day hike
		Increase swimming endurance	1 endurance workout and 1 masters session added
		Spring duathlon (C-priority)	

continued >

TABLE 12.1 CONTINUED

		GOALS	TACTICS
BASE 3	**Strength SM** **Weeks to Race 4–7**	Increase cycling endurance	Century is key long ride; weeks before and after are moderate rides
		Increase running endurance	Complete 2 trail runs of 1 hour, 45 min., and 2 hours' duration
		Start with moderate muscular endurance training	Add weekly indoor training muscular endurance session
		Maintain swim endurance	Continue as per previous block
		Century ride (C-priority)	
PEAK	**Strength SM** **Weeks to Race 2–3**	Specific race preparation	1 race-simulation brick per week
			Add 1 muscular endurance swim per week
RACE	**Weeks to Race 1**	**Half-Ironman (A-priority)**	
TRANS	**Weeks to Race 16**	Race recovery	Total rest
BASE 1	**Strength AA1** **Weeks to Race 12–15**	Ensure race recovery	1st week very easy, 2nd week moderate, 3rd week normal, followed by recovery week
		Start to rebuild strength	Start very light with single set of each exercise; build from there to AA1 levels
		Maintain aerobic pathways	Focus on workout frequency; resist urge to add lots of endurance
		Maintain skills	Weekly skills session in each sport
		2-mile open water (C-priority)	

continued >

TABLE 12.1 CONTINUED

		GOALS	TACTICS
BASE 2	**Strength** AA2 **Weeks to Race** 8–11	Increase cycling endurance	Weekly long rides, with focus on extending comfortable aerobar ride time
		Increase running endurance	Weekly long run
		Maintain swimming endurance	1 masters session, 1 endurance swim per week; other swimming technique-oriented
		Century ride (C-priority) **Olympic (B-priority)**	
BASE 3	**Strength** AA3 **Weeks to Race** 4–7	Race-specific cycling endurance work	Weekly moderate-intensity hill ride
		Maintain running endurance	Weekly long run
		Increase strength	AA3 strength training
		Specific race preparation	1 race-simulation brick per week Add weekly open-water swim
PEAK	**Strength** SM **Weeks to Race** 2–3	**Sprint (C-priority)**	
RACE	**Weeks to Race** 1	Rejuvenation **Ironman (AAA-priority)**	

TABLE 12.2 NOVICE NICK'S BASE TRAINING, EARLY SEASON

BASE 2, WEEK 1		TRAINING	NOTES	DAILY TIME (HOURS)
Monday	AM	Bike 90 min.	Aerobic ride	2.50
	PM	Swim 60 min.	Technique swim	
Tuesday		Run 30 min.	Speed skills	2.00
		Strength 60 min.	Strength maintenance	
		Bike 30 min.	Easy spin	
Wednesday	AM	Bike 75 min.	Muscular endurance on trainer	2.30
	PM	Swim 60 min.	Masters swim	
Thursday		Bike 75 min.	Aerobic maintenance brick, including cycling speed skills	2.00
		Run 45 min.		
Friday		Swim 90 min.	Endurance swim	1.50
Saturday	AM	Run 1 hour, 45 min.	Endurance trail run	2.50
	PM	Bike 45 min.	Easy spin	
Sunday		Day off		0.00
Weekly total				**12.80**

BASE 2, WEEK 2				
Monday	AM	Bike 60 min.	Aerobic maintenance brick	2.50
		Run 30 min.		
	PM	Swim 60 min.	Technique swim	
Tuesday		Run 30 min.	Speed skills	2.00
		Strength 60 min.	Strength maintenance	
		Bike 30 min.	Easy spin	
Wednesday	AM	Bike 75 min.	Muscular endurance on trainer	2.30
	PM	Swim 60 min.	Masters swim	
Thursday		Run 90 min.	Endurance run on rolling terrain	1.50
Friday		Swim 90 min.	Endurance swim	1.50
Saturday		Bike 5 hours, 40 min.	**Century ride**	6.00
		Run 20 min.	Easy transition run	
Sunday		Day off		0.00
Weekly total				**15.80**

Note: ▨ = Strength training sessions   ▨ = Brick workouts

TABLE 12.3 NOVICE NICK'S BASE TRAINING, LATE SEASON

BASE 3, WEEK 1		TRAINING	NOTES	DAILY TIME (HOURS)
Monday	AM	Bike 60 min.	Aerobic maintenance brick	2.50
		Run 30 min.		
	PM	Swim 60 min.	Masters swim	
Tuesday		Run 30 min.	Speed skills	1.75
		Strength 60 min.	Strength maintenance	
		Bike 15 min.	Easy spin	
Wednesday	AM	Bike 90 min.	Hilly ride	2.50
	PM	Swim 60 min.	Technique swim	
Thursday		Run 1 hour, 45 min.	Endurance: 45 min. easy, 60 min. steady	1.80
Friday		Swim 90 min.	Endurance swim	1.50
Saturday		Bike 3 hours	Steady BT ride	3.50
		Run 30 min.	Transition run	
Sunday		Day off		0.00
Weekly total				**13.55**

BASE 3, WEEK 2				
Monday	AM	Run 90 min.	Endurance run	2.50
	PM	Swim 60 min.	Masters swim	
Tuesday		Run 30 min.	Speed skills	1.75
		Strength 60 min.	Strength maintenance	
		Bike 15 min.	Easy spin	
Wednesday	AM	Bike 90 min.	Hilly ride	2.50
	PM	Swim 60 min.	Technique swim	
Thursday		Bike 90 min.	Speed skills, easy ride	2.00
		Run 30 min.	Steady pace off bike	
Friday		Swim 90 min.	Endurance swim	1.50
Saturday		Bike 4 hours	Steady BT ride	4.50
		Run 30 min.	Easy transition run	
Sunday		Day off		0.00
Weekly total				**14.75**

Note: ▢ = Strength training sessions   ▢ = Brick workouts

TABLE 12.4 NOVICE NICK'S PEAK TRAINING

PEAK, WEEK 1		TRAINING	NOTES	DAILY TIME (HOURS)
Monday	AM	Bike 60 min.	Steady ride	2.00
	PM	Swim 60 min.	Open-water swim	
Tuesday		Run 30 min.	Speed skills	1.75
		Strength 60 min.	Strength maintenance	
		Bike 15 min.	Easy spin	
Wednesday	AM	Swim 1 hour, 15 min.	Hilly ride	1.25
Thursday		Bike 1 hour, 45 min.	Aerobic maintenance brick	2.50
		Run 45 min.		
Friday		Swim 90 min.	Endurance swim	1.50
Saturday		Bike 2 hours, 30 min.	Race-simulation brick	3.50
		Run 60 min.		
Sunday		Day off		0.00
Weekly total				**12.50**

PEAK, WEEK 2				
Monday	AM	Bike 45 min.	Steady ride	1.75
	PM	Swim 60 min.	Open-water swim	
Tuesday		Run 30 min.	Speed skills	1.75
		Strength 60 min.	Strength maintenance	
		Bike 15 min.	Easy spin	
Wednesday	PM	Swim 1 hour, 15 min.	Muscular endurance swim	1.25
Thursday		Bike 1 hour, 15 min.	Aerobic maintenance brick	1.75
		Run 30 min.		
Friday		Swim 90 min.	Endurance swim	1.50
Saturday		Bike 90 min.	Race-simulation brick	2.00
		Run 30 min.		
Sunday		Day off		0.00
Weekly total				**10.00**

Note: ▢ = Strength training sessions   ▢ = Brick workouts

THE RUNNER

Rachel the Runner has been running for most of her adult life. She has done a number of marathons and has qualified for the Boston Marathon. Her running endurance is excellent. She has done a few triathlons, including a half-Ironman-distance race last season. She managed to get through her half-Ironman-distance race, but it hurt! Her legs were completely dead coming off the bike, and her run time was 30 min. slower than she expected.

Over the years, Rachel has had a wide range of overuse injuries, but she is proud of her ability to train through anything. Her swimming results have been solid, but she has noticed that her average heart rate by sport tends to decline as the race progresses. She has a good cycling endurance base but lacks the power to push a big gear or to do anything other than spin up hills. This is a major concern for her because she has heard that the bike course on her goal race is tough.

Rachel's season will be built around the bike because her key limiter is muscular endurance on the bike. Given her injury history, Rachel is going to be very cautious with her run volume and frequency.

Running races will be used to ensure that she maintains her subthreshold speed. To train her legs to run off the bike, frequent bricks will be scheduled throughout the year. Rachel is very goal-oriented and will purchase a power meter so that her progress can be tracked with regular testing.

Rachel has experience with strength training, but when she's honest with herself, she realizes that she has tended to focus more on cosmetic lifting than on sport-specific work. Given her limited experience with lower-body strength training, she will skip the max strength phase this season. See Tables 12.5–12.8 for Rachel's training.

TABLE 12.5 RACHEL THE RUNNER'S ANNUAL TRAINING PLAN AND TACTICS

		GOALS	TACTICS
PREP 1	**Strength** AA1 **Weeks to Race** 28–31	Reestablish structured training	Workout frequency
		Improve strength training technique	1 session/week with personal trainer to learn technique
		Improve technical skills	Twice-weekly swim and bike skills sessions
PREP 2	**Strength** AA2 **Weeks to Race** 24–27	Improve swim technique	Attend weekend swim clinic
		Improve ability to run off bike	4 rides/week; short run following every ride
		Build overall endurance	Use bike-run sessions to build endurance and improve transitions
		Half-marathon (C-priority)	
PREP 3	**Strength** AA3 **Weeks to Race** 20–23	Stay healthy and injury-free	Reduce running; no racing; increase long-ride duration
		Improve cycling-specific strength	Steady increases in cycling-specific gym work
		Build run endurance	Gradually extend endurance to 1 hour, 40 min. duration
BASE 1	**Strength** AA1 **Weeks to Race** 16–19	Start building bike muscular endurance	Start 8-week protocol for early-season bike muscular endurance
		Extend overall endurance	Ride long 3 of 4 weeks
		Build run endurance	Weekly long run includes cruise intervals to maintain leg speed
		Century ride (C-priority)	
		Half-marathon (C-priority)	
BASE 2	**Strength** AA2 **Weeks to Race** 12–15	Continue to build bike muscular endurance	Use moderate muscular endurance training; save the toughest sessions for later in the season
		Build subthreshold run speed	Weekly tempo run session to complement endurance running
		Maintain swim endurance	Regular attendance at masters swim
		Olympic (C-priority)	

continued >

		GOALS	TACTICS
BASE 3	**Strength** AA3 **Weeks to Race** 9–11	Maximize cycling-specific gym strength	2 strength sessions/week: 1st session tough, 2nd session moderate
		Prepare for half-Ironman race	2 weeks out: 4.5-hour race-simulation brick; cautious running thereafter
		10K (C-priority)	
		Half-Ironman (B-priority)	
TRANS	**Weeks to Race** 8	Rejuvenation	Week of unstructured training
EASY	**Weeks to Race** 7	Avoid temptation to return too soon	Week of easy training
BUILD	**Strength** SM **Weeks to Race** 4–6	Build race-specific muscular endurance	Race-simulation bricks in weeks 23 and 24; focus on TT through the rolling hills
		Midweek bike muscular endurance session	
		Century ride (B-priority)	Target large negative split on century ride; maximize time on the aerobars
PEAK	**Strength** SM **Weeks to Race** 2–3	Specific race preparation	2 race-simulation bricks per week
			Add weekly open-water swim
RACE		**Ironman (AAA-priority)**	
OFF			

TABLE 12.5 CONTINUED

TABLE 12.6 RACHEL THE RUNNER'S BASE TRAINING

BASE 2, WEEK 2		TRAINING	NOTES	DAILY TIME (HOURS)
Monday		Run 30 min.	Speed skills	2.00
		Strength 1 hour	Strength maintenance	
		Bike 30 min.	Easy spin	
Tuesday	AM	Swim 1 hour, 15 min.	Masters swim	2.50
	PM	Run 1 hour, 15 min.	Aerobic run	
Wednesday	AM	Bike 1 hour, 30 min.	Muscular endurance bike on trainer	2.50
	PM	Run 1 hour	Tempo run	
Thursday		Swim 45 min.	Technique swim	0.75
Friday		Run 30 min.	Speed skills	2.25
		Strength 1 hour	Strength maintenance	
		Bike 45 min.	Easy spin	
Saturday	AM	Swim 1 hour, 30 min.	Masters swim	7.00
	PM	Bike 5 hours	Endurance ride	
		Run 30 min.	Easy transition run	
Sunday		Day off		0.00
Weekly total				**17.00**

BASE 2, WEEK 3				
Monday		Run 30 min.	Speed skills	1.75
		Strength 60 min.	Strength maintenance	
		Bike 15 min.	Easy spin	
Tuesday	AM	Swim 1 hour, 15 min.	Masters swim	3.00
	PM	Bike 1 hour, 45 min.	Aerobic ride	
Wednesday	AM	Bike 1 hour, 30 min.	Muscular endurance bike on trainer	2.50
	PM	Run 1 hour	Tempo run	
Thursday	AM	Bike 30 min.	Speed skills	3.00
		Strength 1 hour	Strength maintenance	
		Bike 15 min.	Easy spin	
	PM	Swim 1 hour, 15 min.	Technique swim	
Friday		Day off		0.00
Saturday		Swim 45 min.	Open-water swim	1.50
		Bike 30 min.	Easy spin	
		Run 15 min.	Easy run	
Sunday		**Olympic-distance triathlon**		TBD
Weekly total				**11.75**

Note: ▭ = Strength training sessions   ▭ = Brick workouts

TABLE 12.7 RACHEL THE RUNNER'S BUILD TRAINING

BUILD, WEEK 1		TRAINING	NOTES	DAILY TIME (HOURS)
Monday		Run 30 min.	Speed skills	1.75
		Strength 1 hour	Strength maintenance	
		Bike 15 min.	Easy spin	
Tuesday	AM	Swim 1 hour, 15 min.	Masters swim	2.75
	PM	Bike 1 hour, 30 min.	Steady ride	
Wednesday		Bike 2 hours, 30 min.	Steady brick	3.00
		Run 30 min.		
Thursday	AM	Swim 60 min.	Masters swim	2.50
	PM	Bike 1 hour, 30 min.	Muscular endurance bike	
Friday		Day off		0.00
Saturday	AM	Swim 1 hour, 30 min.	Masters swim	2.25
	PM	Bike 45 min.	Speed skills	
Sunday		Bike 3 hours	Race-simulation brick	4.50
		Run 1 hour, 30 min.		
Weekly total				**16.75**

BUILD, WEEK 2				
Monday		Bike 15 min.	Easy spin to warm up	1.50
		Strength 1 hour	Strength maintenance	
		Bike 15 min.	Easy spin	
Tuesday		Swim 1 hour, 15 min.	Masters swim	1.25
Wednesday		Bike 2 hours	Steady brick	3.00
		Run 1 hour		
Thursday	AM	Bike 1 hour, 30 min.	Masters swim	2.75
	PM	Swim 1 hour, 15 min.	Muscular endurance bike	
Friday		Run 1 hour, 15 min.	Tempo run	1.25
Saturday		Swim 1 hour, 30 min.	Masters swim	1.50
Sunday		Bike 4 hours	Race-simulation brick	5.00
		Run 1 hour	Steady ride BT	
Weekly total				**16.25**

Note: ▨ = Strength training sessions ▨ = Brick workouts

TABLE 12.8 RACHEL THE RUNNER'S PEAK TRAINING

PEAK, WEEK 1		TRAINING	NOTES	DAILY TIME (HOURS)
Monday	AM	Swim 1 hour, 15 min.	Masters swim	2.25
	PM	Run 1 hour	Speed skills	
Tuesday		Bike 15 min.	Easy spin to warm up	1.25
		Strength 45 min.	Strength maintenance	
		Bike 15 min.	Easy spin	
Wednesday	AM	Swim 45 min.	Technique swim	3.00
	PM	Bike 1 hour, 30 min.	Race-simulation brick	
		Run 45 min.		
Thursday		Day off		0.00
Friday	AM	Swim 1 hour, 15 min.	Masters swim	2.75
	PM	Bike 1 hour, 30 min.	Aerobic maintenance ride	
Saturday		Bike 3 hours	Race-simulation brick	4.00
		Run 1 hour		
Sunday		Swim 45 min.	Open-water swim	0.75
Weekly total				**14.00**

PEAK, WEEK 2				
Monday	AM	Swim 1 hour, 15 min.	Masters swim	2.00
	PM	Run 45 min.	Speed skills	
Tuesday		Bike 15 min.	Easy spin to warm up	1.25
		Strength 45 min.	Strength maintenance	
		Bike 15 min.	Easy spin	
Wednesday	AM	Swim 1 hour	Technique swim	3.00
	PM	Bike 1 hour, 30 min.	Race-simulation brick	
		Run 30 min.		
Thursday		Day off		0.00
Friday	AM	Swim 1 hour, 15 min.	Masters swim	2.25
	PM	Bike 1 hour	Aerobic maintenance ride	
Saturday		Bike 1 hour, 15 min.	Race-simulation brick	2.00
		Run 45 min.		
Sunday		Swim 1 hour	Open-water swim	1.00
Weekly total				**11.50**

Note: [   ] = Strength training sessions   [   ] = Brick workouts

THE VETERAN

Kona Ken has been in the sport of triathlon for a number of years. His sole focus for the upcoming season is to qualify for Ironman Hawaii. He came painfully close to a rolldown slot this past season, missing by less than 15 min. (At every qualifying race for the World Championship, slots not taken by the top performers "roll down" to the slower athletes in each race division. Many athletes have come within minutes of earning a ticket to the World Championship.) He is a well-balanced athlete, and his times are consistently in the top 25 percent for all three sports. He loves to ride and has excellent overall endurance. He works full-time but has significant flexibility with his schedule.

Ken has read a number of training guides and has a good understanding of all aspects of training. He's had a few minor injuries over the years but is biomechanically sound. His work ethic is well-known in the local triathlon community, and he prides himself on his ability to train hard year-round. Last season he had excellent performance in his early races but was disappointed when his early results didn't translate to late-season Ironman-distance performance. In reviewing his past season, Ken realizes that he was likely tired for most of the summer.

Ken's race season is geared toward giving him the maximum opportunity to qualify. Ken lives in a climate that enables him to ride outdoors year-round, and he has plenty of buddies who are up for a tough session at any time. Ken's season is built around two Ironman-distance races. If he manages to qualify at his first Ironman-distance race of the year, then he plans on skipping the second to focus on Ironman Hawaii.

In order to ensure freshness through the season, Ken is going to limit his group training until he is in the Build period for his first Ironman-distance race. Following that race, he has scheduled two weeks completely off, followed by two transition weeks. When he returns to training after his midseason break, he is going to repeat Base 1 and Base 2 but shorten them to three-week periods. To ensure that he maintains his overall strength, he is going to repeat the Prep period of his strength program.

Ken's qualification strategy is to use specific race-simulation workouts to better guide his race day pacing, specifically his early bike efforts. Improved pacing, better recovery, and avoiding last year's burnout should give him the boost that he wants to get to the Big Show. If he makes it to Kona, then he's promised himself to enjoy the day and celebrate the hard work that it took to get there.

With his swimming, Ken is going to focus on two key workouts per week: his long endurance session and a challenging muscular endurance workout. In order to prepare his body to ride after a long swim, Ken will occasionally swim prior to his long ride. Ken's focus for his running will be volume built through consistency. The bulk of his "fast" running will be done in his B- and C-priority races. Given his prior experience with going flat during the season, he needs to be careful not to overuse high-intensity training.

Tables 12.9–12.12 show Ken's training regimen.

TABLE 12.9 KONA KEN'S ANNUAL TRAINING PLAN AND TACTICS

		GOALS	TACTICS
PREP 1	**Strength AA1** **Weeks to Race 24–27**	Reestablish structured training	Workout frequency
		Improve strength training	1 session/week with personal trainer to learn proper technique
		Improve technical skills	Swim and bike skills training 2 times/week
PREP 2	**Strength AA2** **Weeks to Race 20–23**	Build swim endurance	Swim a lane down in masters; focus on perfect technique
		Stay fresh	Avoid group training; limit riding to small chainring only
		Increase functional strength	Learn new strength training techniques (Swiss Ball, medicine ball)
BASE 1	**Strength AA3** **Weeks to Race 16–19**	Build run endurance prior to MS lifting	Weekly endurance run session
		Stay fresh	Continue to avoid group training
		Build bike endurance	Weekly long ride and cycling frequency focus
BASE 2	**Strength MS** **Weeks to Race 12–15**	Get strong	Achieve life-best strength in key lifts
		Stay healthy	Show caution with run volume
		Build bike endurance	Build long-ride volume and focus on cycling frequency
BASE 3	**Strength SM** **Weeks to Race 8–11**	Start muscular endurance bike training	1st 4 weeks of 8-week bike muscular endurance program
		Increase bike endurance	1 stretch week with cycling volume focus
		Test aerobic run speed	Half-marathon race at end of recovery week
		Half-marathon (B-priority)	
BUILD	**Strength SM** **Weeks to Race 4–7**	Specific race preparation	Run-pacing BT to determine appropriate run speed
			Use steady-ride BT to determine appropriate bike effort
			Use race-specific muscular endurance BTs to prepare for specific race terrain
			Strength training takes backseat to sport-specific work
		Olympic (C-priority)	

continued >

TABLE 12.9 CONTINUED

		GOALS	TACTICS
PEAK	**Strength** SM **Weeks to Race** 2–3	Specific race preparation	2 race-simulation bricks/week
			Add weekly open-water swim
RACE	**Weeks to Race** 1	**Ironman (A-priority)**	
OFF	**Weeks to Race** 21	Rejuvenation	No training at all
OFF	**Weeks to Race** 20		
TRANS	**Strength** AA1 **Weeks to Race** 18–19	Rejuvenation	Skills and light aerobic training only
			Return to gym for high-repetition, low-intensity training
BASE 1	**Strength** AA1 **Weeks to Race** 15–17	Stimulate aerobic systems	Focus on workout frequency
		Target a late-season peak	Limited use of muscular endurance training; interval duration kept short
		Maintain quickness in all sports **Olympic (C-priority)**	Weekly speed-skills sessions
BASE 2	**Strength** AA2 **Weeks to Race** 12–14	Reestablish race-specific endurance	Increase steady-state training in all sports
		Stay fresh **Olympic (C-priority)**	Show caution with group training
BASE 3	**Strength** AA3 **Weeks to Race** 8–11	Build race-specific muscular endurance	Steady-state endurance training with moderate muscular endurance inserts
		Complete overall endurance focus	2 stretch weeks with bike volume focus
		Check overall fitness	Use half-Ironman race to test fitness and guide final prep
		Half-Ironman (B-priority)	

continued >

TABLE 12.9 CONTINUED

		GOALS	TACTICS
TRANS	Weeks to Race 7		
BUILD	Strength SM Weeks to Race 4–6	Specific race preparation	No racing to focus on race-simulation training Same tactics as previous Build period Apply lessons from training and racing to date
PEAK	Strength SM Weeks to Race 2–3	Specific race preparation	2 race-simulation bricks/week Add weekly open-water swim
RACE	Weeks to Race 1	**Ironman (AAA-priority)**	
TRANS	Strength SM Weeks to Race 4–6	Rejuvenation	
PEAK	Strength SM Weeks to Race 2–3	Ensure freshness on race day	Repeat previous Peak period but eliminate all high-intensity work
RACE		**Ironman (fun)**	

TABLE 12.10 KONA KEN'S MIDSEASON BASE TRAINING

BASE 3, WEEK 1		TRAINING	NOTES	DAILY TIME (HOURS)
Monday	AM	Run 30 min.	Run speed skills	3.00
		Strength 1 hour	Strength maintenance	
		Bike 15 min.	Easy spin	
	PM	Swim 1 hour, 15 min.	Masters swim	
Tuesday		Bike 3 hours	Easy ride	3.00
Wednesday	AM	Bike 2 hours, 30 min.	Steady brick with short muscular endurance intervals	4.25
		Run 30 min.		
	PM	Swim 1 hour, 15 min.	Masters swim	
Thursday	AM	Bike 1 hour, 45 min.	Steady ride	3.25
	PM	Run 1 hour, 30 min.	Endurance run	
Friday		Swim 1 hour, 30 min.	Endurance swim	1.50
Saturday		Bike 5 hours	Endurance ride	5.50
		Run 30 min.	Easy transition run	
Sunday		Day off		0.00
Weekly total				**20.50**

BASE 3, WEEK 2				
Monday	AM	Run 30 min.	Speed skills	3.00
		Strength 1 hour	Strength maintenance	
		Bike 15 min.	Easy spin	
	PM	Swim 1 hour, 15 min.	Masters swim	
Tuesday		Bike 2 hours	Easy ride	2.00
Wednesday	AM	Run 2 hours	Endurance run	3.25
	PM	Swim 1 hour, 15 min.	Masters swim	
Thursday		Bike 30 min.	Easy spin to warm up	1.75
		Strength 1 hour	Strength maintenance	
		Bike 15 min.	Easy spin	
Friday		Swim 1 hour, 30 min.	Endurance swim	1.50
Saturday		Bike 5 hours	Endurance ride	5.50
		Run 30 min.	Easy transition run	
Sunday		Day off		0.00
Weekly total				**17.00**

Note: ▨ = Strength training sessions　▨ = Brick workouts

TABLE 12.11 KONA KEN'S BUILD TRAINING

BUILD, WEEK 1		TRAINING	NOTES	DAILY TIME (HOURS)
Monday		Bike 3 hours	Race-simulation brick	4.50
		Run 1 hour, 30 min.		
Tuesday		Day off		0.00
Wednesday	AM	Bike 15 min.	Easy spin	2.75
		Strength 45 min.	Strength maintenance	
		Bike 15 min.	Easy spin	
	PM	Swim 1 hour, 30 min.	Endurance swim	
Thursday		Bike 4 hours	Steady BT ride	4.50
		Run 30 min.	Easy run	
Friday		Swim 1 hour	Technique swim	1.00
Saturday		Run 45 min.	Speed skills	2.00
		Strength 45 min.	Strength maintenance	
		Bike 30 min.	Easy spin	
Sunday	AM	Swim 1 hour, 30 min.	Muscular endurance swim	3.50
	PM	Run 2 hours	Run-pacing BT	
Weekly total				**18.25**

BUILD, WEEK 2				
Monday		Day off		0.00
Tuesday	AM	Bike 1 hour, 30 min.	Endurance ride	3.00
	PM	Swim 1 hour, 30 min.	Endurance swim	
Wednesday		Bike 4 hours	Race-simulation brick	5.00
		Run 1 hour		
Thursday		Bike 15 min.	Easy spin to warm up	1.25
		Strength 45 min.	Strength maintenance	
		Bike 15 min.	Easy spin	
Friday		Swim 1 hour, 30 min.	Muscular endurance swim	1.50
Saturday		Bike 2 hours, 30 min.	Race-simulation brick	4.00
		Run 1 hour, 30 min.		
Sunday		Swim 45 min.	Technique swim	0.75
Weekly total				**15.50**

Note: ▨ = Strength training sessions   ▨ = Brick workouts

TABLE 12.12 KONA KEN'S PEAK TRAINING

PEAK, WEEK 1		TRAINING	NOTES	DAILY TIME (HOURS)
Monday		Swim 1 hour, 15 min.	Technique swim	1.25
Tuesday		Run 30 min.	Speed skills	1.75
		Strength 45 min.	Strength maintenance	
		Bike 30 min.	Easy spin	
Wednesday	AM	Swim 45 min.	Technique swim	4.25
	PM	Bike 2 hours, 15 min.	Race-simulation brick	
		Run 1 hour, 15 min.		
Thursday		Day off		0.00
Friday	AM	Bike 1 hour, 15 min.	Aerobic maintenance brick	3.00
		Run 15 min.		
	PM	Swim 1 hour, 30 min.	Muscular endurance swim	
Saturday		Bike 2 hours, 30 min.	Race-simulation brick	3.50
		Run 1 hour		
Sunday		Swim 1 hour, 15 min.	Open-water swim	1.25
Weekly total				**15.00**

PEAK, WEEK 2				
Monday		Run 30 min.	Speed skills	1.50
		Strength 45 min.	Strength maintenance	
		Bike 15 min.	Easy spin	
Tuesday	AM	Bike 45 min.	Easy spin	2.00
	PM	Swim 1 hour, 15 min.	Endurance swim	
Wednesday		Bike 1 hour, 45 min.	Race-simulation brick	2.50
		Run 45 min.		
Thursday		Day off		0.00
Friday	AM	Bike 1 hour, 15 min.	Aerobic maintenance brick	2.75
		Run 15 min.		
	PM	Swim 1 hour, 15 min.	Muscular endurance swim	
Saturday		Bike 1 hour, 45 min.	Race-simulation brick	2.25
		Run 30 min.		
Sunday		Swim 1 hour	Open-water swim	1.00
Weekly total				**12.00**

Note: ▨ = Strength training sessions   ▨ = Brick workouts

THE WORKING ATHLETE

One of the challenges of using a traditional periodization model is that the cycles of volume don't always fit with the realities of your life. Put another way, when you use a periodization table to determine your training schedule, you may be doing either too little or too much. As you now know, of these two situations, doing too much is the most risky. What follows is an alternative approach that may help you achieve greater consistency and satisfaction with your training.

- *Ultimate goal:* To maximize training consistency over multiple months and seasons. By aiming for a "little less" each week, you will achieve more over the long run.
- *Weekday training:* Determined by the reality of your life situation, primarily your obligations to work and family.
- *Weekend training:* Split between an endurance day (typically Saturday) and a family day (typically Sunday).
- *Endurance day:* Training shifts based on your experience, fitness, goal event, and time of year. The nature of your endurance day will progress gradually and in harmony with daylight, climate, and your fitness. In your early Base period, the purpose of this session is to build endurance. As the season progresses, your focus shifts toward the ability to perform across your desired race duration.
- *Family day:* Make the people who support your athletic goals your top priority. This improves your emotional harmony and gives you a break from athletics. Another positive benefit is that you arrive at work on Monday feeling fresh—meaning that you remain happily employed and ready to increase the quality of your weekday sessions.

By working out a training schedule with input from all the key players in your life, you remove the constant struggle to "squeeze in" and "juggle" training sessions. You have an agreed-upon structure that you'll repeat over the long term. This is a holistic approach that fits your training into the larger goal of a successful lifestyle.

When you plan your training schedule, aim for a structure that you can complete "no sweat" for forty weeks per year. Also, while the structure of the training week remains similar, deliberately vary your training protocol (what you do in each session) every six to eight weeks according to the guidelines in this book.

The two sample weeks shown in Table 12.13 provide an excellent starting point for applying this concept.

TABLE 12.13 WORKING ATHLETE'S TRAINING PLAN, SAMPLE WEEKS

STANDARD PROGRAM			
Monday	Bike/run		
Tuesday	Swim/strength		
Wednesday	Second-longest bike/run		
Thursday	Long run		
Friday	Long swim		
Saturday	Endurance day		
Sunday	Nontriathlon day		

ADVANCED PROGRAM		
Monday	AM	Swim/strength
	PM	Bike/run
Tuesday	AM	Long run
	PM	[Spin/yoga]
Wednesday	AM	Swim
	PM	[Spin]
Thursday	AM	Second-longest bike/run
	PM	[Yoga]
Friday		Long swim/strength
Saturday		Endurance day
Sunday		Nontriathlon day

Note: Workouts in square brackets are optional.

Taking the concept further, how can you apply the concepts of the basic week to your own program? Start by asking yourself the following questions:

- What is your number-one goal event for this year?
- When is it?
- How long do you expect to take to finish? If you make an error in this estimation, it is better to assume a little too long than too short for the duration of the race.
- How many events that long, or longer, have you completed in the last two years?

These first four questions help you focus on the most appropriate training for the bulk of your year. Nearly every athlete lining up for an Ironman-distance race will benefit from placing his or her training focus on Base-oriented workouts and using the Build period for race-simulation (rather than high-intensity) workouts.

- What is your preferred day for your longest training day of the week? We recommend a nonwork day. Please choose a specific day of the week.
- Do you like to have a total rest day (no training at all)?

These questions enable you to place your "anchor" workout on the most important day of your training week. In the examples shown in Table 12.13, this day is assumed to be Saturday. However, the exact day of the week is not important. Simply mark your preferred day "endurance day" and mark the day after as your easiest day of the week ("nontriathlon day" in the example). If you prefer a total rest day, then your nontriathlon day will be free of exercise. If you prefer light activity, then a technique swim, light yoga session, or easy spin would be appropriate.

In the winter and early spring, your endurance day can consist of crosstraining or a mix of activities the main goal of which is to build your endurance. As the weather improves and your race approaches, your endurance day should gradually shift toward more specific training and eventually include your race-simulation workouts.

The rest of your workouts can be placed using the template in Table 12.13. Remember that you are much more likely to be successful if you aim for a little less than you think possible. You will receive a big mental boost each week from giving yourself room to outperform.

Use the information in Part II of this book to create workouts for the rest of the week. Keep the structure of your workouts simple, and focus on the key elements of long-course racing (endurance and muscular endurance). You will find that consistent application of your basic week is far more important than the fine detail contained in the exact training protocol that you plan to use.

Finally, ensure that you schedule recovery within each week, each training block, and each series of blocks. Voluntarily unloading training stress will keep your program enjoyable and greatly reduce the risks associated with injury, burnout, and excessive fatigue.

Finishing Strong

PART IV

CHAPTER 13

RECOVERY AND WELLNESS

WITH JEFF SHILT, MD

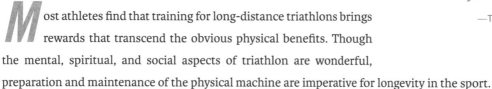

> *Do what you can, with what you have, where you are.*
> —THEODORE ROOSEVELT

Most athletes find that training for long-distance triathlons brings rewards that transcend the obvious physical benefits. Though the mental, spiritual, and social aspects of triathlon are wonderful, preparation and maintenance of the physical machine are imperative for longevity in the sport.

Much like training protocols and nutrition, health care maintenance for endurance athletes is evolving. Within the medical community, awareness of injury prevention and treatment lags behind advances in endurance training protocols. The following recommendations will serve as guidelines for anyone seeking a healthy approach to endurance training.

HEALTH BASELINE

Establishing a personal health baseline with a physical exam and blood work is important for two reasons. First and foremost, the standard health guidelines that pertain to the general population are not likely to be relevant because of the increased physical demands you are placing on your body and the nutritional constraints that accompany such an effort. Furthermore, the extreme physical stress of training can reveal chronic conditions that might otherwise go unnoticed. By completing a baseline exam in your Prep period (a step we recommend for athletes at all levels), you will have a better understanding of what is normal and healthy for your body before you put it through the test of training for an Ironman.

Blood work results are considered normal within a wide range of values in order to include the majority of the healthy population. Because "normal" is so broadly defined, it is not the most useful standard for most endurance athletes. Your healthy baseline is the optimal basis for comparison.

FERRITIN LEVELS SHOULD BE CLOSELY MONITORED and ideally maintained above 80 ng/ml in females and 100 ng/ml in males. Should your baseline ferritin level fluctuate more than 25 percent, with a corresponding decrease in serum iron and iron saturation and a concomitant rise in total iron binding capacity, it could be an indication that you need treatment. Excessive fatigue and poor performance can be the result of low iron stores, or anemia.

Ideally, a medical care provider knowledgeable about endurance training and familiar with your personal health baseline will interpret your tests. Lab results must be considered in relation to your training, previous test values, and other personal demographic variables.

Demographic variables are important, and both age and sex can alter the normal values. Intense training periods (generally in the final twelve weeks before an A-priority event) will elevate levels of certain enzymes and other indicators of muscle damage or inflammation.

Younger triathletes and those with several years' experience in endurance sports will naturally have higher baseline values for testosterone, luteinizing hormone, and platelet levels. These possible variations by age and sex are additional reasons to establish your individual healthy baseline.

Table 13.1 lists the recommended laboratory tests, some of which assess your general health status. The Comprehensive Metabolic Panel (CMP) is composed of fourteen separate measures of organ function and muscle inflammation. Creatinine, ALT, and AST are the only components of CMP that should be tested on a quarterly basis; however, the test is often ordered as a complete panel. The CBC is a panel that looks more closely at bone marrow function and can provide indicators of problems such as immune function disorders or anemia.

Repeat blood work should be done quarterly, ideally at the start of the Prep, Base, Build, and Peak periods. Nearly all blood parameters elevated by intense exercise sessions studied in the routine profile should return to normal during this period of time. By timing your recovery periods in this way, you will optimize the benefits of your important training cycles.

If your values do not fall within your baseline, many things should be considered. Statistical variability can play a role, and up to 5 percent of normal values will be incorrectly

TABLE 13.1 RECOMMENDED LABORATORY TESTS

BLOOD TEST	BASELINE	QUARTERLY/ SYMPTOMATIC	WHAT TEST MEASURES
Cortisol	X	X	Body's response to stress
Free testosterone	X	X	Level of male hormone
Lipid profile	X		Level of circulating fat
Cholesterol		X	
HDL			Good cholesterol
LDL			Bad cholesterol
Triglycerides			
CBCs	X	X	Oxygen-carrying capacity of blood and platelet count
Iron with TIBC	X		Iron status in body
Transferrin	X		Nutrition and liver status
Ferritin	X	X	Amount of stored iron (best test for iron deficiency)
Vitamin B12	X		Levels of one of the eight subtypes of vitamin B (diagnoses macrocytic anemia)
Folic acid	X		Levels of one of the eight subtypes of vitamin B (diagnoses macrocytic anemia)
CMP*	X	X	Organ function (panel includes 14 tests)
TSH	X		Thyroid function
CRP or ESR	X	X	Levels of inflammation

Notes: * indicates that test does not need to be repeated unless symptoms suggest otherwise. HDL = high-density lipoprotein; LDL = low-density lipoprotein; CBC = complete blood count; TSC = thyroid-stimulating hormone; CMP = comprehensive metabolic panel

Normal values are not included for the lab tests. We recommend that you consult the physician ordering and evaluating the tests.

reported "out of range." You can request that the test be repeated on the same blood sample, and sometimes the result will then be within the normal range. Before drawing conclusions about abnormal results or contemplating treatment, you should always do another test. Many facilities maintain their own reference ranges, so it is ideal to have your blood work done in the same location. Some tests have a very high degree of consistency from location to location, so these results can be compared without concern.

If an abnormal result is confirmed, it may indicate a problem and warrant further investigation. A physician familiar with endurance training is invaluable in determining the significance of a result that deviates from your baseline.

ACTIVE RECOVERY

To improve your fitness, you will apply and absorb varying amounts of physical stress. However, your training must be balanced by appropriate recovery. When this delicate balance is upset, overuse injuries occur.

Most physicians recommend that overuse injuries be treated with rest, ice, compression, and elevation (RICE). This approach is frustrating to the highly motivated athlete. Long periods of rest lead to significant musculoskeletal deconditioning; a longer recovery period; and the most damaging result, depression. When used appropriately, active recovery facilitates a faster return to training and can stave off the negative aspects that accompany long periods of rest.

Active recovery is not a magic bullet, and before embarking on it, you must consider the underlying cause of overuse injuries. Successful application of this approach requires patience and diligence. Accelerating the process beyond your body's ability to heal can cause further damage or prolong your injured state.

Before applying the principles of active recovery, an accurate diagnosis is imperative. Misdiagnosis can worsen your actual condition, resulting in extended, and additional, treatment. Carefully review the conditions appropriate for active recovery in Table 13.2. If you think that you may have a condition that requires medical evaluation or intervention, you should immediately see a health care professional.

> **AVOID INJURY AND ACCELERATE RECOVERY**
>
> Active recovery can be preventive: By incorporating low-intensity exercise following workouts, you will speed the musculoskeletal rebuilding phase and recharge your body for the next training session. Active recovery should be used during the cool-down phase of a workout and should be composed of 10–15 min. of activity at heart rate Zone 1.
>
> Additionally, active recovery should be included in the 48 hours following a competition or BT workout. Active recovery workouts are part of periodized training, so this is in keeping with the guidelines for planning your week and training periods. Limit recovery sessions to 1 hour or less, and keep them very easy.

■ *Treating Overuse Injuries*

Active rest is gaining popularity in injury recovery. Like active recovery, this method involves low-intensity exercises to stimulate blood flow to the musculoskeletal system. However, active rest maintains intensity below that of your steady training zones. Though little is known regarding the exact processes responsible for healing, the results of this approach are superior to those of the commonly applied RICE program. Though the other components of the RICE method are likely beneficial in all approaches, complete immobilization, or rest, is often counterproductive to healing soft-tissue injury.

TABLE 13.2 INJURIES, SYMPTOMS, AND APPROPRIATE RESPONSES

CONDITION	LAYPERSON'S TERM	COMMON SYMPTOMS
Diagnoses responding to active recovery		
Achilles tendinitis		Pain in tendon above heel
Plantar fasciitis	Heel spurs	Pain in heel
Patellofemoral syndrome/ quadriceps or patellar tendinopathy	Runner's knee	Pain in kneecap
Hamstring tendinopathy		Pain along tendon in back of thigh by buttock or knee
Iliotibial band syndrome	Lateral runner's knee	Ache/pain/burning along outside of knee
Piriformis syndrome		Pain, numbness, or tingling in buttock and back of leg
Rotator cuff tendinopathy	Swimmer's shoulder	Pain when beginning the pull phase of the swim stroke
Diagnoses requiring medical evaluation		
Tibial periostitis	Shin splints	Pain along the shin bone
Morton's neuroma		Pain or tingling, usually between third and fourth toes
Acromioclavicular injuries		Bump and pain after fall on shoulder
Rotator cuff tears		Shoulder pain, common with overhead injuries
Diagnoses requiring medical intervention		
Exertional compartment syndrome		Pain in calf with exercise
Stress fractures	Broken bone	Pain in affected bone
Fractures	Broken bone	Pain in affected bone
Meniscal tears	Torn cartilage in knee	Painful catching or popping in knee

In order to accelerate the healing process and reduce lost time from exercise, it helps to carefully apply an active rehabilitation process. We recommend three phases to accomplish this goal.

Active rest. Begin with activity modification. This means eliminating the sport or training pattern that initiated or aggravated your symptoms. You can treat any pain and swelling with ice and nonsteroidal anti-inflammatory drugs (NSAIDs). Keep in mind that NSAIDs are an excellent treatment for inflammation and discomfort after hard training sessions and races;

however, there is no scientific evidence that their use during training or races will lead to improvement in performance or reduction in pain. In fact, during sustained exercise, NSAIDs may actually cause health problems (see sidebar, "Ibuprofen and Other NSAIDs"). As soon as reasonably possible, begin active motion (motion performed by you) of the injured area. Avoid painful passive motion (motion performed by others). When possible, initiate an eccentric exercise program, as described in the next section. During this period, continue cardiovascular fitness with aerobic activities that do not involve the injured area. Institute soft-tissue therapy to loosen up knots and tight areas.

Reconditioning. Once you obtain full (pain-free) range of motion, further gains in strength should be sought to correct deficits created by the injury. These gains are accomplished with progressive loads, stretching, and proprioceptive training.

Resumption of sport. After you reach your preinjury strength, complete a short Base period to ensure that you can withstand increased training load. Depending upon your time in the sport and the severity of your injury, this Base period can be as short as four weeks. It is common to require twelve weeks (or more) with more severe injuries. If you are a novice, you should be conservative and plan on a longer Base period.

■ *Eccentric Exercise*

An eccentric strengthening program places the muscle under load while lengthening, in contrast to the more common concentric contraction, in which the muscle is under load while being shortened. This approach helps increase the durability of the muscle so that it becomes more resistant to injury. As you progress with the exercises, you can begin to increase the speed of the eccentric contraction. This results in increased power to the exercised muscle. You should wait a minimum of three weeks after an injury before seeking specific strength gains through the rehabilitation process.

A general description of an eccentric program is listed below. These principles can be applied to any muscle group.

1. Maintain a static stretch of the affected muscle for 15–30 sec. Repeat this stretch three to five times consecutively.
2. Perform the eccentric exercise slowly on the first two days and increase the speed gradually over the next five days. By day seven, the exercise should be performed quickly. Expect muscle soreness during the first one to two weeks of training.

Ibuprofen and Other NSAIDs

Ibuprofen and other nonsteroidal anti-inflammatory drugs (NSAIDs), such as Naprosyn, Aleve, and Motrin, are excellent treatment options for inflammation and pain and can be very helpful after intense training sessions or races. However, they should be avoided during such sessions because they have been shown to negatively affect kidney and liver function by restricting blood flow and filtration rates. This effect has the potential to promote hyponatremia (low sodium levels) and dehydration. In sustained exercise, these problems can not only reduce performance but also threaten health.

Some reports noted a connection between NSAIDs and numerous cases of symptomatic hyponatremia several years ago at Ironman® Canada. Many athletes were hospitalized after this event, and in review, it was discovered that most of them had been using NSAIDs for several days prior to the race or were using them during the race. NSAID-induced hyponatremia is related to impairment in antidiuretic hormone release. In addition, NSAIDs can cause acute renal failure in dehydrated athletes and can also lead to NSAID toxicity and rhabdomyolysis (skeletal muscle breakdown after repetitive muscle trauma, for example pavement pounding).

Acetaminophen, such as Tylenol, has a less dramatic effect on these functions and may relieve discomfort just as well as ibuprofen. Acetaminophen, however, is not an anti-inflammatory. There are also concerns about its long-term health consequences for those who use it regularly.

Another reason not to use NSAIDs during race situations is their effect on the gut. Many endurance athletes and weekend warriors find themselves being treated for gastrointestinal bleeding. The decreased blood supply to the gut during endurance events may increase the risk of bleeding, and those who have experienced side stitches after ingesting food or carbohydrate-replacement solutions during exertion can be sure that their blood supply to the gut is less than optimal.

If you are taking any NSAIDs for pain, avoid taking any for at least forty-eight hours prior to a race as well as during the race. It is best not to use any medications, including over-the-counter drugs, unless under a doctor's direction.

3. After reaching full speed, increase the resistance. It is essential to limit the load on the muscle to isolate the target muscle group. Excessive added weight commonly requires assistance by additional muscle groups, diluting the benefit of the program.

4. Repeat the static stretch as initially described.

Athletes who patiently and consistently apply eccentric exercise programs experience excellent pain relief and faster return to function. This process outperforms traditional approaches of concentric exercise, stretching, splinting, friction massage, and ultrasound.

Eccentric exercise is highly effective when using active recovery techniques for treating tendinitis. For tendinitis, a two-step treatment approach is optimal. Warm up with a flexibility routine to increase the resting length of the affected muscle-tendon unit, thereby reducing stresses on the joint. Then, in the same session, continue on to an eccentric exercise program that uses progressively increasing loads. Discomfort is common during the progression of the program, and exercise should continue as long as it can be tolerated.

Excellent protocols have been established for the most common issues facing triathletes—rotator cuff tendinopathy, Achilles tendinopathy/plantar fasciitis, patellofemoral syndrome/patellar and quadriceps tendinopathy, hamstring tendinopathy, iliotibial band syndrome, and piriformis syndrome—all of which are described in more detail in the following sections. For each of these exercises, perform three sets of fifteen repetitions (twice daily) for twelve weeks.

Rotator Cuff (Supraspinatus) Tendinopathy

The athlete slowly lowers the arm from a position parallel to the ground (see Figure 13.1a) to one in which the arm is nearly perpendicular to the ground. The arm is in 30 degrees of abduction and the thumb is pointed toward the ground (see Figure 13.1b). The unaffected arm should be used to assist the affected or injured arm back to a perpendicular position.

Weight is slowly added to the exercise when the motion is performed without pain. The weight is gradually increased by adding a small amount of weight, each time reaching a new level of slightly painful training.

Use great caution when adding weight during rotator cuff training. If excessive weight is added, the deltoid will compensate for the weak rotator cuff, and the exercise will no longer be effective. It is rare to require more than 10 pounds for this exercise; 5 pounds is most commonly used.

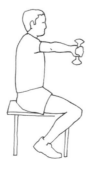

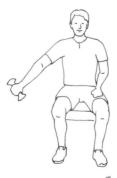

FIGURE *13.1a*   FIGURE *13.1b*

Achilles Tendinopathy/Plantar Fasciitis

The Achilles is a conjoined tendon of the gastrocnemius and soleus muscles. Therefore, the calf muscle is eccentrically loaded both with the knee straight and bent. When straight, the gastrocnemius is primarily activated; when bent, activation of the soleus muscle occurs.

Initially, the load should consist of body weight alone, with the athlete standing on a step. Movement is achieved by using both legs to lift (up on two legs). The exercise is performed eccentrically by the injured leg providing all resistance for the extension phase (down on one leg). As the athlete progresses, the protocol shifts from a count of "up on two, down on one" to "up on one, down on one," with the injured leg taking the full load throughout the exercise cycle.

Figures 13.2a–13.2c show the starting and ending points of this exercise. Expect some discomfort during it. After you are able to complete the progression without pain, you may choose to add weight to further build strength (see Figure 13.3).

It is also recommended that you wear a night splint that maintains the foot at 90 degrees while you are sleeping. If your injury is slow to heal, shock-wave therapy may be beneficial. Finally, make certain your running shoes and bicycle cleats are not excessively worn. Excessive wear can result in excessive pathologic motion. Replacing worn shoes and cleats is helpful.

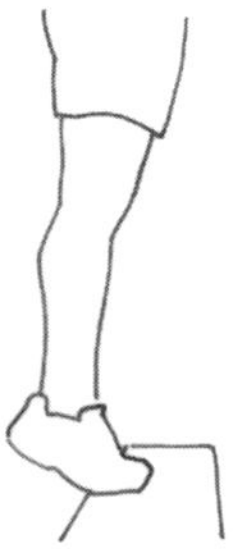

FIGURE *13.2a*
START, GASTROCNEMIUS

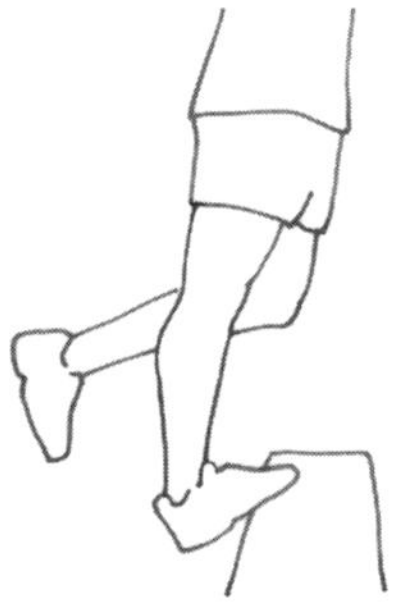

FIGURE *13.2b*
FINISH, GASTROCNEMIUS

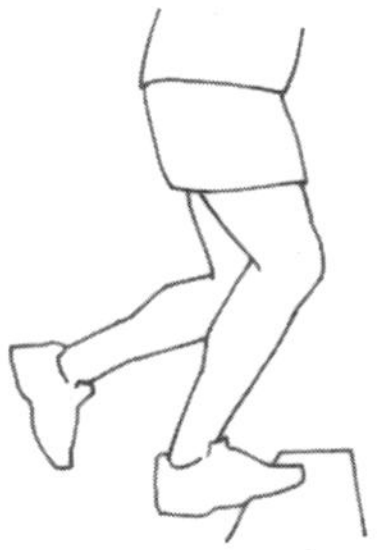

FIGURE *13.2c*
FINISH, SOLEUS

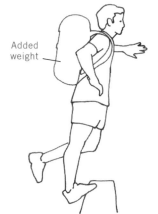

Added weight

FIGURE *13.3*

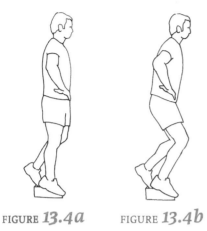

FIGURE *13.4a*   FIGURE *13.4b*

Patellofemoral Syndrome/Patellar and Quadriceps Tendinopathy

Stand on a 25-degree decline board with the entire weight on the injured leg and the knee extended, as shown in Figure 13.4a. From this position, slowly flex the knee to 70 degrees (Figure 13.4b). Return to the starting position using the unaffected leg to fully extend.

Hamstring Tendinopathy

As seen in Figures 13.5a and 13.5b, a stability ball is used in this exercise. Lie on your back with your feet on the ball. Keep your knees, hips, and shoulders in a straight line. Your elbows should be spread wide (at shoulder level) to maintain stability. While keeping the spine and pelvis straight, roll the ball back and forth by bending your knees. Increase the difficulty level by folding your arms over your chest and lifting one leg off the ball (see Figures 13.6a and 13.6b).

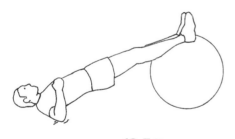

FIGURE *13.5a*

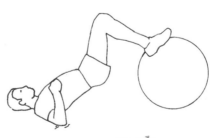

FIGURE *13.5b*

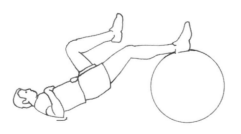

FIGURE *13.6a*

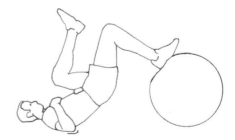

FIGURE *13.6b*

Alternatively, use a hamstring curl machine with a partner. Your partner will raise your leg 90 degrees while you lie on your stomach. Extend your knee slowly.

In later stages, hamstring lowers can be performed. Begin by kneeling on the floor. Your partner places his or her weight on your ankles. You then lower your body slowly to the floor while your partner keeps your feet on the ground (Figures 13.7a and 13.7b). To reduce the stress on the hamstrings, you can use your arms (Figure 13.17c).

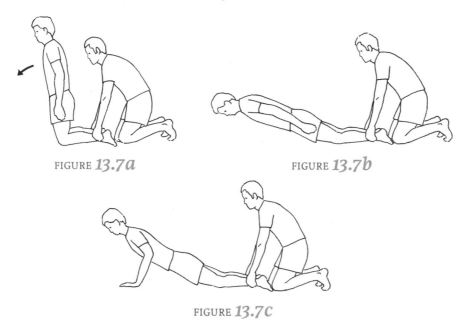

FIGURE *13.7a*   FIGURE *13.7b*

FIGURE *13.7c*

Iliotibial Band (Gluteus Medius) Syndrome

Two exercises are recommended for ITB syndrome: the pelvic drop and the frontal plane lunge.

To begin the pelvic drop exercise, stand on the affected leg on a step. By dropping your pelvis on that side, your unaffected foot dangles off the step and descends toward the floor (Figures 13.8a and 13.8b). Your affected gluteal muscle is stretched during this effort. Bring your foot and pelvis to level position. You may choose to place your hand on a wall for balance.

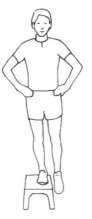
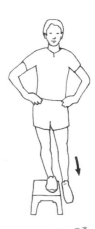

FIGURE *13.8a*   FIGURE *13.8b*

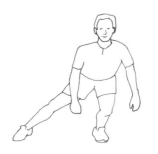

FIGURE **13.9**

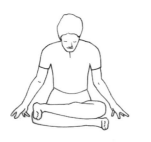

FIGURE **13.10**

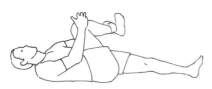

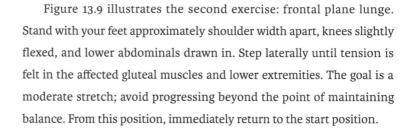

Figure 13.9 illustrates the second exercise: frontal plane lunge. Stand with your feet approximately shoulder width apart, knees slightly flexed, and lower abdominals drawn in. Step laterally until tension is felt in the affected gluteal muscles and lower extremities. The goal is a moderate stretch; avoid progressing beyond the point of maintaining balance. From this position, immediately return to the start position.

Piriformis Syndrome

This syndrome is difficult to diagnose because the pain is vague and often confused with the symptoms of a herniated disk. Pain commonly occurs in the buttock and back of the thigh. The symptoms are exacerbated by flexing the hip, moving the knee toward the midline, and internally rotating the leg (see Figure 13.10). The area just below the mid-buttock is painful to the touch. The pain is generally worse when sitting than standing, although the injury is commonly caused by running.

Unfortunately, no specific eccentric exercise can be recommended for this injury. Treatment is directed at stretching the piriformis and strengthening the hip external rotators.

Yoga has been helpful in addressing symptoms, particularly the following poses: Agnistambhasana (fire log pose; see Figure 13.11), Janusirsasana (head-to-knee forward bend; see Figures 13.12a and 13.12b), and Matsyendrasana (half lord of the fishes; see Figure 13.13). These poses can be achieved by most triathletes slowly and with a little persistence.

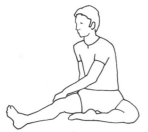

FIGURE **13.11**

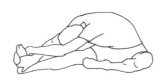

FIGURE **13.12*a***

FIGURE **13.12*b***

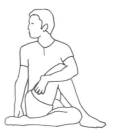

FIGURE **13.13**

Injection of corticosteroids and Botox® has been successful when more conservative measures fail. Although surgery can relieve compression of the sciatic nerve, it is recommended only as a salvage procedure and should be a last resort.

ENHANCING ACTIVE RECOVERY

Many treatment options can enhance your approach to active recovery. The options include heat, cryotherapy, therapeutic ultrasound, Active Release Techniques® (ART), deep-tissue massage, foam rollers, and a variety of more invasive approaches.

Cryotherapy (icing) is an effective early means for reducing inflammation, swelling, and pain. Ice should be your first treatment option following intense exercise sessions and acute injury. You should apply ice to the affected area two or three times per day for 12–20 min. at a time.

Applying heat before flexibility training of muscle-tendon injuries increases the effectiveness of the sessions by maintaining flexibility gain for longer periods of time than in cases when you don't warm up first.

Soft-tissue therapy is a mainstay of many athletes. By eliminating myofascial restrictions (including trigger points, muscle tightness, and knots) prior to eccentric strengthening, its effectiveness can be enhanced. Deep-tissue massage using devices such as foam rollers or tennis balls is an excellent tool to alleviate these issues. These devices apply direct pressure to the affected areas and serve as an effective means of self-massage, often proving successful in eliminating pain.

Low-energy shock-wave therapy delivered on a weekly basis has also demonstrated success. This treatment can be particularly useful for Achilles tendinitis that has been resistant to eccentric training programs.

If such treatments are unsuccessful, more invasive approaches are available. Prilotherapy, platelet gel injections, neuromuscular blockade (Botox), Aprotinin, heparin, dextrose, and corticosteroid injections have all been used for difficult cases that don't respond to the treatments outlined earlier. Prilotherapy and platelet gel injections work by providing growth factors, which increase the healing potential for injured tissues. Botox injections partially weaken the affected muscle, thereby reducing tension on the healing tissue. Corticosteroid injections work well to reduce inflammation in joints, but their use in tendinopathy should be approached with caution. Aprotinin has demonstrated success in small trials and is believed to work by blocking the enzymatic breakdown of affected tissue.

OVERTRAINING/UNDERPERFORMANCE SYNDROME

Continual improvement in performance requires a delicate balance between overload and recovery. Extending the volume, frequency, and number of sessions beyond your body's ability to recover may result in overtraining, or underperformance syndrome. This syndrome, though well recognized, is poorly described in objective terms. Collectively, both physical and psychological symptoms are present and likely the result of adrenal collapse. This generally accepted form of diagnosis is one of exclusion, meaning that all other causes of poor performance have been ruled out.

Common warning signs of overtraining include:

- Feeling drained despite adequate rest
- Sudden drop in performance
- Reduction in capacity to absorb training volume or intensity
- Increased episodes of illness
- Change in sleep pattern (disrupted, greatly increased, or greatly reduced)
- Headaches
- Excessive mood swings or depression
- Loss of enthusiasm for the sport
- Change in appetite (increased, decreased, or cravings for sugar)

Although there are no specific tests for overtraining, if you are experiencing several of these warning signs, it is an indication that you need to immediately reduce training stress.

For athletes who have the benefit of baseline blood testing, an elevated ratio of cortisol over testosterone is a physiological warning sign. Your physician can also look for decreased salivary IgA levels, increased alpha-1 antitrypsin, and increased creatine phosphate (CRP) levels.

Initial treatment of this disorder is a long period of rest until energy levels are restored and laboratory values are normalized. This can be a career-ending illness, so the warning signs must be taken seriously and addressed early.

OTHER COMMON ACHES AND PAINS

A variety of common issues can develop owing to the nature of endurance athletes' training and racing. Although many problems are easily prevented, left unattended they can develop into serious injuries.

These are some of the most common issues faced in training and racing long. We offer some simple advice on how to prevent them and care for them when they do occur.

■ Swim Vertigo

Many athletes experience swim vertigo, or dizziness, when swimming in open water. One cause may be the chop and bump from waves (seasickness); however, most often they become dizzy when colder water gets into their ears, affecting their equilibrium.

To prevent this problem, try swimming with earplugs and increasing your open-water swimming workouts. The more experienced and comfortable you get in open water, the less likely you are to suffer swim vertigo.

■ Abdominal Pain

Abdominal pain, common among endurance athletes, can be especially acute when running. Aside from stitches, which are discussed later, stressed gastrointestinal (GI) symptoms appear in such forms as belching, nausea, vomiting, diarrhea, bloating, intestinal cramps, and stomachache. A major contributor to GI problems is dehydration. This becomes even more of an issue when an athlete loses more than 4 percent of his or her body weight during a race. Pre-race meals are another contributor to GI stress. Meals within 30 min. of a race start and meals high in fat or protein content have been shown to cause vomiting, and meals high in fiber have been shown to cause intestinal cramps. Finally, attempting to consume calories during periods of excessive intensity and the resulting high heart rate can cause gastrointestinal shutdown. Pre-race and race diets are discussed in detail in Chapter 15.

Many GI problems can be prevented by ensuring proper hydration. This is best done by drinking appropriate quantities of a 6–8 percent carbohydrate solution. Cooler beverages have been shown to empty from the stomach at a faster rate. If you are using bars or gels, consume them with plenty of water because gastric emptying slows once the fluids in your gut have a greater than 10 percent carbohydrate content.

If you experience severe or progressive GI symptoms, visit your doctor to eliminate the possibility of a more serious underlying problem. If you experience GI problems in a race, remember the golden rule of digestive distress: Slow down. Quite often a seemingly insurmountable issue will sort itself out during a 10- to 15-min. "stand-down," or period of lower-intensity racing.

■ *Bloating*

Generally common in races, stomach bloating is often the result of going too hard, which forces your stomach to "shut down," meaning it stops clearing liquids and foods. This throws your electrolytes out of balance, causing further problems. The best method to reverse this condition is to slow down, relax, and consume only plain water. To prevent bloating from happening, know your sodium needs from training and previous racing, and remember to stick with what worked in your long workouts and previous races.

■ *Side Stitches*

Almost every athlete has experienced side stitches—a sharp pain just under the rib cage. What actually causes stitches is unknown. However, it is commonly believed that they are caused by a cramp in the diaphragm muscle, exercising too soon after eating, or training at too high an intensity without a proper warm-up. Some research has shown fewer side stitches in athletes with better aerobic fitness.

The frequency of side stitches can be reduced by not eating closer than one to two hours prior to a workout or two to three hours prior to a race, including side stretches in your warm-up routine, and ensuring that you are properly hydrated. To relieve a side stitch, breathe rhythmically and deeply, exhaling forcefully when the foot opposite the stitched side strikes the ground. For example, with a right-side stitch while running, you may find that exhaling when your left foot strikes the ground and inhaling on your right-foot strike will cause it to go away. If you ease the pace a little, a stitch will generally subside.

Side stitches are particularly common for runners; it is unusual to get a side stitch on the bike unless the course is quite rough for an extended time and there is some sort of jostling. Cyclists are more likely to experience intestinal angina—pain from too intense an effort while food is being absorbed.

■ *Muscle Cramps*

Every endurance athlete has experienced muscle cramps. Although they can affect any muscle, calves, hamstrings, and quadriceps are most common. Pain from muscle cramps can vary in intensity and duration.

As with side stitches, the precise causes of cramps are unknown. The common theories are exercising or racing in heat, dehydration and overexertion leading to electrolyte depletion or imbalance, poor stretching routines, muscle fatigue, poor posture, poor conditioning, and inefficient biomechanics.

Measures to prevent or reduce the frequency of muscle cramps include regular stretching and flexibility exercises before and after workouts, strengthening of muscles prone to cramping along with their antagonistic muscles, improving biomechanics, hydrating regularly, and consuming a sports drink while training or racing in heat for longer than one hour. Training that incorporates downhill running and eccentric quad exercises can increase the durability of the quadriceps muscles and help prevent cramping.

The day before and the morning of a long race, it may be a good idea to use table salt more liberally on your food to increase the body's sodium levels. On race day, the sports drink used for the race should also provide adequate levels of sodium, and eating salty foods may also help prevent cramping. Race day nutrition is discussed in more detail in Chapter 15.

■ Neck Pain

Athletes often suffer from stiff, sore necks and shoulders on long rides. If there is no actual pathology in the neck or shoulders, time in the saddle goes a long way toward strengthening these areas. Ensuring correct bike setup can help prevent this problem, and so can flattening your back and relaxing more on the aerobars. Some athletes may find that they are doing a "crunch" for the whole ride.

Nothing may be wrong with your bike setup, but many people have a tendency to ride with a death grip on the bars. Once you learn to relax your upper body, the pain will likely disappear. Upper-body relaxation starts with your face and jaw. Making sure that your face and jaw are always relaxed will reduce upper-body tension and increase your economy in all sports. An excessively aggressive aerodynamic position without adequate hamstring and low-back flexibility may create excessive strain on the head and neck as you crane to see "up the road." Strengthening the neck extensors can improve these symptoms, but if the pain persists, a less aggressive position may be required to eliminate the pain.

■ Back Pain

Low-back pain is common when logging long hours on the bike, especially in the aero position. The majority of lower-back problems begin with tight hamstrings and weak core musculature; however, they are exacerbated when cycling. Many athletes tend to round the lower back, stressing ligaments along the spine that provide support and stability. This stress causes irritation and inflammation of the ligaments, which leads to lower-back pain. Rotating your pelvis forward on the saddle and dropping your stomach toward the top tube to maintain a flat back can alleviate these stresses. More important is ensuring that your bike is correctly set up.

If you are susceptible to lower-back pain, you may wish to avoid standing when climbing, as this position places additional strain on the lower back. However, if the back pain is caused by a herniated or ruptured disk, standing may be helpful because sitting places the disk under the most strain. Experiment to find the position most likely to alleviate your symptoms. In addition, be very careful with the effort level of all climbs, particularly those early in the race.

A regular stretching and strengthening routine, including supporting muscles of the back (abs, hamstrings, hip flexors, shoulders) as well as the lower back itself, will improve flexibility and posture, thereby reducing lower-back pain. Hamstring-stretching routines will reduce the stress on the pelvis and lower back, and a core strengthening routine will improve the strength of the muscles that support the spine. Many of these exercises are discussed in Chapter 9.

Numb Feet and Hands

It's not uncommon for cyclists to experience numbness in their hands and feet. Pedals with small platforms, shoes that are too small or narrow, and shoes that allow too much flex in the sole often cause numb feet. Shoes that are too small or narrow squeeze the toes together, thereby putting pressure on the nerves in the feet. Platforms that are too small, combined with shoes that are too flexible, can produce uneven pressure on the feet, thereby causing numbness.

To prevent foot numbness, ensure that your shoes are properly fitted to your feet, that the soles are strong, and that your platforms are suitable. Shift your feet and roll your toes regularly while riding to help keep the blood moving.

Cyclists often experience numbness or tingling sensations in their hands. This is called "cyclist's palsy" and is generally caused by compression of the ulnar or median nerve.

Hand numbness can be prevented by correct bike setup, adjusting the aerobars, wearing cycling gloves with gel padding, using aero pads with gel padding, switching hand positions often during a ride, and stretching your wrists after all rides. If the symptoms persist beyond the completion of your bike rides, night wrist splints can be helpful. If this fails, seek medical advice.

Saddle Sores

More common than numbness while cycling are saddle sores. Irritated skin, blocked pores, and friction from pressure points on the saddle are the common causes. Heat and moisture within cycling shorts also allow bacteria into the pores, causing pimples and blisters.

Saddle sores need to be cleaned, and an antibiotic ointment, such as Polysporin or Neosporin, should be applied. The area should then be kept dry when not riding by applying talcum powder daily after showers. This will help prevent a bacteria-friendly environment.

Using a lubricant such as Body Glide or Chamois Butter directly on the shorts will help to prevent saddle sores caused by friction. Be sure that your shorts are cleaned after every ride and replaced when they become worn, and choose shorts with padding that doesn't have excessive stitching. Avoid wearing anything under your shorts, as seams from cotton or nylon underwear can cause friction and irritate the skin. Clean the area immediately following every ride, using a gentle soap. Don't use alcohol, as it will dry out and irritate your skin more. If you are unable to clean the area right away, change into a pair of loose-fitting, dry shorts to allow the skin to breathe.

The right saddle will also help in preventing saddle sores. There are many ergonomic saddles on the market. Find one that fits your anatomy and is comfortable for long periods of time. Standing out of the saddle frequently on long rides will also help to relieve pressure.

Black Toenails

Very common among long-distance runners, black toenails are caused when your toes repeatedly hit the front of your running shoe, causing bruising and bleeding beneath the nail. This happens when your shoes are too tight, fit poorly, or have a toe box that is the wrong shape for your foot. The bruised toenail will turn black and eventually fall off as a new nail grows underneath.

To prevent black toenails, choose running shoes for racing that are a half size too large and the correct shape for your foot. This will leave enough room for your toes to slide without hitting the front of the toe box. Another solution for some is to wear extra-thin socks with normal-sized running shoes. Keeping your toenails trimmed evenly and straight across the tops of the toes will also help.

If you feel pain or excessive pressure beneath the toenail, we recommend a visit to your doctor, who can alleviate the pressure by making a small hole in the nail.

■ *Blisters*

Another common problem for long-distance runners, blisters are generally caused by poorly fitting shoes, swollen feet, running in wet shoes and socks, or friction from poor sock choices.

Small blisters are best left alone, but large blisters should be drained to relieve pressure. This can be done with a safety pin or sewing needle after heating it over a flame until it is glowing red. Once it cools, puncture and gently drain the blister. Apply an antibiotic ointment such as Polysporin or Neosporin to the area and cover with a bandage.

To prevent blisters, ensure that your shoes are the right size and shape for your foot. Choose socks made from synthetic blends, and avoid socks with thick seams or stitching. Applying petroleum jelly or talcum powder to your feet can aid in reducing friction. Do your best to avoid getting your shoes and socks wet during races. If repeated blisters occur, loosely taping those areas helps alleviate discomfort.

■ *Calluses*

Another ailment of long-distance running is calluses—areas of thick, hard skin caused by pressure or friction from running, poorly fitting shoes, flat or high-arched feet, or a bony prominence in the foot.

Calluses can be removed by gently filing them with a pumice stone or other gentle abrasive surface after either a bath or soaking the feet in a bucket of warm water and Epsom salts. Avoid letting calluses get large, as the skin can crack, which may lead to infection.

To prevent calluses, regularly apply moisturizers to keep the skin supple. Choose shoes with good arch support and shock absorption. When running, wear thicker socks to reduce friction, apply moleskin to friction areas, or use an insole that absorbs shock inside the shoe.

■ *Chafing*

Chafing is another common problem owing to friction during swimming, cycling, and running. Chafing can occur during the swim if your wetsuit rubs against the back of your neck. A sleeveless wetsuit may cause chafing under the arms. Inner thighs may become chafed on the bike by shorts that are too short, allowing your skin to rub against the nose of your bike seat. On the run, you may experience chafing on the inner thighs if your legs rub against each other, or under the arms if you wear a racing singlet.

The best way to prevent chafing is to apply a lubricant, such as Body Glide or petroleum jelly, to the skin in areas where friction is common.

SPECIAL CONSIDERATIONS

■ Masters Athletes

As triathlon ages, so do its participants. Though most elite-level athletes are in their second or third decade, the largest group of participants is 35- to 50-year-old master athletes. This trend is continuing, and participants well into their 70s are completing Ironman-distance events on a regular basis. As a result of the aging of event participants, we have seen people with total hip replacements complete the Ironman Triathlon World Championship in Kona, records for oldest female and male finishers advance, and many age-group records shattered every year. As the popularity of the sport increases, so will the older athlete contingent. As one might expect, this population has unique needs. Flexibility and strength training are important to maintain range of motion and lean muscle mass. These factors and others that go along with aging must be carefully monitored during training.

■ Challenged Athletes

Participation in triathlon by physically challenged athletes is increasing as well. Advances in prosthetics, orthotics, wheelchairs, and equipment modifications have made such endeavors not only possible but more effective in terms of performance. Marc Herremans is one example. He competed successfully as a professional able-bodied athlete, but after a tragic cycling accident resulted in thoracic-level paraplegia, he went on to race at the highest level in triathlon in the challenged athletes division. Some challenged athletes, such as Sarah Reinertsen, were born with congenital defects. Sarah has met challenge after challenge to become the first above-knee amputee to complete Ironman Hawaii.

Special consideration should be given to these athletes regarding observation and care during triathlons. In particular, buoyancy and thermoregulation can be a significant challenge during the swim. Assistance with prosthetics, clothing, and gear changes should be available during the bike and run. Adequate sunscreen and lubricant for areas prone to blisters and friction should be encouraged and applied. Additional information can be found at www.challengedathletes.org.

CONCLUSION

It is inevitable that you will encounter some obstacles in your training. By treating small issues seriously—while they are still small—you can tackle problems before they derail your training plans. With patience, most problems can be prevented or successfully treated.

Dr. Jeff Shilt is an orthopedic surgeon and multiple Ironman finisher. Having raced in nine Ironman-distance triathlons and qualified for the Ironman Triathlon World Championship in Hawaii, he brings unique insight to triathlon. He served as the U.S. team physician for the International Triathlon Union Triathlon World Championships in 2003 and 2005, working with elite, age-group, and physically challenged triathletes. Dr. Shilt has a particular interest in helping athletes with medical conditions or limitations.

CHAPTER 14

PEAKING FOR YOUR IRONMAN

 In the final three weeks, always keep one gear in reserve. Save your best for race day.

—DAVE SCOTT,
SIX-TIME IRONMAN WORLD CHAMPION

Probably the greatest misconception about tapering for an Ironman-distance race is that all an athlete needs to do is kick back and drop the volume, and a peak performance will result. This is far from the truth. There are three components to a successful taper:

1. Recovering from the specific preparation of the Build period (see Chapter 5)
2. Building energy inward by freshening mentally as well as physically
3. The use of specific BT workouts to maintain endurance with race-specific training

During your taper, consider the mental and physical state that you want to have on the morning of the race: fit, fresh, and focused. Many triathletes end their Build period on edge. Be wary of tipping yourself over the edge with excessive intensity or volume in the Peak period. You have spent many months preparing for race day, so give yourself every chance to succeed.

THE PEAK PERIOD

The two most important elements of the Peak period are intensity and recovery. Because of the reduced volume during this period, it is important to maintain intensity. Basically, you are trading a little endurance for what you hope will be a significant improvement in race performance.

Always consider intensity in light of your average race effort. The most valuable form of intensity is a mixture of moderately hard efforts (Zone 3) within steady (Zone 2) main sets. Many athletes have ruined months of preparation by excessive Zone 4 and 5 training in the final weeks of their preparation.

Remember that the overriding goal for the Peak period is to prepare to race. As well as eliminating all training fatigue, reduce (ideally, remove) as much nontraining stress as possible. The ideal Peak period schedule has you eager to complete each workout and worried that you are not doing enough. If you are fresh for every session, you are on track. If you are arriving at your breakthrough workouts tired, additional recovery should be your highest priority.

■ Peak Period Workouts

Most athletes will have completed a race-simulation BT on the weekend before the start of Peak Week 1 (see sidebar in Chapter 5, "Finishing Your Build Period"). For this reason, the start of the week should be light in terms of both volume and intensity. Begin your Peak period by ensuring that you have recovered from all residual Build period fatigue.

The Build period contains workouts that are specific to the demands of the course—most important are race-simulation bike rides in conditions and terrain similar to those of race day. The Build period ends with a recovery week (which starts four weeks before race day and ends three weeks before race day). The recovery week should be similar to your normal training week with three important changes: (1) workout duration at 40–60 percent of normal levels; (2) from Monday to Thursday (at least), no training above heart rate Zone 2; and (3) no physiological testing.

The weekend that is three weeks before the race day should include more recovery (if required) or a moderate race-simulation workout.

The Peak period is the two weeks prior to Race Week, and Race Week is the week that ends with race day.

Breakthrough Workouts

You will do a race-intensity or mini-race-simulation workout every 72–96 hours in the Peak period, so there will typically be two race-simulation breakthrough workouts planned for each week. Working athletes are likely to be under time constraints during the week, and therefore Week 1's longer breakthrough (BT) workout should be scheduled for the weekend.

BT1 (Peak Week 1, no. 1). Scheduled for Wednesday or Thursday, this session is normally the shorter breakthrough workout of the week and lasts 2–3.5 hours, depending on recovery. As the shorter session, this workout should incorporate an element of maintenance for your key strengths. If you have not fully recovered from the Build period, this session should be changed to an aerobic maintenance workout (recommended for athletes at all levels). Normally, the running aspect of the race-simulation brick is limited to 30–45 min. with a tempo finish (heart rate Zone 3, or close to half-Ironman-distance race pace).

NOVICE ATHLETES (OR ATHLETES WITH ENDURANCE AS THEIR GREATEST LIMITER) WILL LIKELY BENEFIT FROM REDUCING THE LENGTH of (or eliminating completely) the midweek breakthrough workout and extending the length of the first Peak Week weekend breakthrough workout to 4.5 hours. In order to compensate for the additional volume of this weekend workout, reduce its average intensity. Typically, this session would start in heart rate Zone 1 and build to Zone 2.

N   **NOVICE**

Keep in mind that the goal of the entire Peak period is to build energy inward by freshening mentally as well as physically. Any session that feels draining, or starts to leave you "flat," should be reduced in duration and intensity. The hard work is done—what matters is absorbing the training done prior to the Peak period. If you make a mistake, it should be on the side of doing too little and being "too fresh" for your event. In this period, active rest is much better than total rest.

BT2 (Peak Week 1, no. 2). Scheduled for Saturday or Sunday, this is the key breakthrough workout of the Peak period. It is likely the last opportunity to add material fitness and therefore should address your greatest personal limiter. This session is normally 3–4 hours long with 45–60 min. of running. After you establish your running legs, the workout should build to a tempo finish, similar to BT1.

BT3 (Peak Week 2, no. 1). Scheduled for Wednesday or Thursday of Week 2, this workout should be done at goal Ironman-distance race pace (or slightly faster). If you are recovering well, you will benefit from inserting blocks of 10–30 min. of heart rate Zone 3 efforts into the bike and run legs. The total duration of this session is normally 2–3 hours, with 30–45 min. of running—it is likely to be counterproductive to run longer than 45 min.

BT4 (Peak Week 2, no. 2). This workout is scheduled for the final weekend before the race. It is normally done with full race setup (clothing, wheels, etc.) and includes a large percentage of muscular endurance work. Typical duration is 90–120 min., including 30 min. of running—again, running longer is likely to be counterproductive.

Table 14.1 summarizes BT workouts for Peak Weeks 1 and 2.

TABLE 14.1 BREAKTHROUGH WORKOUTS FOR PEAK WEEKS 1 AND 2

		TRAINING	NOTES	SPECIAL INSTRUCTION
PEAK WEEK 1	**Monday**			
	Tuesday			
	Wednesday	BT1 workout, 2–3.5 hours Purpose: Maintenance for key strengths	Bike 1.5–3 hours Run 30–45 min. Tempo finish, HR Zone 3, close to half-IM race pace.	Novice: Reduce or eliminate BT1
	Thursday	Recovery		
	Friday			
	Saturday	BT2 workout, 3–4 hours Purpose: Address greatest personal limiter	Bike: Include 10- to 15-min. HR Zone 3–4 effort at end of bike leg. Run 45–60 min.: Build to tempo finish	Novice: Increase BT2 to 4.5 hours; reduce intensity to HR Zones 1–2.
	Sunday	Recovery		
PEAK WEEK 2	**Monday**			
	Tuesday			
	Wednesday	BT3 workout, 2–3 hours Purpose: Practice goal IM race pace or slightly faster	Intervals of 10–30 min. HR Zone 3 effort on bike and run legs. Run 30–45 min.	
	Thursday	Recovery		
	Friday			
	Saturday	BT4 workout, 1.5–2 hours Purpose: Primarily muscle endurance work	Bike: Include 10–15 min. HR Zone 3–4 effort at end of bike leg. Run 30 min.: Use full race setup.	
	Sunday	Recovery		

Note: BT workouts could also be scheduled on Thursdays and Sundays.

If you have had problems holding back early in the race, you should schedule one break-through workout per week in which the bike is done at target Ironman-distance effort. The run in this session could be a faster, muscular endurance–oriented session. Typically, the longer breakthrough workout each week should be done in terrain that closely mimics the race venue. The exception is if you have a critical limiter in one particular area (for example, hill climbing, rollers, or flat riding). You would likely achieve greater benefits from focusing your longer breakthrough session on your critical limiter.

The day after every breakthrough workout should be either a total rest day or a very light, technique-oriented day. No weights or hard swimming should be scheduled for this day. Sleep is an important element of recovery, and many athletes experience sleep disruption during the Peak period.

Swimming and Strength Workouts

If you have been doing regular strength maintenance work during the season, continue to lift once a week during the Peak period. Schedule strength training in such a way that it does not impair the quality of the breakthrough sessions. The final strength session in Peak Week 2 should be lighter than usual—perhaps only one set of each exercise.

Most athletes will benefit from maintaining their "normal" swimming schedule during the Peak period (one longer swim, one faster swim, one technique swim). Athletes swimming four times a week or more should incorporate at least one open-water swim per week. Those swimming three times per week or less should incorporate an open-water swim into Peak Week 2. Athletes who have difficulty with open-water swims should continue with the weekly open-water swims that were started during the Build period. Open-water swims (that are nonrecovery in nature) should include 20- to 45-min. blocks of continuous swimming at goal Ironman-distance effort. These workouts are an excellent time to work on your drafting technique as well as sighting skills.

All other workouts in the Peak period are secondary to the goals of maintaining intensity and ensuring recovery. Additional training load beyond the breakthrough workouts outlined earlier will prove counterproductive—trust your training and resist the urge to test yourself prior to race day.

■ Important Peak Week Considerations

All workouts should start with a period of heart rate Zone 1 effort. This allows you to warm up and simulates the discipline that will be required at the start of the Ironman-distance bike leg. Typically, this "easier" period lasts for the first 20–25 percent of the scheduled bike leg. All workouts should also incorporate an element of sub-lactate-threshold muscular endurance work. For most athletes, heart rate Zone 3 intensity is sufficient.

Hydrate at the level you wish to consume during a race. This is particularly important for athletes living in cooler climates who may be racing in hot weather.

The overall goal of the breakthrough workouts is to prepare the body to race, so many athletes wonder if it makes sense to train in the hottest part of the day. There is a trade-off between slower breakthrough sessions owing to the heat and the acclimatization benefit of midday training. Most athletes will have sufficient heat training from the Build period so that, on balance, it makes sense to avoid the hottest part of the day and maximize average training speed.

As the race draws near, if you are feeling tired before or during a session, eliminate the session or cut it short. It is essential that you be totally fresh at the end of Peak Week 2.

In order to simulate the "heavy legs" sensation experienced at the start of the marathon, you should include 10–15 min. of harder effort (HR Zones 3–4) at the end of the bike for at least two of the race-simulation breakthrough workouts. All transitions should be as quick as possible, with transition gear laid out in race fashion (typically bagged). At the start of the run leg of each race-simulation breakthrough workout, focus on cadence and maintaining good form. The goal of the first 10–15 min. of the transition run should be to establish a steady, comfortable tempo.

> **IT CAN BE HARD TO GET A GOOD NIGHT'S SLEEP** as race day approaches. Here are a few tips to help you rest more soundly.
> - Reduce daily caffeine intake.
> - Don't exercise late in the day.
> - Take a hot shower or bath before bed.
> - Go for a short evening walk, followed by a gentle stretching session.
> - Slightly increase your carbohydrate intake for dinner.
> - Wake up at the same time each day.

■ *Common Issues During the Peak Period*

Many athletes have a very strong urge to get one last megasession completed. If this training period is working as intended, you will start to feel fresh and have high energy levels. At this stage, it can be tempting for the highly motivated athlete to go long. This is a mistake—it is far better to go fast than to go long. Save your energy for race day.

Probably the most dangerous urge is the desire to run long. Running is the most physically stressful of all three sports and therefore should be approached with the most caution. If you have running endurance as a key limiter, it might make sense to plan a 90- to 120-min. run for BT1. For most athletes, a long run less than sixteen to eighteen days before an Ironman-distance race is counterproductive.

As training volume is reduced, you will want to focus on your nutrition and lower your overall caloric intake. This practice is particularly relevant for Peak Week 2. Most athletes will have become used to a high intake of food during the Build period. Considerable discipline can be required to ensure that you arrive at Race Week with your desired body composition. Replacing energy-dense food sources with fresh fruits and vegetables can be one strategy for dealing with appetite challenges. Great care should be taken with the nutrition strategy for the period before, during, and after key breakthrough sessions. These sessions are very important, and you should ensure that you have sufficient carbohydrates in your diet for optimal performance and recovery.

Almost all athletes will experience doubt about their training and potential race performance. This feeling comes from a variety of sources, including residual fatigue from the Build period, pre-race nerves, and the normal anxiety everyone experiences from time to time. A good strategy for combating these fears is to review your training log and remember the large number of quality sessions that you have completed.

RACE WEEK

All athletes share one goal for Race Week: to arrive at the start line in the best condition possible. Recovery is paramount in all decisions made during Race Week.

■ *Race Week Workouts*

What follows is an outline of a standard Race Week strategy for a Sunday race. Athletes racing on a Saturday should adjust backward by one day.

Day 1. Following the completion of the final breakthrough workout on the weekend before Race Week, you will likely want to take a break from cycling and running on Monday. For this reason, it is typically best to schedule a swim of 45–60 min. Ideally, this will be an open-water swim at the race venue. The main set of this workout should be six intervals of 90 sec. The intervals should be swum at threshold pace on a rest interval of 30–60 sec. In addition, the workout should include 10–20 min. of continuous swimming at target race effort. The rest of the workout should include technique work that focuses on balance and stroke-length drills.

Day 2. The main workout on Tuesday is a run session lasting 30–45 min. This workout should include an easy warm-up followed by four to eight strides with walking recoveries. The main set of this workout should be five intervals of 90 sec. duration. The intervals should be run at threshold pace on a rest interval of 3 min. Focus on maintaining perfect form and a smooth cadence at all times during this workout.

The secondary workout for Tuesday is a light spin that is completed before the evening meal. This workout is optional, and its intensity should be low.

Day 3. On Wednesday, the main workout is a 30- to 45-min. bike session. This should be an easy ride that includes four threshold intervals of 90 sec. duration. Recovery should consist of easy riding. These intervals can be spread throughout the ride or done on 30- to 60-sec. recovery intervals.

The secondary workout for Wednesday is an easy swim of 30–45 min. If you are already at the race venue, you should swim on the course, ideally at the race start time. This workout should be used to note landmarks as well as the swim exit. Be sure to note any underwater hazards at the swim start and finish.

Day 4. Thursday's key session is an easy brick that includes 4 threshold intervals of 90 sec. duration. The intervals should be evenly split between the bike and the run. The duration of the brick should be 60–90 min. This session is an excellent opportunity to ride the run course and note any significant climbs. As on Wednesday, the secondary workout is an optional 20- to 40-min. easy swim.

Day 5. Friday should be a very light day (total rest for most) on which you take care of registration formalities, final equipment checks, and race briefings. This is a good day to get away from the crowds by driving the bike and run courses.

Day 6. Following the break on Friday, you should schedule a swim, bike, and run session that lasts 45–60 min. (total). This session is best done in the morning on Saturday. The entire session should be done at an easy pace with three to four 30-sec. pickups (brief faster work) inserted into the bike and the run. The purpose of the pickups is to stimulate fast-twitch muscle fibers and ensure that you feel fresh on race day. After this workout, tighten all bolts on your bike. This is a good day to focus on rest. Restful activities include watching television, going to a movie matinee, and taking a guided bus tour of the area.

Day 7. Sunday is race day, and some important considerations for race day are discussed later in this chapter. Table 14.2 outlines these Race Week workouts.

> **ATHLETES WHO FEEL FATIGUED DURING RACE WEEK** should consider eliminating the optional 1 bike, 1 swim sessions and training at the low end of indicated workout duration.
>
> If you arrive early at the race venue, you will likely benefit from the acclimatization effect of the additional morning swims, but the duration should be kept short and the intensity low.
>
> Athletes doing their first Ironman-distance race should keep their time goals, if any, to themselves. Without any previous race experience over the distance, it is hard to accurately predict race performance. Most athletes are 1 to 2 hours slower than they anticipate. Race strategies are discussed in detail in Chapter 15.
>
> **N**   NOVICE

■ *Important Race Week Considerations*

Ideally, you should arrive at the race site four to seven days before racing. This schedule allows plenty of time to recover from the journey and prepare for the race. Athletes traveling across time zones should allow one day for each time zone crossed. See the "Pre-race Checklist and Race Day Checklist" sidebar for preparation tips.

Maintain your normal hydration routine. If you are flying to the race venue, be sure to remain hydrated on your flight because the lack of humidity on aircraft can result in dehydration.

TABLE 14.2 WORKOUTS FOR RACE WEEK

		TRAINING	NOTES	SPECIAL INSTRUCTION
RACE WEEK	**Monday**	Swim 45–60 min. Purpose: Ideally an open-water swim at the race venue	6 x 90 sec. at threshold pace (RI 30–60 sec.) 10–20 min. at race pace	Add drills to swim to work on balance and stroke length
	Tuesday	Run 30–45 min. Purpose: Focus on perfect form and smooth cadence	Easy warm-up 4–8 strides with walking recoveries 5 x 90 sec. at threshold pace (RI 3 min.)	
		Easy spin (optional)	Best before your evening meal	
	Wednesday	Bike 30–45 min.	Include 4 x 90 sec. at threshold pace (RI 30–60 sec.)	
		Easy swim 30–45 min. Purpose: Ideally an open-water swim at the race venue and at race start time		Look for landmarks and hazards
	Thursday	Easy brick 60–90 min.	Bike includes 2 x 90 sec. at threshold pace Run includes 2 x 90 sec. at threshold pace	Try to bike the run racecourse
		Easy swim 20–40 min. (optional)		
	Friday	REST	Drive the bike and run courses. Final equipment check. Handle registration details.	
	Saturday	Swim, bike, or run 45–60 min.	Include 4 x 30-sec. pickups	Best in the morning
	Sunday	RACE DAY		

Race Week training volume is likely to be one-quarter to one-third of normal workloads. For this reason, you will be best served by reducing your caloric intake. Here are some ideas for achieving this result.

- Use only water during Race Week sessions—avoid sports drinks, energy bars, and gels.
- When hungry, increase consumption of fresh fruits and vegetables that are low on the glycemic index.
- Eat smaller, more frequent meals.
- Reduce consumption of energy-dense foods, typically those with a high sugar and fat content or dry carbohydrate foods such as crackers and pretzels.
- Don't overeat at the pre-race dinner—save it for the awards banquet.

Bike maintenance is best carried out during the Peak period, well before arrival at the race site. To ensure that everything is in working order, all Race Week workouts should be done using full race setup (wheels and all accessories). If you arrive at the race venue late in the week, you should schedule an additional easy ride to ensure that your bike is fully functional.

Spend at least 15 min. per day mentally running through your race strategy as well as visualizing a positive outcome to any anticipated race day challenges.

Use your spare time during Race Week to increase the amount of stretching you do. Stretching should be gentle and targeted at keeping you limber. It is most important to stretch during the period of travel to the race site (particularly when long periods of sitting are required).

Two days before the race start, begin increasing your sodium intake if you are racing in a hot climate. Approximately eighteen hours before the race start, move to a low-fiber diet.

PRE-RACE CHECKLIST

- Take your bike to the local bike shop for a checkup.
- Ensure that all supplies are stocked in advance.
- Take care of any last-minute emergencies.
- Pack all transition bags.
- Pack all special-needs bags.

RACE DAY CHECKLIST

- Wake up three to four hours before race start.
- Eat breakfast and begin mental preparations.
- Double-check special-needs bags.
- Gather swim start gear.
- Prepare post-race recovery drink for dry-clothes bag.
- Add anything you'll want post-race to dry-clothes bag.
- Double-check bike and transition bags.
- Find a quiet place to collect your thoughts prior to the race start.
- Smile and enjoy the day ahead.

See the detailed "Race Day Checklist" in Chapter 15.

DOUBT IS NORMAL. Most athletes will experience periods of self-doubt during Race Week. Here are some tips for counteracting self-doubt:

- Make a list of issues. Beside each issue, write out a strategy for dealing with it.
- Think back to key breakthrough sessions. Remember the hard work and preparation you have done.
- Know that an element of doubt is normal. Acknowledge the feeling, but remain focused on the weeks of preparation you have completed.
- Discuss your concerns with experienced athletes. Veterans of previous races are an excellent source of information as well as coping strategies.

See Chapter 11 for more on mental preparation for race day.

■ *Common Issues During the Peak Period*

Most athletes will experience a change in their sleep pattern during Race Week. Some will have a desire to sleep more, and others will experience a significant reduction in their need for sleep. Owing to reduced training volume, most athletes will be best served by eliminating all naps. This approach will make it easier to maintain normal sleeping patterns. Even if you can't sleep at night, it is beneficial to spend the time lying down—visualization and relaxation exercises are an excellent way to pass the time.

Keep your workout intensity in check. If the taper has worked as intended, you will feel very strong during the final workouts of Race Week. It is essential to avoid the urge to increase the duration and intensity of Race Week sessions. Energy is best saved for race day, and it is not possible to add any fitness.

Try to avoid crowds. Many athletes find it draining to spend time in large groups of people during Race Week. The constant nervous tension surrounding most competitors can be emotionally and physically exhausting. Consider allocating a block of quiet time each day. Reading a book, watching a movie, or engaging in some other activity away from the race venue can help maintain your energy levels.

Be aware of goal inflation, and maintain perspective regarding your race goals. The taper, the crowds, and the general race zatmosphere can lead to goal inflation. Remember your goals when you started your journey as well as the enjoyment the months of preparation have brought to your life.

Keep your daily schedules light. Do your best to minimize all work and social commitments during Race Week. Stressful and fatiguing situations (and people) should be avoided as much as possible.

CHAPTER 15

RACING LONG

ronman-distance racing is the greatest physical challenge most athletes will undertake. Many excellent athletes have been humbled by this awesome event. The following series of tips is designed to help you get the most out of a day that should be one of the most memorable experiences of your life.

> *You've done all this training; you've been out there for hours; for heaven's sake, don't let it slip away.*
>
> —HEATHER FUHR, IRONMAN WORLD CHAMPION

BEFORE YOU START

Ideally, you will arrive a few days in advance of the race so you can become familiar with the venue. Even if you have less time, you can still use this checklist.

Swim start. Review the swim start area; early morning is best as winds and chop are more likely to be light. Review the swim exit area, if possible.

Transition areas. Walk the transition areas to familiarize yourself with their layout.

Personal time. Carve out a few hours each day to relax and review your written race plan. By leaving yourself underscheduled during Race Week, you will reduce the pressure on yourself.

Strategy review. When you are relaxed, spend some time doing an honest review of the likely average effort you will be able to sustain across the day. Remember that your overall result will be fastest by building your effort across the day.

Race Day Checklist

The day before your race, you will be required to drop off your bike and your swim-to-bike and bike-to-run transition bags. Following are basic gear and accessory suggestions.

SWIM-TO-BIKE (T1)

- Towel (optional)
- Cycling shoes (can be on bike)
- Cycling helmet
- Cycling jersey (optional if using a trisuit; can be worn under wetsuit)
- Sunglasses
- Sunscreen (applied pre-race)
- Cycling gloves (optional)
- Cycling socks (optional)
- Sports bar/gels/salt tabs (held together with elastic band and/or secured to bike)
- Race belt

BIKE-TO-RUN (T2)

- Running shorts (optional if using trisuit or Speedo)
- Running socks (very risky to run without socks)
- Hat or visor (useful for placing other items inside and wrapping with elastic to save time)
- Sunscreen (applied by race volunteers)
- Vaseline (small tube for start of run)
- Sports bar/gels/salt tabs
- Race belt

SPECIAL-NEEDS BAGS

On race morning, you will be required to drop off your special-needs bags. There is one bag for the bike and one bag for the run. It's up to you what you put in these bags—remember that in most races, the bags will not be returned. Here are a few common ideas:

- Favorite snack food
- Extra sport bars/gels/salt tabs
- Extra bike tube and CO_2 cartridge
- Extra running shirt for warmth if running into the night
- Letters of encouragement from friends

Nutrition. In anticipation of race day, it can be difficult to control your nutrition. Some athletes find themselves rushed and either miss a meal or eat something out of the ordinary. Others can overeat in their effort to make sure they have enough stored energy for race day. Your first priority should be to eat normally. This requires careful planning, but it is the first step to optimal performance. Here are a few tips for your pre-race menu:

- Increase table salt intake for 48 hours prior to race day.
- Hydrate normally with water. Drinking gallons of water is not required.
- The day before the race, eat small meals frequently.
- Go to a low-fiber diet 18 hours before the race start.

On race morning, you should consume 600–1,000 calories 3–4 hours before the start. Target breakfast completion for 2.5–3 hours before race start. Two hours is okay unless you are eating a high-fat breakfast that will digest slowly (which is not recommended).

THE SWIM

The swim start can be crazy, with many people in close proximity. Remember to keep breathing and don't "engage" other swimmers. It is a long day, and you'll simply waste energy by fighting for position. Aggressive swimmers can provide excellent drafting opportunities for the intelligent athlete.

Athletes who expect to swim in less than an hour should seed themselves toward the front. Athletes who expect to swim longer than 75 min. should be toward the back. Everyone else should be in the middle. For your first Ironman-distance swim, it is best to be a bit wide and a little farther back than you think may be necessary.

The swim should feel very easy to you. The combination of race adrenaline and the taper will impair your pace judgment. Athletes almost always believe they are swimming very easy. However, if you wear a heart rate monitor, you will be able to see (after the fact) that you were working quite hard. Once you have established yourself with a good draft, it is best to relax and enjoy the ride. No matter what speed you swim, you want to "cruise" this part of the race.

If you find yourself struggling from starting too hard, use a little backstroke to relax your breathing. Then swim into some clear water and regain your composure. Once you have settled, get back into the flow and look for a draft to take you around the course.

The turns are key points for any race. Most swimmers will slow as they come into the turn. In races that have a long distance before the first turn, swimmers are all forced together at the turning buoy. These two reactions provide the intelligent racer with an opportunity to improve his or her position by finding a faster draft or bridging forward to a faster group.

> **AT EACH RACE, EXPERIENCED ATHLETES WILL BE A VALUABLE SOURCE** of information for the best place to start. Seek these veterans out before the race and have them explain their thoughts about the course. With the size of the fields in many Ironman-distance races, it is worth remembering that there is no clean water available for most of the field. "Taking it out hard" will leave you overextended in a very crowded environment—not a good place to be early in the day.
>
> **N   NOVICE**

> **STRONG SWIMMERS CAN GAIN TIME** by bridging from pack to pack as the swim establishes itself. Be wary of bridging, as even a short distance can prove challenging. This skill should first be practiced in B- and C-priority races as well as in training. Knowing the distance you can bridge is a valuable skill for open water. Bridging is appropriate for only the very strongest triathlon swimmers. Even then, it is likely best to save your effort for the marathon.
>
> **I   INTERMEDIATE**

Remember that it is pointless to swim hard at any stage. Most swimmers are best served by staying relaxed and enjoying the draft around the course. Enjoy the swim, as it should be the easiest part of your day.

SWIM-TO-BIKE TRANSITION

As part of your race preparations, you should have walked the transition areas and rehearsed your swim exit. You should also have mentally and physically rehearsed what you are going to do during your first transition. This preparation should make transition straightforward as you execute your race strategy.

Many athletes race through transitions. Because you will have been horizontal for an hour or more, you will achieve the fastest and least stressful transition by walking. Going from the swim to fast running is hard on the body, and you will have to soft-pedal for a long time to recover. Rushing transition can put an undue strain on your low back, hamstrings, and digestive system. Move smoothly to your bike and settle into your ride.

> IN THE MONTHS PRIOR TO THE RACE, it is useful to ride the course, in whole or in sections, in order to gain an understanding of the bike leg. If you are unable to ride the course in advance, be sure to drive it prior to race day. Note landmarks around the 30-, 60-, and 90-mile marks to help you remember to control your effort during the race.
>
> You should plan ahead for the weather you may face. Even in summer, and even in many races in temperate climates, it is possible to have cold and wet conditions. In the tropics, it is important to keep your clothing wet during the bike to stay cool. In locations where the sun is fierce, wear UV-protective clothing and a water-based sunscreen that does not impair your ability to sweat.

THE BIKE

Your goals for the early part of the bike should be to settle into your cycling rhythm and start replenishing the energy that was used in the swim. Specific hydration and nutrition recommendations are discussed later in the chapter.

Early in the bike you will likely feel better than at any time in the previous three months. Many races are blown in the first 90 min. of the bike leg. You will be rested, energized, and very strong. It is crucial that you avoid riding too hard. You have a long day ahead, and the first five to six hours of the race should feel comfortable and controlled. If you feel you are "racing" at any time early in the race, you are going far too hard.

Proper early bike pacing enables you to establish your nutrition and hydration strategies. This is the key benefit of early race control. Almost all athletes find that as the race progresses, it becomes more and more difficult to motivate themselves to eat. In addition, it is much easier for your body to digest food and drink while riding than while running.

Ironman-distance racing is not a bike race, and it is essential to respect the marathon that lies ahead. Given the aerodynamics of cycling (fast-moving air) versus running (slow-moving air), your fastest time will result when you are able to place your greatest output in the marathon leg.

So how should an athlete approach the bike portion of the event? Table 15.1 offers some guidelines for your effort level and heart rate. You should adjust these guidelines based on the results of your honest (and most realistic) race-simulation rides.

For power guidelines, see Table 15.2. These should be used to help guide your race-simulation and key bike workouts. If you make a mistake, then start each leg of the race a little too easy.

Whether you race on wattage, heart rate, or perceived exertion, use your effort wisely. Show control when you are feeling strong, and keep your focus when you experience bad patches. Hills and headwinds present unique challenges and will tempt you to ride harder than you had planned. Many athletes who race the best relative to their training note that they never exceed heart rate Zone 2 on the bike. The entire ride is done in the lower end of their aerobic range. This is a conservative strategy that works for many athletes, particularly those concerned about their endurance and how they might perform in the run.

Many athletes find they run more comfortably if they ease off on solid food for the last 20–30 min. of the bike. If you have experienced stomach problems early in the run before, then this could be a good idea. However, it is essential that you continue to consume calories, so a liquid or gel food source should be substituted.

Finally, there will likely be one or more periods on the bike during which you experience doubt about your race. This feeling is normal, and overcoming these challenges is a key part of what makes the race so special. These bad patches never last long, and it is important to maintain your cycling momentum when faced with mental and physical challenges. Breaking the ride into smaller and smaller mental segments is a great way to get through it without feeling the "hugeness" of such a long period of effort.

> STRONG CYCLISTS WILL ALMOST ALWAYS BE TEMPTED to use their bike leg as a "weapon." This is a serious mistake because difficulties in the run are very costly in terms of time lost. Most often 5–10 min. on the bike can be the difference between being able to put together a solid run and having to walk. Your fastest race will result from adopting a conservative bike strategy and putting any surplus energy into the second half of the run.
>
> **I** **INTERMEDIATE**

TABLE 15.1 PACING GUIDELINES

SEGMENT	EFFORT GUIDELINES	HEART RATE GUIDELINES	NOTES
Miles 1–30	Pace should feel easy. Goals: Settle into a comfortable cycling rhythm; establish food and drink strategy.	Once the heart rate has settled from the swim, typically upper Zone 1.	You should be holding back through this whole segment.
Miles 31–60	Pace should feel steady. Goals: A continued emphasis on nutrition and hydration as well as an overall assessment of how the day is progressing.	Typically, Zone 2 effort.	The goal of this stage is to maintain a steady effort at goal Ironman-distance bike pace.
Miles 61–90	Pace should feel steady. Hills and rollers will see efforts up to mod-hard intensity. Avoid threshold intensity. Goals: This is the meat of the ride. Here is where early ride pacing pays off or takes its toll. Goal should be to work a little harder than goal effort. If you have paced properly you will begin to move up the field.	Typically, upper Zone 2 effort with short periods of Zone 3 effort when climbing.	This is the key stage and where you will have to concentrate to maintain your focus. Early ride pacing starts to pay off, and you will receive a mental boost as you start to move through the field.
Miles 91–112	Pace should feel steady to mod-hard. There will be fatigue and stiffness, but these should be manageable. Goals: Maintain your cycling momentum and continue to eat. Chances are, you will have lost your appetite, but continued nutrition is essential for a strong run.	Zone 2 effort with periods of Zone 3 effort when climbing.	Maintain your focus on pacing, nutrition, and aero position. Race fatigue can cause your mind to wander. Maintain task orientation.

TABLE 15.2 APPROPRIATE PACING WITH POWER

BIKE SPLIT \ INTENSITY FACTOR	67%	68%	69%	70%	71%	72%	73%	74%	75%	76%	77%	78%	79%	80%
6:30	292	301	309	319	328	337	346							
6:20	284	293	302	310	319	328	338	347						
6:10	277	285	294	302	311	320	329	338	347					
6:00	269	277	286	294	302	311	320	329	338	347				
5:50	262	270	278	286	294	302	311	319	328	337	346			
5:40	254	262	270	278	286	294	302	310	319	327	336	345		
5:30	247	254	262	270	277	285	293	301	309	318	326	335	343	352
5:20	239	247	254	261	269	276	284	292	300	308	316	324	333	341
5:10	232	239	246	253	260	268	275	283	291	298	306	314	322	331
5:00		231	238	245	252	259	266	274	281	289	296	304	312	320
4:50			230	237	244	251	258	265	272	279	287	294	392	309
4:40				229	235	242	249	256	263	270	277	284	291	299
4:30					227	233	240	246	253	260	267	274	281	288

Note: Intensity factor = average normalized power divided by functional threshold power.
Source: Copyright 2008 by Rick Ashburn.

	Left a little on the table
	Safe zone for unsure runners and novices
	Good range for most age-group athletes with good preparation
	For proven strong Ironman runners only
	Run a few miles, then walk it in
	You are likely blown; try again next year

The numbers shown above are the training stress scores (TSS) associated with the relevant bike split and intensity factor. They are included here to help guide your race-simulation rides and target race pacing. For more information on power analysis, visit www.TrainingPeaks.com. Specific reference material can be found at www.cyclingpeakssoftware.com/power411/.

Racing with Power

Ironman-distance race performance is maximized when marathon speed is optimized. In other words, the fastest Ironman-distance race performances result from events in which the athlete ran well relative to his or her training potential. Racing with power provides you with an additional tool to effectively manage your bike effort.

General guidelines. Do not spend any material time near functional threshold power. If you are standing, riding over rollers, or climbing, then start backing off as you approach functional threshold power.

Never hit VO_2max power, even for a second. The physiological cost associated with riding at VO_2max significantly exceeds the expected time benefit.

Half-Ironman-distance benchmarking. A half-Ironman-distance race can provide valuable data for use in an Ironman-distance race. In order to consider the race data valid, it is important that you were able to run well off the bike. We define running well as being able to run within 7 percent of your open half-marathon time. If you were not able to achieve this run performance, then assume that you rode too hard on the bike leg.

Armed with a valid half-Ironman race result, review the average power (not normalized) and average heart rate from the bike leg. Use the data as follows:

- The average heart rate from the bike leg becomes the absolute maximum heart rate cap. Do not exceed this cap for any reason, even when climbing. On the flats, you should be 10–20 bpm below this benchmark.
- The average power (not normalized) from the bike leg becomes a maximum power cap for riding on the flats (not a target).

Race-simulation workouts. Ultimately, your goal effort for the bike leg should come from honest race-simulation rides. As a starting point, target a power output of 10 percent under half-Ironman-distance effort. Remember that your best training performance provides a maximum reference point rather than a base reference point.

Physically, a well-trained athlete can exceed these guidelines. However, the metabolic cost far exceeds the small benefit that accrues to the bike split.

These guidelines have helped the best athletes in the sport run to their potential.

BIKE-TO-RUN TRANSITION

Many athletes spend a long time in the second transition. Unless you have a medical problem, you should move through the transition area steadily and efficiently. Even if you are walking on the run course, you are making better time than if you were sitting in transition.

If you are racing in conditions where the sun is strong, take advantage of the sunscreen available in the transition area. In all races, be sure to use a lubricant on sensitive areas. Carrying a small tube of Body Glide or Vaseline can save time and enable on-the-fly lubrication.

THE RUN

After winning Ironman New Zealand in 2002, Cameron Brown described the marathon as "twenty miles of hope and six miles of reality." This is an excellent approach to the run.

A few minutes of power walking is an excellent way to start your marathon, reduce the stress on your digestion, and establish your cadence. Many marathons have been ruined by an overexuberant opening 3 miles.

If you have executed your race strategy according to plan, then once you have found your running legs, you will feel strong in the early part of the run. Many athletes find that they are able to run very fast in the early part of the marathon. Again, having patience and holding back is essential. Early in the run, athletes should focus on maintaining a relaxed pace while doing their best to ensure that their nutrition and hydration needs are being met.

In general, you should be able to maintain a pace that is 40–90 sec. per mile slower than what you have run in a half-Ironman-distance race. Better-conditioned and better-paced athletes will be at the lower end of this range. Another common run prediction formula is that a properly trained and paced athlete should be able to run within 20 min. of a recent stand-alone marathon time.

Although it can be interesting to develop a pacing strategy in advance, most athletes will find that they are left with few options on race day. Once you leave your bike, it is best to run with a little in reserve until at least mile 16 of the marathon. Whether you are racing for prize money, for a slot at the World Championships, or simply for the joy of finishing, you will find that huge amounts of time can be made up, or lost, between miles 14 and 20.

The race really begins somewhere near the end of the first half of the marathon. By this stage, everyone is feeling tired, and the race is starting to grind down people's resolve. The second half of the marathon is when you will find out the results of your training, pacing, nutrition, and hydration efforts. It is also when you will discover whether you have the toughness to push well beyond your comfort zone. Athletes who are looking to achieve their very best should bring all of their mental strength to bear on the final half of the marathon. It is essential to continue to eat, drink, and push right to the finish line. You never know what is happening

Gordo's Top 10 Mistakes in Ironman Racing

10 Did too much in the week leading up to the race.

9 Ate too much in the week leading up to the race.

8 Didn't check race setup until 60 min. before bike check-in closed (there were problems).

7 Drank a bottle of extra-strength sports drink before the swim start.

6 Forgot that it is normal to feel bad sometimes during the race.

5 Ate a sports bar in T1 (water or nothing now).

4 Mixed sports drink too strong.

3 Hung on to the feet of a faster swimmer for far too long.

2 Went anaerobic in the first 400 m of the swim.

1 Rode too hard in the first 90 min. of the bike.

with your competitors up the road, and it is possible to make up substantial time and placings in the final stages of the race. Even if you are having problems, continue to press onward, as you could recover very quickly. There are many examples of athletes coming back when their prospects appeared bleak at various times during the race.

It is recommended that all athletes experiment with a run/walk strategy in training and consider using it on race day. If you think there is a chance that you will walk during any part of the marathon, then create a plan to get the most out of your walking. Start at the beginning of the marathon and stick to the pattern you've rehearsed in training. This is a proven method that has helped athletes of all abilities. You will find more information on run/walk strategies in the "Run/Walk Protocol" section in Chapter 8.

Break the run into pieces if it gets challenging: A good strategy can be to run from aid station to aid station. The next aid station becomes the key objective, and you are rewarded with a walking break, which you can use for effective eating and drinking.

Wear clothing that will see you through the heat of the late afternoon and keep you warm in the evening. Your first Ironman-distance experience is not a race; it is a test of how much patience you are prepared to exercise so that you do not expire during the marathon.

Training for and racing in an Ironman triathlon are a large undertaking. The training involves long hours laced with numerous trials and tribulations. Race day is the icing on the cake, but even the icing runs from time to time. It's a long day out there, and anything can happen at any time.

In order to prevent some of the more common errors in training, do your best to learn from the common mistakes of others. The best way to overcome race day mishaps is to prevent them from the beginning and remain calm while dealing with them if they come up.

MENTAL TOUGHNESS

Odds are that sometime during the day, you are going to feel really, really bad. This feeling is normal, and things will get better if you persevere to the end. Finish at all costs, and you will thank yourself later.

Even on a good day, things will go wrong—the race has no respect for previous results. If your last race was good, then the next one could be a challenge. Start with a series of objectives in mind, and if one is not achievable, drop down to the next. Remember to keep everything in perspective and continually move toward the finish line. If your wheels come off, then regroup by slowing down (or even stopping) and focusing on your nutrition and hydration. Many athletes have taken breaks of 30–60 min., eaten some real food, and finished comfortably within the cutoff.

RACE DAY NUTRITION

You have probably come across some wildly different guidelines for the number of calories you need on race day. Keep in mind that such estimates are highly variable from one athlete to another. Some Ironman triathletes can consume up to 600 calories per hour without difficulty, whereas others top out at 225 per hour. It is very important to practice what your body can handle during training and C-priority races. Rehearse your nutrition and hydration strategy under race-type conditions in the months before your A-priority race. Do not try anything new in your most important race. Make the race as normal as possible for your body.

You can modify this timeline according to your personal nutrition needs for race day:

Five to 8 min. prior to race start. Drink 10–16 ounces of sports drink (slightly diluted), or consume one gel with half a bottle of water. You will not consume anything else until your heart rate has settled to below your early race target.

On the bike. Drink half a bike bottle of water before starting to eat—it settles the stomach and ensures that the food is more easily absorbed. Once your heart rate has settled, begin consuming gels, sports bars, and sports drinks as required. Remember to drink water to aid absorption of gels and bars.

Common Race Day Errors

Here are the classic errors many athletes make in a race situation.

Trying something new on race day. The number-one rule on race day is "nothing new." You have spent many months training and preparing for race day. Waking up on race morning and deciding you are going to try this new sports drink your friends swear by, or throwing on a brand-new pair of running shoes, is not the wisest choice. Always go with what you have proven in training and what works for you—from nutrition to equipment to clothing.

Starting too fast on the swim. Many athletes get caught up in the mass energy at the race start and hit the water full speed ahead. The start can be crazy with so many people so close, and you can easily find yourself 300 m off the beach gasping for breath with your heart rate over the top. You aren't going to win the race by winning the swim, but you can certainly lose it.

Aim for a pace that feels very comfortable; keep your strokes long and your breath relaxed. After a full taper and pumped with adrenaline, you might feel as if you are taking it easy when in fact you are swimming moderately hard to hard. Pick up a draft and ride a set of feet through the swim. Drafting will enable you to take minutes off your swim time without any extra effort. The key thing to remember during the swim is to stay relaxed with a smooth stroke. If you stay aerobic, draft well, and maintain your stroke mechanics, a pleasant surprise will likely await you at the swim exit.

Starting too fast on the bike. We keep repeating this one, so it must be important. At the start of the bike, ride easy and let your body and, specifically, your heart rate settle. Early on, you may feel fantastic and can easily push the pace. It will be tough to let a few people drop you, but you must let your system settle and start to take in the nutrition. Pushing too hard too soon can leave you with nothing in the tank late in the day.

The race is supposed to feel comfortable for the first three to four hours. Don't be fooled. It will get tough later, and there is no need to rush this process. By conserving on the bike, you will put yourself in a position to run the marathon. The mental benefit of passing people on the run far outweighs the few minutes you might save by pushing on the bike. A solid pacing strategy will see you to T2 in good shape.

Blowing up in the first half of the run. Stick to your pre-race plan and hold back until at least mile 16 of the run. Think of it as a test of how much patience you are prepared to exercise so that you don't expire or explode before the second half of the marathon—which is where the real race begins.

Misjudging Mother Nature. You may have had a top-notch taper. Nutrition and pacing may be spot-on. You may be feeling unstoppable. However, the one formidable force you forgot to prepare for was the elements. The race goes on, rain or shine. Being unprepared for heat and glaring sun or rain and cold can ruin what would otherwise be a perfect day out. In hot races, remember to use a water-based sunscreen as well as reflective clothing. If there is a chance of rain, pack more clothing than you think you need—arm warmers, leggings, gloves, and socks.

You can test and adapt this example of nutrition for the bike leg based on your needs and how much time you think you'll need:

- 0–20 min.: Water only
- 20–40 min.: 150 calories
- 40–60 min.: 150 calories
- 60–120 min.: Target 150 calories per 20 min.

The above schedule would provide 750 calories in the first two hours—this figure would be an appropriate starting point for an average male competitor but must be tested extensively prior to race day. Appetites and concentration can lapse later in the day, so it is beneficial to have a little nutrition in the bank. If you target 450 calories per hour, you'll probably end up with 375 to 425 calories. Smaller male athletes and women will need to reduce these quantities. Always base your race day caloric intake on what you learned during training.

> **BOTH YOUR BODY WEIGHT AND YOUR ANTICIPATED TIME** on the course will affect your nutrition plan. Middle-of-the-pack or back-of-the-pack Clydesdale men are going to need to eat significantly more than will a 165-pound athlete. In general, most men should target 450 calories per hour and most women 200–300 calories per hour.

Eat right up to the end of the bike. Anything can happen on the run, so it is wise to have a calorie buffer.

In T2. Consume one or two gels if you can stomach them, followed by water.

On the run. Alternate between cola/water and sports drink/water at every aid station. Start on the cola immediately. If you are peeing a lot, drop the water, but keep alternating between cola and sports drink. Many athletes can never eat anything solid or semisolid during the run.

Finally, as a general rule, don't plan on anything other than liquid "survival" calories during the run, and try to consume 60 percent of your bike calories in the first half of the ride.

RACE DAY HYDRATION

On the bike, drink only water until your heart rate has settled, then drink one to two bike bottles of water alternating with sports drink per hour. If you are peeing more than once an hour, back off on the water and switch to sports drink. If you aren't peeing at all, slow down and increase your hydration to ensure that you finish the bike well hydrated. By the time you feel thirsty, you are most likely dehydrated. Stay slightly ahead of your needs when it comes to hydration. If you find yourself dehydrated, then slow your effort immediately and increase overall hydration; the time you lose will be more than compensated for by improved late-race performance.

On a hot day, you should be looking at consuming more than 1 quart per hour, though personal needs are highly variable here. Target a minimum of 1 quart per hour, and ease off if you start peeing more than once an hour. If your food on the bike consists of gels, bars, and a liquid carbohydrate source, a higher water intake early in the bike is essential because of the concentrated nature of your food.

If you are having problems with bloating on the run and you are peeing, switch to sports drink/cola only. If you feel bloated and are not peeing, take an electrolyte tablet, slow down, and switch to water only.

Athletes should look at sodium supplementation as insurance. Most athletes probably don't need it, but they feel better taking it. There are, however, certain athletes who may experience significant troubles if they don't supplement. If you think you might benefit from sodium supplementation, you should experiment during your long sessions in training. Such experimentation is highly recommended if you are new to Ironman-distance racing.

Another factor to bear in mind is the sports drink you are planning to use. Some athletes use a sports drink that contains no sodium, but to race long on that beverage (alone) would be pretty risky. In general, 400 mg of sodium per hour is enough for most athletes. Some athletes require up to 1,000 mg of sodium per hour, and others require no supplementation at all.

If you plan to supplement, you should start as soon as you start drinking water on the bike. How much extra sodium you take in depends on how much sodium is in the sports drink and food you are consuming. By reading labels and using simple math, you can determine the quantity weeks in advance of the race. There are many commercial electrolyte sources available. Be wary of chronic sodium supplementation, as you may be placing yourself on a high-sodium diet without realizing it. Consult your health care professional if you are in doubt.

IMMEDIATE TRANSITION GUIDELINES

Immediately after your race, put your priorities in this order:

1. Remove all heat stress; reestablish normal hydration levels.
2. Consume recovery foods.
3. Remove all heat from legs.
4. Undertake a flexibility routine.

POST-RACE GUIDELINES

We highly recommend that there be no efforts above heart rate Zone 1 for the first four days after a half-Ironman-distance race and for ten days after an Ironman-distance race. After this window, sustained efforts above Zone 2 should be done only in the pool (if at all). If you have completed your final race of the season, then there is no rush to get back to training, and you should consider an extended period of little to no training.

Sleep as much as you want (and more than normal). Sleep is far more important than training during this time.

Eat high-quality foods. Your training volume will be low, so avoid sugars and high-GI carbohydrates. Focus on nutrient-dense foods such as whole fruits, fresh vegetables, and lean protein. Note that lean protein does not mean fat-free processed meat. Whole cuts of "real" (ideally free-range) meat are superior.

Walk and stretch as much as you want. Easy spinning for 15–30 min. prior to a stretching session promotes circulation and mobility in sore muscle groups and will speed recovery. Massages and yoga are other active-recovery activities that will enhance your recovery.

Do no running for at least four days after a half-Ironman-distance race and twelve days after an Ironman-distance race. As an additional guideline, you should not start running until you feel you are able to hold a steady pace on the bike. If you are unable to elevate your heart rate on the bike or feel breathless very quickly (in any session), then you need more recovery and total rest.

Somewhere in the four- to fourteen-day post-race window, you will likely start to feel better. At this stage, you can begin to test your recovery with steady aerobic efforts (heart rate Zone 2) on the bike. Resist the urge to hammer yourself, and be very cautious in group situations. Such caution is especially essential if you had a disappointing race because your mind will try to convince you to "redeem" yourself. Save your energy for preparing for next time rather than blowing your recovery period. Remember that, for many reasons, race recovery for

> **TAKE RESPONSIBILITY** for your own recovery, race smart, and plan ahead.
>
> - You can remove heat stress and leg heat by standing in cold water up to your waist (i.e., return to the swim start).
> - If you feel faint, elevate your legs, eat recovery food, and drink fluids. This will likely help you more than taking an IV.
> - Avoid deep-tissue massages and hot tubs in the first twenty-four hours after the race. Although they may feel good, these treatments are likely to cause further muscle trauma. A sports massage is better timed for the two- to five-day period directly after the race.

any distance can take up to four months. Keep resting until you feel ready to go. Rushing your race recovery is a false economy.

At all times, remember that if you feel like doing nothing, then doing nothing is okay. When you are tired, focus on low-impact active recovery. The deeper your base, the more likely you will benefit from active recovery. If you are completely nuked, then total rest is the best way to go.

IRONMAN-DISTANCE RACE RECOVERY

One of the most common mistakes athletes make is coming back too quickly after an ultraendurance event. Many athletes have pushed themselves into a deeply overtrained state by following an Ironman-distance race with a series of short-course races. If your body is not ready to start training again, you will receive numerous warning signals. Ignoring these signals and continuing to push will likely end in either injury or illness.

Recovery time varies from person to person and from season to season. In general, most athletes will find that they require at least two months before they are able to race or train hard again. The recovery period is highly variable—it can be as short as a month or as long as six months. Additional recovery guidelines are described in Chapter 5.

One of the best methods to promote recovery is frequent massage. Although research typically doesn't support this, there is little doubt in the minds of those who use it that it is effective. Massage helps to relieve muscle tension, removes metabolic waste products, and may reduce muscle soreness following strenuous training. Most effective for your body is one massage every week throughout the year and two massages per week during your key Build periods. Acupressure and Rolfing may also be beneficial.

RETURNING TO TRAINING

If you are deeply fatigued, then keep resting and focusing on low-impact active recovery. Watch your morning heart rate. It will give you a clue to your recovery. Continue to make sleep the number-one priority throughout this period.

As a trained athlete, you will likely recover fastest with low-intensity work. There will come a point when you need to help yourself with light activity. If you have a job where you sit a lot, then get up at least every 90 min. to stretch. Walking, a few side bends, a few knee bends—these help year-round but even more when you have post-race stiffness. After you have been feeling eager to train for at least five days, it is time to begin tapering back into training. When you feel ready to train again, keep in mind that maintaining your skills inventory is a year-round priority—as you pick up swimming, cycling, and running, always focus on form.

As swimming is the most skill-oriented of our sports, your first priority is to get back in the water. Frequent, moderate, and skill-oriented swims are best. Be very cautious with any muscular endurance work. Sustained high-intensity swimming is the most risky form of training at this time.

Help preserve your aerobic pathways by getting back on your bike. Choose some favorite rides, and keep your pace and intensity low. On at least one ride, insert 15–30 min. of steady riding at heart rate Zone 2 to "test" your recovery. Your steady pace in this stage should be based on rating of perceived exertion (RPE)—don't drill yourself!

Your taper, the race, and the subsequent break mean that your strength will be close to a season low. Head to the gym and ease back into strength training. It is very important that you do not try to add any strength. For at least the first three strength training sessions, limit yourself to a single set of each exercise, twenty-five to thirty repetitions at an intensity that is "embarrassingly light."

If your swimming and cycling are going well, then it is time to add an easy run. Again, choose a favorite route and stay flexible on duration. If you are feeling good, then a moderate run is okay—otherwise, keep it short. It is normal to have an elevated heart rate when coming back to running. Use your heart rate monitor and insert walking breaks to ensure that you don't overdo it.

You now have the benefit of a little distance from your race. Sit down and spend some time reviewing your race, and season, performance. Write down the lessons you learned for the future. You should also consider your key limiters for achieving your future goals.

Finally, consider your goals: Do they represent what you want to do with your life? Are they appropriate and achievable? Are you committed to doing what it takes to achieve them? We race and train for ourselves. Be 100 percent honest with yourself. If your heart is not in long-distance racing, recognizing it will be the best choice for you.

EPILOGUE BY JOE FRIEL

Triathlon is a challenging and fulfilling sport made all the more enjoyable when success accompanies participation. Going long is the biggest challenge in triathlon. I hope you have found this book to be helpful as you prepare for your next Ironman-distance race. Please let us know what you discovered, as we are always interested in hearing from real athletes like you. To contact me, go to my Web site at www.TrainingPeaks.com. I look forward to hearing of your success in long-distance triathlon racing.

EPILOGUE BY GORDON BYRN

Our goal in creating the second edition of this book was to bring the text up-to-date with the latest information, primarily with respect to nutrition, power-based training, and our best advice for achieving your athletic potential. Although there are material changes in the text, the fundamentals of endurance success remain the same—a consistent, moderate protocol applied over time.

For more information and further updates, visit my personal Web site at www.Endurance Corner.com.

APPENDIX A

DEFINING YOUR TRAINING ZONES BY SPORT

The following tables will help you define your training zones throughout the season for swimming, cycling, and running. To find your personal training zones you will locate your average functional threshold (FT) pace or your FT heart rate (FTHR). Tables A.1 and A.4 estimate your swimming and running training zones based on pace. In the case of swimming, this approach is preferable due to the limitations of using a heart rate monitor in the pool. To use pace to define your running zones, it is important that you use your time for a 5km or 10km race, not triathlon splits, which would be slower.

You will notice that there is not a pace-based table for cycling—power is a better measurement. You can also refer to the power-based cycling tests in Chapter 7 to establish your training zones for cycling.

Tables A.2 and A.3 use FT heart rate to pinpoint your training zones for cycling and running, respectively. You will need to first complete the Bike and Run FTHR Test in Appendix B.

TABLE A.1 ESTIMATED SWIMMING ZONES

Use your average split time for a 1,000-meter or 1,000-yard time trial.

1,000 M/YD	ZONE 1 Active Recovery	ZONE 2 Extensive Endurance	ZONE 3 Intensive Endurance	ZONE 4 Threshold Training	ZONE 5A Threshold Training	ZONE 5B VO$_2$max Intervals	ZONE 5C Anaerobic Repetitions
9:35–9:45	1:13+	1:09–1:12	1:04–1:08	1:01–1:03	0:58–1:00	0:54–0:57	0:53–max
9:46–9:55	1:15+	1:11–1:14	1:06–1:10	1:02–1:05	0:59–1:01	0:55–0:58	0:54–max
9:56–10:06	1:16+	1:12–1:15	1:07–1:11	1:03–1:06	1:00–1:02	0:56–0:59	0:55–max
10:18–10:28	1:18+	1:14–1:17	1:09–1:13	1:05–1:08	1:02–1:04	0:58–1:01	0:57–max
10:29–10:40	1:20+	1:15–1:19	1:10–1:14	1:06–1:09	1:03–1:05	0:58–1:02	0:57–max
10:41–10:53	1:22+	1:17–1:21	1:12–1:16	1:08–1:11	1:05–1:07	1:00–1:04	0:59–max
10:54–11:06	1:23+	1:19–1:22	1:13–1:18	1:09–1:12	1:06–1:08	1:01–1:05	1:00–max
11:07–11:18	1:24+	1:20–1:23	1:14–1:19	1:10–1:13	1:07–1:09	1:02–1:06	1:01–max

continued >

TABLE A.1 ESTIMATED SWIMMING ZONES, CONTINUED

1,000 M/YD	ZONE 1 Active Recovery	ZONE 2 Extensive Endurance	ZONE 3 Intensive Endurance	ZONE 4 Threshold Training	ZONE 5A Threshold Training	ZONE 5B VO$_2$max Intervals	ZONE 5C Anaerobic Repetitions
11:19–11:32	1:26+	1:21–1:25	1:15–1:20	1:11–1:14	1:08–1:10	1:03–1:07	1:02–max
11:33–11:47	1:28+	1:23–1:27	1:17–1:22	1:13–1:16	1:10–1:12	1:05–1:09	1:04–max
11:48–12:03	1:29+	1:24–1:28	1:18–1:23	1:14–1:17	1:11–1:13	1:06–1:10	1:05–max
12:04–12:17	1:32+	1:26–1:31	1:20–1:25	1:16–1:19	1:13–1:15	1:07–1:12	1:06–max
12:18–12:30	1:33+	1:28–1:32	1:22–1:27	1:17–1:21	1:14–1:16	1:08–1:13	1:07–max
12:31–12:52	1:35+	1:30–1:34	1:24–1:29	1:19–1:23	1:16–1:18	1:10–1:15	1:09–max
12:53–13:02	1:38+	1:32–1:37	1:26–1:31	1:21–1:25	1:18–1:20	1:12–1:17	1:11–max
13:03–13:28	1:40+	1:34–1:39	1:28–1:33	1:23–1:27	1:20–1:22	1:14–1:19	1:13–max
13:29–13:47	1:41+	1:36–1:40	1:29–1:35	1:24–1:28	1:21–1:23	1:15–1:20	1:14–max
13:48–14:08	1:45+	1:39–1:44	1:32–1:38	1:27–1:31	1:23–1:26	1:17–1:22	1:16–max
14:09–14:30	1:46+	1:40–1:45	1:33–1:39	1:28–1:32	1:24–1:27	1:18–1:23	1:17–max
14:31–14:51	1:50+	1:44–1:49	1:36–1:35	1:31–1:35	1:27–1:30	1:21–1:26	1:20–max
14:52–15:13	1:52+	1:46–1:51	1:39–1:45	1:33–1:38	1:29–1:32	1:23–1:28	1:22–max
15:14–15:52	1:56+	1:49–1:55	1:42–1:48	1:36–1:41	1:32–1:35	1:25–1:31	1:24–max
15:43–16:08	1:58+	1:52–1:57	1:44–1:51	1:38–1:43	1:34–1:37	1:27–1:33	1:26–max
16:09–16:38	2:02+	1:55–2:01	1:47–1:54	1:41–1:46	1:37–1:40	1:30–1:36	1:29–max
16:39–17:06	2:04+	1:57–2:03	1:49–1:56	1:43–1:48	1:39–1:42	1:32–1:38	1:31–max
17:07–17:38	2:09+	2:02–2:08	1:53–2:01	1:47–1:52	1:43–1:46	1:35–1:42	1:34–max
17:39–18:12	2:13+	2:05–2:12	1:57–2:04	1:50–1:56	1:46–1:49	1:38–1:45	1:37–max
18:13–18:48	2:18+	2:10–2:17	2:01–2:09	1:54–2:00	1:50–1:53	1:42–1:49	1:41–max
18:49–19:26	2:21+	2:13–2:20	2:04–2:12	1:57–2:03	1:53–1:56	1:44–1:52	1:43–max
19:27–20:06	2:26+	2:18–2:25	2:08–2:17	2:01–2:07	1:56–2:00	1:48–1:55	1:47–max
20:07–20:50	2:31+	2:22–2:30	2:12–2:21	2:05–2:11	2:00–2:04	1:52–1:59	1:51–max
20:51–21:37	2:37+	2:28–2:36	2:18–2:27	2:10–2:17	2:05–2:09	1:56–2:04	1:55–max
21:38–22:27	2:42+	2:33–2:41	2:22–2:32	2:14–2:21	2:09–2:13	2:00–2:08	1:59–max
22:38–23:22	2:48+	2:38–2:47	2:27–2:37	2:19–2:26	2:14–2:18	2:04–2:13	2:03–max
23:23–24:31	2:55+	2:45–2:54	2:34–2:44	2:25–2:33	2:20–2:24	2:10–2:19	2:09–max
24:32–25:21	3:02+	2:52–3:01	2:40–2:51	2:31–2:39	2:25–2:30	2:15–2:24	2:14–max

TABLE A.2 CYCLING HEART RATE ZONES

Find your FT pulse (bold) in the Zone 5a column. Read across, left and right, for cycling training zones.

ZONE 1 Active Recovery	ZONE 2 Extensive Endurance	ZONE 3 Intensive Endurance	ZONE 4 Threshold Training	ZONE 5A Threshold Training	ZONE 5B VO$_2$max Intervals	ZONE 5C Anaerobic Repetitions
<109	109–122	123–128	129–136	**137**–140	141–145	146+
<110	110–123	124–129	130–137	**138**–141	142–146	147+
<110	110–124	125–130	131–138	**139**–142	143–147	148+
<111	111–125	126–130	131–139	**140**–143	144–147	148+
<112	112–125	126–131	132–140	**141**–144	145–148	149+
<113	113–126	127–132	133–141	**142**–145	146–149	150+
<113	113–127	128–133	134–142	**143**–145	146–150	151+
<114	114–128	129–134	135–143	**144**–147	148–151	152+
<115	115–129	130–135	136–144	**145**–148	149–152	153+
<116	116–130	131–136	137–145	**146**–149	150–154	155+
<117	117–131	132–137	138–146	**147**–150	151–155	156+
<118	118–132	133–138	139–147	**148**–151	152–156	157+
<119	119–133	134–139	140–148	**149**–152	153–157	158+
<120	120–134	135–140	141–149	**150**–153	154–158	159+
<121	121–134	135–141	142–150	**151**–154	155–159	160+
<122	122–135	136–142	143–151	**152**–155	156–160	161+
<123	123–136	137–142	143–152	**153**–156	157–161	162+
<124	124–137	138–143	144–153	**154**–157	158–162	163+
<125	125–138	139–144	145–154	**155**–158	159–163	164+
<126	126–138	139–145	146–155	**156**–159	160–164	165+
<127	127–140	141–146	147–156	**157**–160	161–165	166+
<128	128–141	142–147	148–157	**158**–161	162–167	168+
<129	129–142	143–148	149–158	**159**–162	163–168	169+
<130	130–143	144–148	149–159	**160**–163	164–169	170+
<130	130–143	144–150	151–160	**161**–164	165–170	171+
<131	131–144	145–151	152–161	**162**–165	166–171	172+

continued >

TABLE A.2 CYCLING HEART RATE ZONES, CONTINUED

ZONE 1 Active Recovery	ZONE 2 Extensive Endurance	ZONE 3 Intensive Endurance	ZONE 4 Threshold Training	ZONE 5A Threshold Training	ZONE 5B VO$_2$max Intervals	ZONE 5C Anaerobic Repetitions
<132	132–145	146–152	153–162	**163**–166	167–172	173+
<133	133–146	147–153	154–163	**164**–167	168–173	174+
<134	134–147	148–154	155–164	**165**–168	169–174	175+
<135	135–148	149–154	155–165	**166**–169	170–175	176+
<136	136–149	150–155	156–166	**167**–170	171–176	177+
<137	137–150	151–156	157–167	**168**–171	172–177	178+
<138	138–151	152–157	158–168	**169**–172	173–178	179+
<139	139–151	152–158	159–169	**170**–173	174–179	180+
<140	140–152	153–160	161–170	**171**–174	175–180	181+
<141	141–153	154–160	161–171	**172**–175	176–181	182+
<142	142–154	155–161	162–172	**173**–176	177–182	183+
<143	143–155	156–162	163–173	**174**–177	178–183	184+
<144	144–156	157–163	164–174	**175**–178	179–184	185+
<145	145–157	158–164	165–175	**176**–179	180–185	186+
<146	146–158	159–165	166–176	**177**–180	181–186	187+
<147	147–159	160–166	167–177	**178**–181	182–187	188+
<148	148–160	161–166	167–178	**179**–182	183–188	189+
<149	149–160	161–167	168–179	**180**–183	184–190	191+
<150	150–161	162–168	169–180	**181**–184	185–191	192+
<151	151–162	163–170	171–181	**182**–185	186–192	193+
<152	152–163	164–171	172–182	**183**–186	187–193	194+
<153	153–164	165–172	173–183	**184**–187	188–194	195+
<154	154–165	166–172	173–184	**185**–188	186–195	196+
<155	155–166	167–173	174–185	**186**–189	190–196	197+
<156	156–167	168–174	175–186	**187**–190	191–197	198+
<157	157–168	169–175	176–187	**188**–191	192–198	199+
<158	158–169	170–176	177–188	**189**–192	193–199	200+

continued >

TABLE A.2 CYCLING HEART RATE ZONES, CONTINUED

ZONE 1 Active Recovery	ZONE 2 Extensive Endurance	ZONE 3 Intensive Endurance	ZONE 4 Threshold Training	ZONE 5A Threshold Training	ZONE 5B VO$_2$max Intervals	ZONE 5C Anaerobic Repetitions
<159	159–170	171–177	178–189	**190**–193	194–200	201+
<160	160–170	171–178	179–190	**191**–194	195–201	202+
<161	161–171	172–178	179–191	**192**–195	196–202	203+
<162	162–172	173–179	180–192	**193**–196	197–203	204+
<163	163–173	174–180	181–193	**194**–197	198–204	205+
<164	164–174	175–183	182–194	**195**–198	199–205	206+

TABLE A.3 RUNNING HEART RATE ZONES

Find your FT pulse (bold) in the Zone 5a column. Read across, left and right, for training zones.

ZONE 1 Active Recovery	ZONE 2 Extensive Endurance	ZONE 3 Intensive Endurance	ZONE 4 Threshold Training	ZONE 5A Threshold Training	ZONE 5B VO$_2$max Intervals	ZONE 5C Anaerobic Repetitions
<120	120–126	127–133	134–139	**140**–143	144–149	150+
<120	120–127	128–134	135–140	**141**–144	145–150	151+
<121	121–129	130–135	136–141	**142**–145	146–151	152+
<122	122–130	131–136	137–142	**143**–146	147–152	153+
<123	123–131	132–137	138–143	**144**–147	148–153	154+
<124	124–132	133–138	139–144	**145**–148	149–154	155+
<125	125–133	134–139	140–145	**146**–149	150–155	156+
<125	125–134	135–140	141–146	**147**–150	151–156	157+
<126	126–135	136–141	142–147	**148**–151	152–157	158+
<127	127–135	136–142	143–148	**149**–152	153–158	159+
<128	128–136	137–143	144–149	**150**–153	154–158	159+
<129	129–137	138–144	145–150	**151**–154	155–159	160+
<130	130–138	139–145	146–151	**152**–155	156–160	161+
<131	131–139	140–146	147–152	**153**–156	157–161	162+
<132	132–140	141–147	148–153	**154**–157	158–162	163+
<132	132–141	142–148	149–154	**155**–158	159–164	165+
<133	133–142	143–149	150–155	**156**–159	160–165	166+
<134	134–143	144–150	151–156	**157**–160	161–166	167+
<135	135–143	144–151	152–157	**158**–161	162–167	168+
<136	136–144	145–152	153–158	**159**–162	163–168	169+
<137	137–145	146–153	154–159	**160**–163	164–169	170+
<137	137–146	147–154	155–160	**161**–164	165–170	171+
<138	138–147	148–155	156–161	**162**–165	166–171	172+
<139	139–148	149–155	156–162	**163**–166	167–172	173+
<140	140–149	150–156	157–163	**164**–167	168–174	175+

continued >

TABLE A.3 RUNNING HEART RATE ZONES, CONTINUED

ZONE 1 Active Recovery	ZONE 2 Extensive Endurance	ZONE 3 Intensive Endurance	ZONE 4 Threshold Training	ZONE 5A Threshold Training	ZONE 5B VO$_2$max Intervals	ZONE 5C Anaerobic Repetitions
<141	141–150	151–157	158–164	**165**–168	169–175	176+
<142	142–151	152–158	159–165	**166**–169	170–176	177+
<142	142–152	153–159	160–166	**167**–170	171–177	178+
<143	143–153	154–160	161–167	**168**–171	172–178	179+
<144	144–154	155–161	162–168	**169**–172	173–179	180+
<145	145–155	156–162	163–169	**170**–173	174–179	180+
<146	146–156	157–163	164–170	**171**–174	175–180	181+
<146	146–156	157–164	165–171	**172**–175	176–182	183+
<147	147–157	158–165	166–172	**173**–176	177–183	184+
<148	148–157	158–166	167–173	**174**–177	178–184	185+
<149	149–158	159–167	168–174	**175**–178	179–185	186+
<150	150–159	160–168	169–175	**176**–179	180–186	187+
<151	151–160	161–169	170–176	**177**–180	181–187	188+
<152	152–161	162–170	171–177	**178**–181	182–188	189+
<153	153–162	163–171	172–178	**179**–182	183–189	190+
<154	154–163	164–172	173–179	**180**–183	184–190	191+
<155	155–164	165–173	174–180	**181**–184	185–192	193+
<155	155–165	166–174	175–181	**182**–185	186–193	194+
<156	156–166	167–175	176–182	**183**–186	187–194	195+
<157	157–167	168–176	177–183	**184**–187	188–195	196+
<158	158–168	169–177	178–184	**185**–188	189–196	197+
<159	159–169	170–178	179–185	**186**–189	190–197	198+
<160	160–170	171–179	180–186	**187**–190	191–198	199+
<160	160–170	171–179	180–187	**188**–191	192–199	200+
<161	161–171	172–180	181–188	**189**–192	193–200	201+
<162	162–172	173–181	182–189	**190**–193	194–201	202+

continued >

TABLE A.3 RUNNING HEART RATE ZONES, CONTINUED

ZONE 1 Active Recovery	ZONE 2 Extensive Endurance	ZONE 3 Intensive Endurance	ZONE 4 Threshold Training	ZONE 5A Threshold Training	ZONE 5B VO$_2$max Intervals	ZONE 5C Anaerobic Repetitions
<163	163–173	174–182	183–190	**191**–194	195–201	202+
<164	164–174	175–183	184–191	**192**–195	196–202	203+
<165	165–175	176–184	185–192	**193**–196	197–203	204+
<166	166–176	177–185	186–193	**194**–197	198–204	205+
<166	166–177	178–186	187–194	**195**–198	199–205	206+
<167	167–178	179–187	188–195	**196**–199	200–206	207+
<168	168–178	179–188	189–196	**197**–198	199–207	208+
<169	169–179	180–189	190–197	**198**–201	202–208	209+
<170	170–180	181–190	191–198	**199**–202	203–209	210+
<171	171–181	182–191	192–199	**200**–203	204–210	211+

TABLE A.4 ESTIMATED RUNNING ZONES

Use your time for a 5km or 10km running race (not triathlon split) to estimate your running zones.

5KM	10KM	ZONE 1 Active Recovery	ZONE 2 Extensive Endurance	ZONE 3 Intensive Endurance	ZONE 4 Threshold Training	ZONE 5A Threshold Training	ZONE 5B VO$_2$max Intervals	ZONE 5C Anaerobic Repetitions
14:15	30:00	6:38+	5:52–6:37	5:27–5:51	5:09–5:26	**4:59**–5:08	4:37–4:58	4:36–max
14:45	31:00	6:50+	6:02–6:49	5:37–6:01	5:18–5:36	**5:07**–5:17	4:45–5:06	4:44–max
15:15	32:00	7:02+	6:13–7:01	5:47–6:12	5:27–5:46	**5:16**–5:26	4:53–5:15	4:52–max
15:45	33:00	7:13+	6:23–7:12	5:56–6:22	5:36–5:55	**5:25**–5:35	5:01–5:24	5:00–max
16:10	34:00	7:25+	6:33–7:24	6:06–6:32	5:45–6:05	**5:34**–5:44	5:10–5:33	5:09–max
16:45	35:00	7:36+	6:43–7:35	6:15–6:42	5:54–6:14	**5:42**–5:53	5:18–5:41	5:17–max
17:07	36:00	7:48+	6:54–7:47	6:25–6:53	6:03–6:24	**5:51**–6:02	5:26–5:50	5:25–max
17:35	37:00	8:00+	7:04–7:59	6:34–7:03	6:12–6:33	**6:00**–6:11	5:34–5:59	5:33–max
18:05	38:00	8:11+	7:14–8:10	6:44–7:13	6:21–6:43	**6:09**–6:20	5:42–6:08	5:41–max
18:30	39:00	8:23+	7:24–8:22	6:53–7:23	6:30–6:52	**6:17**–6:29	5:50–6:16	5:49–max
19:00	40:00	8:34+	7:35–8:33	7:03–7:34	6:39–7:02	**6:26**–6:38	5:58–6:25	5:57–max
19:30	41:00	8:46+	7:45–8:45	7:12–7:44	6:48–7:11	**6:35**–6:47	6:06–6:34	6:05–max
19:55	42:00	8:58+	7:55–8:57	7:22–7:54	6:57–7:21	**6:44**–6:56	6:14–6:43	6:13–max
20:25	43:00	9:09+	8:05–9:08	7:31–8:04	7:06–7:30	**6:52**–7:05	6:22–6:51	6:21–max
20:50	44:00	9:21+	8:16–9:20	7:41–8:15	7:15–7:40	**7:01**–7:14	6:31–7:00	6:30–max
21:20	45:00	9:32+	8:26–9:31	7:51–8:25	7:24–7:50	**7:10**–7:23	6:39–7:09	6:38–max
21:50	46:00	9:44+	8:36–9:43	8:00–8:35	7:33–7:59	**7:18**–7:32	6:47–7:17	6:46–max
22:15	47:00	9:56+	8:47–9:55	8:10–8:46	7:42–8:09	**7:27**–7:41	6:55–7:26	6:54–max
22:42	48:00	10:07+	8:57–10:06	8:19–8:56	7:51–8:18	**7:36**–7:50	7:03–7:35	7:02–max
23:10	49:00	10:19+	9:07–10:18	8:29–9:06	8:00–8:28	**7:45**–7:59	7:11–7:44	7:10–max
23:38	50:00	10:31+	9:17–10:30	8:38–9:16	8:09–8:37	**7:53**–8:08	7:19–7:52	7:18–max
24:05	51:00	10:42+	9:28–10:41	8:48–9:27	8:18–8:47	**8:02**–8:17	7:27–8:01	7:26–max
24:35	52:00	10:54+	9:38–10:53	8:57–9:37	8:27–8:56	**8:11**–8:26	7:35–8:10	7:34–max
25:00	53:00	11:05+	9:48–11:04	9:07–9:47	8:36–9:06	**8:20**–8:35	7:43–8:19	7:42–max
25:25	54:00	11:17+	9:58–11:16	9:16–9:57	8:45–9:15	**8:28**–8:44	7:52–8:27	7:51–max

continued >

TABLE A.4 ESTIMATED RUNNING ZONES, CONTINUED

5KM	10KM	ZONE 1 Active Recovery	ZONE 2 Extensive Endurance	ZONE 3 Intensive Endurance	ZONE 4 Threshold Training	ZONE 5A Threshold Training	ZONE 5B VO$_2$max Intervals	ZONE 5C Anaerobic Repetitions
25:55	55:00	11:29+	10:09–11:28	9:26–10:08	8:54–9:25	**8:37**–8:53	8:00–8:36	7:59–max
26:30	56:00	11:40+	10:19–11:39	9:36–10:18	9:03–9:35	**8:46**–9:02	8:08–8:45	8:07–max
26:50	57:00	11:52+	10:29–11:51	9:45–10:28	9:12–9:44	**8:54**–9:11	8:16–8:53	8:15–max
27:20	58:00	12:03+	10:39–12:02	9:55–10:38	9:21–9:54	**9:03**–9:20	8:24–9:02	8:23–max
27:45	59:00	12:15+	10:50–12:14	10:04–10:49	9:30–10:03	**9:12**–9:29	8:32–9:11	8:31–max
28:15	60:00	12:27+	11:00–12:26	10:14–10:59	9:39–10:13	**9:21**–9:38	8:40–9:20	8:39–max

APPENDIX B

TESTING AND WARM-UP PROTOCOLS

Although laboratory tests can provide interesting data, we train in the field, and therefore our experience is that the most useful tests are completed in the field. The tests listed here have been proven to provide a wide range of athletes with accurate intensity zones for their training and racing.

■ A Note on Maximum Heart Rate Tests

Maximum heart rate tests are not recommended, as they are generally inaccurate and extremely stressful on the body. In order to get a true maximum heart rate, you need to push yourself to your absolute limit. This effort can lead to tunnel vision, hearing loss, and near (or actual) collapse. The FT tests outlined in this appendix are much safer and more accurate for the purposes of long-distance training and racing.

■ Swim Functional Threshold Pace Test

Swimming is better tested by pace than by heart rate. In order to determine lactate or functional threshold (FT) pace, start with a deep warm-up (such as the Sample Swim Test Warm-up 1 in this appendix) and then swim a 1,000-meter time trial at the fastest pace you can maintain for the distance. For best results, hold back at the start and build your effort through the test. Your average pace per 100 meters is referred to as your T(1) per 100 pace. Physiologically speaking, your average pace for this test will be above your true functional threshold; however, the training paces contained in Table A.1 (see Appendix A) will accurately define the goals of each training intensity zone.

500s SWIM TEST

The goal of this test is to swim each 500 quicker, descending to your maximum effort. Most swimmers have trouble controlling their pace and reach their maximum effort too quickly. Once you swim the 500s successfully, making each one faster than the last in a balanced manner, your second 500 will be a good estimate of your "steady" pace.

W/U

400 easy on 15 sec. rest
4 x 100 descend on 15 sec. rest
4 x 50 descend on 10 sec. rest

MAIN SET

4 x 500 on 15 sec. rest
Descend to maximum effort with final set

You may also opt to include an additional main set:
200 easy
4 x 200 steady on 15 sec. rest

Cool down.

BEST AVERAGE SWIM TEST

Choose an interval distance (100, 150, 200, or 250) that will take you about three minutes to complete. Swim ten repeats leaving on an interval of 3 min., 30 sec. Aim for your best average pace across the entire workout, keeping pace even from one set to the next. Be sure to note your pace for the initial sets as nearly everyone starts out too fast.

W/U

400 easy on 20 sec. rest
4 x 100 on 15 sec. rest

Set 1: 50 easy, 50 steady
Set 2: 50 steady, 50 mod-hard
Set 3: Easy
Set 4: Fast

4 x 50 easy on 15 sec. rest

MAIN SET

10 x 3 min., leaving on interval of 3 min., 30 sec.

Cool down.

30-MINUTE TIME TRIAL SWIM TEST

For this test, swim for 30 min., aiming for your best average pace. Your first 250 should feel easy. Focus on settling into a steady effort to finish off the first 10 min. Then you will gradually build your effort so the last 15 min. are very close to your average pace for a 1,000 m time trial (T1 pace). Note your average pace for 100 m. To estimate your mod-hard pace, subtract three seconds from your average pace.

W/U

500 easy on 20 sec. rest
4 x 100 descend on 15 sec. rest
4 x 75 done as 25 build, 25 steady, 25 easy on 10 sec. rest
4 x 50 fast on 15 sec. rest
100 easy

MAIN SET

Swim 30 min.

Cool down.

MAX AEROBIC TEST FOR CYCLING

Begin with a deep warm-up (see, for example, the cycling warm-up later in this appendix). For the test, build to the top of Zone 3 over the first 10 min. Then hold that effort for 10 min. You can choose any course for this test, but it is important that you are able to do the test the same way every time. Note your power and pace as appropriate. You can also extend the test to be 40 min., including a 20-min. build to the top of Zone 3, and a 20-min. sustained effort.

BIKE AND RUN FUNCTIONAL THRESHOLD HEART RATE (FTHR) TEST

Following a deep warm-up, perform a 30-min. TT, going at your fastest maintainable pace. After 10 min., hit the lap button on your heart rate receiver. Your average heart rate for the last 20 min. of the TT will roughly be your FTHR—or the bottom of heart rate Zone 5a. Use Tables A.2 and A.3 to find your FTHR for cycling and running, respectively.

Most people go too hard the first time and therefore end up with a lower average heart rate reading for the last 20 min. This is okay because when you are starting, a little low is better than a little high. With time and experience, you will become more accurate.

FTHR testing should be done separately for running and cycling to determine heart rate training zones for each of those sports. These tests are demanding, so you should treat them as breakthrough workouts and ensure proper recovery between tests (allowing at least 48 hours between any two tests is a good rule of thumb).

AEROBIC STEP TEST FOR RUNNING

You might choose to add to your warm-up 20 min. of easy cycling in heart rate Zone 1. Since you will need to conduct this test at the track, it could simply mean hopping on your bike instead of driving.

For this test you will run four laps (1,600 m) at each "step." With each step, you will gradually build to your target heart rate as you run the first two laps, and then hold the target heart rate for the remainder of the step. You will begin the test at 20 bpm below the bottom of your Zone 2 heart rate. With each step, you will increase your target heart rate by 10 bpm. Keep going until you are clearly over your FTHR. (You can choose to keep going and hit your max, but the goal of the test is simply to exceed your FTHR.) To ensure that you are holding an even pace, take splits halfway through each step. At the end of the test, after you cool down, you will want to note times and average and max heart rates for each split.

If you think that your final step will take longer than 8 minutes, reduce all step distances to 1,200 m and build to a target heart rate over the first 600 m of each step.

If you have a portable lactate analyzer, you can test your lactate after the warm-up on the bike, and at the end of each step. This is best done by an experienced tester. Your baseline reading must be less than 1.5 mmol prior to testing. If your initial test shows your lactate level exceeds this, try doing a light activity for ten minutes and then retest. If you are still over the 1.5 mmol, then try again another day. Lactate tests are useful but not essential. An experienced athlete will get a good sense of steady, moderate to moderately hard, and threshold pace and effort from the test.

RUN PACING TEST

This workout can be a useful way to estimate a reasonable pace to target for the running leg of your race. If you are able to hold a steady pace to the end of this workout without significant increases in heart rate or RPE, then it is a good starting point for calculating your target race pace. Your total duration should be 2 hours to 2 hours, 15 min.

Following a thorough warm-up, the first third of your run will be at an easy pace, with little attention given to your mile splits. The second third of the run will be steady. Note your average mile split. For the final third, you will hold the same average pace as you previously held (in the middle third) and notice changes in RPE and average heart rate—both will rise.

Cool down.

VO$_2$MAX TEST FOR RUNNING

Following a deep warm-up (such as the sample running warm-up later in this appendix), run 6 min. at the fastest continuous pace possible. Your goal is to have even or slightly faster splits for each lap.

Note the total distance (in meters) that you complete in the 6 min. VO$_2$max pace is then determined by dividing 142,000 by the total distance run. If you were to cover 1,600 m in 6 min., we would estimate your VO$_2$max pace at 88.75 sec. per 400 m ($142,000 \div 1,600 = 88.75$). Your VO$_2$max pace is also referred to as your sustained speed (SS) pace.

VO$_2$max testing is a maximum-effort test that should be completed only by the strongest athletes who have complete confidence in their ability to finish safely.

Cool down.

> ### TRIPLE BRICK PACE TEST
>
> Like the Run Pacing Test found earlier in this appendix, this test will help to train appropriate pacing. Watch your pace, particularly on the second run interval, so you are able to finish strong.
>
> Do three intervals of 60 min. on the bike, 30 min. running: The first brick should be slower than goal race effort; the second brick should be at goal race effort; the final brick should be faster than goal race effort.
>
> Cool down.

◼ *Sample Swim Test Warm-up*

- 10–20 min. of easy bilateral swimming
- 5–10 min. of steady swimming
- 6 × 50 done as 25 build and 25 easy
- 4 × 50 done as 12.5 sprint and 37.5 easy
- RI between each of the above and after each 50 should be 10–20 sec.

◼ *Shorter Race Warm-up*

This warm-up is good for short races up to Olympic distance and for athletes who are endurance-limited across their race distance.

Ride 15–30 min. easy to warm up your legs. Then do some lower-body stretching for 5–10 min. Following the stretching, walk around, keep your legs warm, and continue to do some light stretching. As close to the race start as possible, do a short skills run consisting of five Strides with walk-backs.

◼ *Deeper Race Warm-up*

This warm-up can be used up to the Olympic distance for most age-group athletes and up to the HIM distance for elite and experience athletes. Strong swimmers (those who can swim an IM-distance swim in 60 min. or less) can use the swim portion of this warm-up for all distances.

Start your warm-up about 75–90 min. pre-race with a 10–15-min. spin on the bike to check gearing and wake up the legs. Return to the transition area, set up, then jog 10–15 min., stretch., and do 4–5 strides. Start swim warm-up at least 35 min. prior to race start with the following:

- 10 min. easy/steady, including 25 backstroke every 100 m. Swim steady to get the arms going, approximately 600 meters. Do a few arm stretches.

- 5 × 100 m on 10-sec. rest intervals as 25 hard stroke, 25 easy, 50 steady (25 stroke done as free, fly, back, fly, free—25 easy and 50 steady are always free)
- 200 steady including 3 pickups, good kick drive on the last pickups
- Stretch arms while waiting for swim start

With most IM-distance races, you will not be able to get your bike out of the transition area. For this reason, a run-swim warm-up combination is recommended for elite and experienced athletes.

■ *Sample Running Warm-up*

Keep in mind that the shorter or more intense your training session or race is, the longer your warm-up should be to maximize performance and guard against injury.

- Run 800 m easy
- Run 1,600–3,000 m with a mix of easy, steady, and running drills
- Eight strides with walk-back recovery (see Chapter 8 for more detail on strides)
- Run 800 m easy, with builds to test effort
- Fully recover for 3–5 min.

APPENDIX C

SWIMMING GLOSSARY

Refer to this glossary for definitions of terms and abbreviations used in the swim workouts in Chapter 6.

3/4 Drill (3/4) Three strokes freestyle, then four strokes backstroke; goal is to keep hips high through transition. Do not start stroking until head and chin have made the transition. Three strokes free, rotate, chin up, four strokes back, rotate, chin down, three strokes free—using this pattern, you will work both rotation directions.

3/5 Alternate between three- and five-stroke breathing unless otherwise noted.

bk Backstroke

b/l Bilateral, three strokes per breath unless otherwise noted

br Breaststroke

Build effort Increase your effort within the interval.

C/D Cool-down

DAB Double-arm backstroke

Descend effort Increase your effort by interval as the set progresses.

DPS Distance per stroke

dr Drill

fly Fly

free Freestyle

IM Individual medley—order is fly, backstroke, breaststroke, then freestyle—if fly is difficult, then you can use polo instead; if your fly or polo form goes, then switch to normal freestyle.

Polo Water-polo swimming, head up freestyle, focus on high elbows

Pull f/g Pull with full gear (band, buoy, paddles)

Pull pads Pull with paddles

RI Rest interval

T(1) Average pace for a 1,000-meter TT

TT Time trial

Wave catch (w/c) One-arm drill where you breathe every two strokes. Staying mainly on your side, focus on recovery up the body line and high elbow on entry, catch, and pull.

W/U Warm-up

APPENDIX D

BRICK WORKOUTS

■ *Indoor Brick Workouts*

These workouts are intended to give you some training ideas for when weather or other factors force you indoors.

INDOOR SESSION 1 (3.25 HOURS)	
W/U	
Run 30 min.	Strides
MAIN SET	
Bike 2 hrs.	1 hr. easy 1 hr. steady
Run 45 min.	15 min. cadence work 15 min. steady 15 min. cadence work
C/D	
15 min. stretching minimum	

INDOOR SESSION 2 (4 HOURS)	
W/U	
Run 30 min.	Strides
MAIN SET	
Bike 75 min.	30 min. easy 15 min. mod-hard 30 min. easy
Run 30 min.	Focus on cadence, head up
Bike 75 min.	25 min. easy 25 min. steady 25 min. mod-hard
Run 30 min.	15 min. of cadence work 15 min. build to mod-hard
C/D	
15 min. stretching minimum	

INDOOR SESSION 3 (3 HOURS)

W/U	
Run 30 min.	Strides with walk-back, otherwise easy

MAIN SET	
Bike 45 min.	Easy with 5 x 20 sec. big gear sprints on 4-min. easy recoveries
Run 30 min.	15 min. steady 15 min. mod-hard
Bike 45 min.	15 min. easy 15 min. steady 15 min. mod-hard
Run 30 min.	Strides with walk-backs, otherwise easy

C/D	
15 min. stretching minimum	

INDOOR SESSION 4 (4 HOURS)

W/U	
Run 30 min.	Strides with walk-backs, otherwise easy

MAIN SET	
Bike 75 min.	20 min. easy 5 x 30 sec. big gear springs on 4-min. easy recoveries Finish steady
Run 30 min.	10 min. smooth cadence, 85–90 rpm 10 min. mod-hard 10 min. steady
Bike 75 min.	30 min. easy 30 min. steady 15 min. mod-hard
Run 30 min.	Strides with walk-backs, otherwise easy

C/D	
15 min. stretching minimum	

INDOOR SESSION 5 (2 HOURS)

W/U

| Run 30 min. | Strides with walk-backs, otherwise easy |

MAIN SET

| Bike 75 min. | 20 min. easy
4 x 30 sec. big-gear sprints on 4-minute easy recoveries
10 min. steady
5 x 1 min. mod-hard at low cadence on 1 min. steady recoveries
Finish steady |
| Run 15 min. | Easy, focus on smooth cadence |

C/D

15 min. stretching minimum

INDOOR SESSION 6 (3 HOURS)

W/U

Easy spinning

MAIN SET

Bike 45 min.	Include 5 x one-leg drills to fatigue with 2 min. spin recoveries
Run 30 min.	Steady
Bike 45 min.	Include 5 x 30 sec. spin-ups, with 2 min., 30 sec. spinning recoveries
Run 30 min.	Steady
Bike 30 min.	Include 5 x 20 sec. big-gear sprints (seated), with 2 min., 40 sec. light spinning recoveries

C/D

15 min. stretching minimum

Note: Rides are easy to steady pace.

■ *Outdoor Brick Workouts*

For more brick workouts, refer to the combined bike/run workouts in Chapter 7.

TRIPLE BRICK

This session helps train appropriate pacing.

MAIN SET

Bike 60 min. Run 30 min.	Slower than goal race effort
Bike 60 min. Run 30 min.	At goal race effort
Bike 60 min. Run 30 min.	Faster than goal race effort

Coach's tip: All transitions should be quick. Watch your pace, particularly on the second run, to be able to finish strong.

BIG-DAY TRAINING

Note: The goal of the brick is to train the body to the demands of an all-day effort. This workout could require as much as 12 hours, including the breaks between the three sessions.

MAIN SET

Swim 45–75 min. Relaxed transition	Easy, negative split
Bike 4–6 hrs. Relaxed transition	Easy, negative split
Run 20–60 min.	Easy, negative split

Coach's tip: The goal of each session is to have a negative split in terms of effort, power, and pace. Transitions should be long and relaxed, including a recovery meal.

REFERENCES AND RECOMMENDED READING

CHAPTER 5

Crouch, Jean. *The Runner's Yoga Book*. Berkeley, CA: Rodmell Press, 1990.

Evans, Mark. *Endurance Athlete's Edge*. Champaign, IL: Human Kinetics, 1997.

Hellemans, Dr. John. *The Training Intensity Handbook*. Napier, New Zealand: KinEli Publishing, 1998.

Personal conversations with coaches Dr. John Hellemans and Mark Elliott, New Zealand Multisport Training Centre run sessions.

Progressions for Athlete and Coach Development. Developed by Human Kinetics for U.S.A. Swimming, 1999.

Romanov, Dr. Nicholas. *The Pose Method of Running* (video). Romanov Academy of Sports Science, 1997.

Scott, Dave. *Dave Scott's Triathlon Training*. New York: Fireside, 1986.

CHAPTER 6

Laughlin, Terry. *Butterfly and Breaststroke the TI Way: Waterproof Drill Guide*. New Paltz, NY: Total Immersion, Inc., 2002.

———. *Swimming Made Easy: The Total Immersion Way for Any Swimmer to Achieve Fluency, Ease, and Speed in Any Stroke*. New Paltz, NY: Swimware, Inc., 2001.

———. *Total Immersion Pool Primer for Freestyle and Backstroke: The TI Way*. New Paltz, NY: Total Immersion, Inc., 2000.

———. *Triathlon Swimming Made Easy: How Anyone Can Succeed in Triathlon (or Open-Water Swimming) with Total Immersion*. New Paltz, NY: Total Immersion, Inc., 2002.

Laughlin, Terry, and John Delves. *Total Immersion: The Revolutionary Way to Swim Better, Faster, and Easier*. New York: Fireside, 1996.

Maglischo, Ernest W. *Swimming Fastest*. Champaign, IL: Human Kinetics, 2003.

CHAPTER 7

Allen, H., and A. Coggan. *Training and Racing with a Power Meter*. VeloPress, 2006.

Baker, A. *The Essential Cyclist*. New York: Lyons Press, 1998.

Bernhardt, G. *The Female Cyclist: Gearing Up a Level*. Boulder, CO: VeloPress, 1999.

Bicycle Gear Inch and Shifting Pattern Calculator: www.panix.com/~jbarrm/cycal/cycal.30f. html.

Bishop, D., and D. G. Jenkins. The Influence of Recovery Duration Between Periods of Exercise on the Critical Power Function. *European Journal of Applied Physiology* 72 (1–2) (1995): 115–120.

Bishop, D., D. G. Jenkins, and A. Howard. The Critical Power Function Is Dependent on the Duration of the Predictive Exercise Tests Chosen. *International Journal of Sports Medicine* 19 (2) (1998): 125–129.

Borysewicz, E. *Bicycle Road Racing*. Brattleboro, VT: VeloNews, 1985.

Boudet, G., E. Albuisson, M. Bedu, and A. Chamoux. Heart Rate–Running Speed Relationships During Exhaustive Bouts in the Laboratory. *Canadian Journal of Applied Physiology* 29 (6) (2004): 731–742.

Burke, E. *Serious Cycling*. Champaign, IL: Human Kinetics, 1995.

Burney, S. *Cyclocross Training and Technique*. Boulder, CO: VeloPress, 1996.

Clingelleffer, A., L. R. McNaughton, and B. Davoren. The Use of Critical Power as a Determinant for Establishing the Onset of Blood Lactate Accumulation. *European Journal of Applied Physiology* 68 (2): 182–187.

Friel, J. *Cycling Past 50*. Champaign, IL: Human Kinetics, 1998.

———. *The Cyclist's Training Bible*. Boulder, CO: VeloPress, 1996.

———. *The Mountain Biker's Training Bible*. Boulder, CO: VeloPress, 2000.

———. *The Triathlete's Training Bible*. Boulder, CO: VeloPress, 1998.

Gaesser, G. A., T. J. Carnevale, A. Garfinkel, et al. Estimation of Critical Power with Nonlinear and Linear Models. *Medicine and Science in Sports and Exercise* 27 (10) (1995): 1430–1438.

Hawley, J. A., and T. D. Noakes. Peak Power Output Predicts Maximal Oxygen Uptake and Performance Time in Trained Cyclists. *European Journal of Applied Physiology* 65 (1) (1992): 79–83.

Herman, E. A., H. G. Knuttgen, P. N. Frykman, and J. F. Patton. Exercise Endurance Time as a Function of Percent Maximal Power Production. *Medicine and Science in Sports and Exercise* 19 (5) (1987): 480–485.

Hill, D. W. The Critical Power: A Review. *Sports Medicine* 16 (4) (1993): 237–254.

Hill, D. W., and J. C. Smith. A Method to Ensure the Accuracy of Estimates of Anaerobic Capacity Derived Using the Critical Power Concept. *Journal of Sports Medicine and Physical Fitness* 34 (1) (1994): 23–37.

Hopkins, S. R., and D. C. McKenzie. The Laboratory Assessment of Endurance Performance in Cyclists. *Canadian Journal of Applied Physiology* 19 (3) (1994): 266–274.

Housh, D. J., T. J. Housh, and S. M. Bauge. The Accuracy of the Critical Power Test for Predicting Time to Exhaustion During Cycle Ergometry. *Ergonomics* 32 (8) (1989): 997–1004.

Housh, T. J., H. A. deVries, D. J. Housh, et al. The Relationship Between Critical Power and the Onset of Blood Lactate Accumulation. *Journal of Sports Medicine and Physical Fitness* 31 (1) (1991): 31–36.

Jenkins, D. G., and B. M. Quigley. Blood Lactate in Trained Cyclists During Cycle Ergometry at Critical Power. *European Journal of Applied Physiology* 61 (3–4) (1990): 278–283.

———. Endurance Training Enhances Critical Power. *Medicine and Science in Sports and Exercise* 24 (11) (1992): 1283–1289.

Lajoie, C., L. Laurencelle, and F. Trudeau. Physiological Responses to Cycling for 60 Minutes at Maximal Lactate Steady State. *Canadian Journal of Applied Physiology* 25 (4) (2000): 250–261.

LeMond, G. *Greg LeMond's Complete Book of Bicycling.* New York: Perigee Books, 1987.

McLellan, T. M., and K. S. Cheung. 1992. A Comparative Evaluation of the Individual Anaerobic Threshold and the Critical Power. *Medicine and Science in Sports and Exercise* 24 (5) (1992): 543–550.

Moritani, T., A. Nagata, H. A. deVries, and M. Muro. Critical Power as a Measure of Physical Work Capacity and Anaerobic Threshold. *Ergonomics* 24 (5) (1981): 339–350.

Morton, R. H. Alternative Forms of the Critical Power Test for Ramp Exercise. *Ergonomics* 40 (5) (1997): 511–514.

———. Critical Power Test for Ramp Exercise. *European Journal of Applied Physiology* 69 (5) (1994): 435–438.

———. Ramp and Constant Power Trials Produce Equivalent Critical Power Estimates. *Medicine and Science in Sports and Exercise* 29 (6) (1997): 833–836.

Mounier, R., V. Pialoux, I. Mischler, J. Coudert, and N. Fellmann. Effect of Hypervolemia on Heart Rate During 4 Days of Prolonged Exercises. *International Journal of Sports Medicine* 24 (7): 523–529.

———. The Relationship Between Power Output and Endurance: A Brief Review. *European Journal of Applied Physiology* 73 (6) (1996): 491–502.

———. A 3-Parameter Critical Power Model. *Ergonomics* 39 (4) (1996): 611–619.

Niles, R. *Time-Saving Training for Multisport Athletes.* Champaign, IL: Human Kinetics, 1997.

Phinney, D., and C. Carpenter. *Training for Cycling.* New York: Perigee Books, 1992.

Skilbeck, P. *Single-Track Mind.* Boulder, CO: VeloPress, 1996.

Sleamaker, R., and R. Browning. *Serious Training for Endurance Athletes.* Champaign, IL: Human Kinetics, 1996.

Vandewalle, H., J. F. Vautier, M. Kachouri, et al. Work-Exhaustion Time Relationships and the Critical Power Concept: A Critical Review. *Journal of Sports Medicine and Physical Fitness* 37 (2) (1997): 89–102.

Vautier, J. F., H. Vandewalle, and H. Monod. Prediction of Exhaustion Time from Heart Rate Drift. *Archives internationales de physiologie, de biochimie et de biophysique* 102 (1) (1994): 61–65.

Wingo, J. E., and K. J. Cureton. Body Cooling Attenuates the Decrease in Maximal Oxygen Uptake Associated with Cardiovascular Drift During Heat Stress. *European Journal of Applied Physiology* 98 (1) (2006): 97–104.

———. Maximal Oxygen Uptake After Attenuation of Cardiovascular Drift During Heat Stress. *Aviation, Space, and Environmental Medicine* 77 (7) (2006): 687–694.

Wingo, J. E., A. J. Lafrenz, M. S. Ganio, G. L. Edwards, and K. J. Cureton. Cardiovascular Drift Is Related to Reduced Maximal Oxygen Uptake During Heat Stress. *Medicine and Science in Sports and Exercise* 37 (2) (2005): 248–255.

CHAPTER 8

Billat, V., B. Flechet, B. Petit, G. Muriaux, and J. P. Koralsztein. Interval Training at VO_2max: Effects on Aerobic Performance and Overtraining Markers. *Medicine and Science in Sports and Exercise* 31 (1) (1999): 156–163.

Daniels, Jack. *Daniels' Running Formula.* Champaign, IL: Human Kinetics, 2005.

McGee, Bobby. *Magical Running: A Unique Path to Running Fulfillment,* 3rd ed. Boulder, CO: Bobbysez Publishing, 2007.

Noakes, Tim. *Lore of Running,* 4th ed. Champaign, IL: Human Kinetics, 2003.

Parker, John L. *Once a Runner.* Tallahassee, FL: Cedarwinds, 1999.

Sandrock, Michael. *Running with the Legends.* Champaign, IL: Human Kinetics, 1996.

Véronique, L. Billat, J. Slawinski, V. Bocquet, A. Demarle, L. Lafitte, P. Chassaing, and J.-P. Koralsztein. Intermittent Runs at the Velocity Associated with Maximal Oxygen Uptake Enables Subjects to Remain at Maximal Oxygen Uptake for a Longer Time Than Intense but Submaximal Runs. *European Journal of Applied Physiology* 81 (3) (2000): 188–196.

CHAPTER 9

Aaberg, Everett. *Resistance Training Instruction.* Champaign, IL: Human Kinetics, 1999.

American Council on Exercises, Personal Trainers Manual. San Diego, CA: American Council on Exercise, 1991.

Friel, Joe. *The Triathlete's Training Bible*, 2nd ed. Boulder, CO: VeloPress, 2004.

Gambetta, Vern, and Steve Odgers. *The Complete Guide to Medicine Ball Training.* Sarasota, FL: Optimum Sports Training, 1991.

CHAPTER 10

Anderson, O. Antioxidants: Do They Really Speed Your Recovery from Strenuous Training? *Running Research News* 13 (4) (1997): 1–5.

Antonio, J., and C. Street. Glutamine: A Potential Useful Supplement for Athletes. *Canadian Journal of Physiology* 24 (1) (1999): 1–14.

Applegate, E. Effective Nutritional Ergogenic Aids. *International Journal of Sports Nutrition* 9 (2) (1999): 229–239.

Blomstrand E., P. Hassmen, B. Ekblom, and E. A. Newsholme. Administration of Branched Chain Amino Acids During Sustained Exercise—Effects on Performance and on Plasma Concentrations of Some Amino Acids. *European Journal of Applied Physiology and Occupational Physiology* 63 (2) (1991): 83–88.

Cerra, F. B., J. E. Mazuski, E. Chute, et al. Branched Chain Metabolic Support: A Prospective, Randomized, Double-Blind Train in Surgical Stress. *Annals of Surgery* 199 (3) (1984): 286–291.

Clarkson, P. M. Antioxidants and Physical Performance. *Critical Reviews in Food Science and Nutrition* 35 (1–2) (1995): 131–141.

Cordain, L., and J. Friel. *The Paleo Diet for Athletes.* Emmaus, PA: Rodale Press, 2005.

Cox, G. R., B. Desbrow, P. G. Montgomery, et al. Effect of Different Protocols of Caffeine Intake on Metabolism and Endurance Performance. *Journal of Applied Physiology* 93 (2002): 990–999.

Doherty, M. The Effects of Caffeine on the Maximal Accumulated Oxygen Deficit and Short-Term Running Performance. *International Journal of Sports Nutrition* 8 (2) (1998): 95–104.

Frassetto, L. A., et al. Effect of Age on Blood Acid-Base Composition in Adult Humans: Role of Age-Related Renal Function Decline. *American Journal of Physiology* 271 (6–2) (1996): F1114–F1122.

———. Potassium Bicarbonate Reduces Urinary Nitrogen Excretion in Postmenopausal Women. *Journal of Endocrinology and Metabolism* 82 (1) (1997): 254–259.

Graham, T. E., E. Hibbert, and P. Sathasivam. Metabolic and Exercise Endurance Effects of Coffee and Caffeine Ingestion. *Journal of Applied Physiology* 85 (3) (1998): 883–889.

———. Caffeine and Exercise: Metabolism, Endurance, and Performance. *Sports Medicine* 31 (11) (2001): 785–807.

Ji, L. L. Oxidative Stress During Exercise: Implication of Antioxidant Nutrients. *Free Radicals in Biology and Medicine* 18 (6) (1995): 1079–1086.

Kleiner, S. M., and M. Greenwood-Robinson. *High-Performance Nutrition.* New York: John Wiley and Sons, 1996.

Kovacs, E. M. R., J. H. C. H. Stegen, and F. Browns. Effects of Caffeinated Drinks on Substrate Metabolism, Caffeine Excretion and Performance. *Journal of Applied Physiology* 85 (2) (1998): 709–715.

Mujika, I., and S. Padilla. Creatine Supplementation as an Ergogenic Aid for Sports Performance in Highly Trained Athletes: A Critical Review. *International Journal of Sports Medicine* 18 (7) (1997): 491–496.

Noakes, Tim. The Low Figure Is for a Fit Acclimatized Athlete and the High Figure Is for an Unfit Non-acclimatized Athlete. *Lore of Running,* 4th ed. Champaign, IL: Human Kinetics, 2002.

Parry-Billings, M., R. Budgett, Y. Koutedakis, et al. Plasma Amino Acid Concentrations in Overtraining Syndrome: Possible Effects on the Immune System. *Medicine and Science in Sports and Exercise* 24 (12) (1992): 1353–1358.

Peyrebrune, M. C., M. E. Nevik, F. J. Donaldson, and D. J. Cosford. The Effects of Oral Creatine Supplementation on Performance in Single and Repeated Sprint Training. *Journal of Sports and Science* 16 (3) (1998): 271–279.

Remer, T., and F. Manz. Potential Renal Acid Load of Foods and Its Influence on Urine pH. *Journal of the American Dietetic Association* 95 (7) (1995): 791–797.

Robertson, J. D., R. J. Maughan, G. G. Duthie, and P. C. Morrice. Increased Blood Antioxidant Systems of Runners in Response to Training Load. *Clinical Science* 80 (6) (1991): 611–618.

Rokitzki, L., E. Logemann, G. Huber, et al. Alpha-tocopherol Supplementation in Racing Cyclists During Extreme Endurance Training. *International Journal of Sport Nutrition* 4 (3) (1994): 253–264.

Schena F., F. Guerrine, P. Tregnaghi, and B. Kayser. Branched-Chain Amino Acid Supplementation During Trekking at High Altitude: The Effects on Loss of Body Mass, Body Composition, and Muscle Power. *European Journal of Applied Physiology and Occupational Physiology* 65 (5) (1992): 394–398.

Sebastian, A., et al. Improved Mineral Balance and Skeletal Metabolism in Postmenopausal Women Treated with Potassium Bicarbonate. *New England Journal of Medicine* 330 (25) (1994): 1776–1781.

Weir, J., T. D. Noakes, K. Myburgh, et al. A High-Carbohydrate Diet Negates the Metabolic Effects of Caffeine During Exercise. *Medicine and Science in Sports and Exercise* 19 (2) (1987): 100–105.

Witt, E. H., E. Z. Reznick, C. A. Viguie, et al. Exercise, Oxidative Damage and Effects of Antioxidant Manipulation. *Journal of Nutrition* 122 (3) (1992): 766–773.

CHAPTER 11

Armstrong, Lance. *It's Not About the Bike: My Journey Back to Life.* New York: G. P. Putnam and Sons, 2000.

Cameron, Julia. *The Artist's Way: A Spiritual Path to Higher Creativity.* New York: Jeremy P. Tarcher/Putnam, 2002.

Hogg, John M. *Mental Skills for Swim Coaches.* Edmonton, Alberta: Sport Excel Publishing, 1995.

Moore, Thomas. *Care of the Soul: A Guide for Cultivating Depth and Sacredness in Everyday Life.* New York: HarperCollins Publishers, 1994.

Tolle, Eckhart. *The Power of Now: A Guide to Spiritual Enlightenment.* Novato, CA: New World Library, 1999.

Wilson, Edward O. *Consilience: The Unity of Knowledge.* New York: Random House, 1999.

CHAPTER 13

Alfredson, Håkan, Tom Pietilä, Per Jonsson, and Ronny Lorentzon. Heavy-Load Eccentric Calf Muscle Training for the Treatment of Chronic Achilles Tendinosis. *American Journal of Sports Medicine* 28 (1998): 360.

Cook, N. J., A. Ng, G. F. Read, B. Harris, and D. Riad-Fahmy. Salivary Cortisol for Monitoring Adrenal Activity During Marathon Runs. *Hormonal Research* 25 (1) (1987): 18–23.

Fallon, K. E. The Acute Phase Response and Exercise: The Ultramarathon as Prototype Exercise. *Clinical Journal of Sports Medicine* 11 (1) (2001): 38–43.

Fredericson, Michael, William Moore, Marc Guillet, and Christopher Beaulieu. High Hamstring Tendinopathy in Runners: Meeting the Challenges of Diagnosis, Treatment, and Rehabilitation. *The Physician and Sports Medicine* 33 (5) (May 2005).

Fredericson, Michael, and Adam Weir. Practical Management of Iliotibial Band Friction Syndrome in Runners. *Clinical Journal of Sports Medicine* 16 (3) (May 2006).

Gleeson, M., G. I. Lancaster, and N. C. Bishop. Nutritional Strategies to Minimise Exercise-Induced Immunosuppression in Athletes. *Canadian Journal of Applied Physiology* 26 (supplement) (2001): S23–S35.

Hug, M., P. E. Mullis, M. Vogt, N. Ventura, and H. Hoppeler. Training Modalities: Over-Reaching and Over-Training in Athletes, Including a Study of the Role of Hormones. *Best Practice and Research Clinical Endocrinology and Metabolism* 17 (2) (2003): 191–209.

Johnson, Darren L., and Scott D. Mair. *Clinical Sports Medicine.* Philadelphia, PA: Mosby, Inc., 2006.

Jonsson, P., and H Alfredson. Superior Results with Eccentric Compared to Concentric Quadriceps Training in Patients with Jumper's Knee: A Prospective Randomised Study. *British Journal of Sports Medicine* 39 (2005): 847–850.

Jonsson, Per, Per Wahlström, Lars Öhberg, and Håkan Alfredson. Eccentric Training in Chronic Painful Impingement Syndrome of the Shoulder: Results of a Pilot Study. *Knee Surgery: Sports Traumatology, Arthroscopy* 14 (2006): 76–81.

Lac, G., and P. Berthon. Changes in Cortisol and Testosterone Levels and T/C Ratio During an Endurance Competition and Recovery. *Journal of Sports Medicine and Physical Fitness* 40 (2) (2000): 139–144.

Nieman, D. C., C. I. Dumke, D. A. Henson, S. R. McAnulty, L. S. McAnulty, R. H. Lind, and J. D. Morrow. Immune and Oxidative Changes During and Following the Western States Endurance Run. *International Journal of Sports Medicine* 24 (7) (2003): 541–547.

Nieman, D. C., and S. L. Nehlsen-Cannarella. The Effects of Acute and Chronic Exercise of Immunoglobulins. *Sports Medicine* 11 (3) (1991):183–201.

Pruitt, Andrew L., and Fred Matheny. *Andy Pruitt's Complete Medical Guide for Cyclists.* Boulder, CO: VeloPress, 2006.

Rompe, J. J. Furia, and N. Maffulli. Eccentric Loading Compared with Shock Wave Treatment for Chronic Insertional Achilles Tendinopathy. *Journal of Bone and Joint Surgery* 90A (1) (2008): 52–61.

Ross, Michael J. *Maximum Performance: Sports Medicine for Endurance Athletes.* Boulder, CO: VeloPress, 2003.

Semple, S. J., L. L. Smith, A. J. McKune, J. Hoyos, B. Mokgethwa, A. F. San Juan, A. Lucia, and A. A. Wadee. Serum Concentrations of C Reactive Protein, Alpha1 Antitrypsin, and Complement (C3, C4, C1 Esterase Inhibitor) Before and During the Vuelta a España. *British Journal of Sports Medicine* 40 (2) (2006): 124–127.

Wu, H. J., K. T. Chen, B. W. Shee, H. C. Chang, Y. J. Huang, and R. S. Yang. Effects of 24 h Ultra-marathon on Biochemical and Hematological Parameters. *World Journal of Gastroenterology* 10 (18) (2004): 2711–2714.

INDEX

A-priority races, 20, 58, 60, 61, 62, 63, 79, 94; demands of, 145; exercise before, 244; goals and, 250

Abdominal pain, preventing/caring for, 293

Acetaminophen, 285

Aches, preventing/caring for, 292–299

Achilles tendinitis, 291

Achilles tendinopathy/plantar fasciitis, 286, 287 (fig.); protocol for, 287

Active Release Techniques (ART), 291

Adaptation, 5, 58, 162, 191, 215, 239; muscular, 191; physical, 59; speeding, 163. *See also* Anatomical Adaptation phase

Advanced obliques, 201, 201 (fig.)

Aero position, 43, 44, 46, 134

Aerobars, 33, 36, 37, 46, 138; back pain and, 41; clip-on, 38; descending and, 137; height of, 465; setup for, 39, 44, 296; time trialing and, 130

Aerobic capacity, 23–24, 25, 85

Aerobic training, 26, 174; weight lifting and, 190; zones, 153, 153 (table)

Aerobics, 15, 58, 59, 62, 65, 76, 79, 126, 182, 192, 221, 284; nonimpact, 95; speed and, 87

Aerodynamics, 37, 44, 45, 142, 158; aggressive, 295; bike position and, 41; importance of, 47, 134; power and, 41

Aggressive fit, 44–47

Air resistance, 46, 134

Allen, Mark: quote of, 13, 82, 251

Alphabets, 86, 86 (fig.)

Alternating leg lift, 202, 202 (fig.)

Anaerobic endurance, 16, 27, 28, 64, 124, 181; training, 78–79, 168, 169

Anatomical Adaptation (AA) phase, 188, 189, 190, 192

Anderson, O., 232

Annual training plan (ATP), 57–58, 63, 89, 251

Antioxidants, 230–232

Anxiety, 249, 308

Arm carriage, 166, 180

Arm coolers, 52

Armstrong, Lance: quote of, 33

Artist's Way, The (Cameron), 237

Back-kick, 102

Back-kick change, 102

Back-kick twist, 102

Back-kick twist down, 102

Back pain, 41; preventing/caring for, 295–296

Backstroke, 121

Backward running, 176

Balance, 104, 133–134, 169, 211, 308; dietary, 215, 219; drills, 99, 101, 110; focus on, 29, 35; improving, 100, 101, 102, 109, 118; maintaining, 135; side-kicking and, 117; swimming and, 97–98, 106

Bands, 35, 36, 113; pros/cons of, 35–36 (table)

Base-leg drive, 206, 206 (fig.)

Base period, 10, 27, 28, 58, 76, 83, 126, 129, 131, 132, 167, 191, 251, 252, 275, 280, 284; crosstraining and, 85; described, 59–60; diet for, 222–223; hydration and, 166; muscular endurance and, 145; planning, 89–94; running, 165; strength training during, 188; trail running and, 165

Basic Week, 275, 276

Basics, getting, 14–17

Bennett, Greg, 45

Bicycles: choosing, 36–40; fitting, 33, 37; maintaining, 311; race-specific/time trial–specific, 38; safety with, 37

Bike and swim emphasis, 65

Bike fit, 42–47, 46 (fig.)

Bike-handling skills, 126, 130, 131, 137

Bike positions, 40–42, 46, 87

Biomechanics, 45, 50, 62, 79, 81, 83, 123, 188, 266, 295

Black toenails, preventing/caring for, 297

Blisters, preventing/caring for, 298

Bloating, preventing/caring for, 294

Blood: acidity/alkalinity of, 221; testing, 281, 292

Body alignment, 166, 170, 170 (fig.)

Body composition, 220, 307; improving, 215, 218; nutrition and, 18

Body Glide, 34, 297, 299

Body mass, 215; climbing and, 136

Body position, 45, 101, 110

Body rotation, 101, 103–104

Borg Scale of Perceived Exertion, 72, 73 (table)

Bottle jump, 134

Bottle pickup, 134

Bounding, 178, 178 (fig.)

Bowden, Lori: quote of, 161

Braking, 135–136, 137

Branch-chain amino acids (BCAA), 233–234

Brazier, Brendan: quote of, 187

Breakdowns, 13, 14, 18

Breakthrough workouts (BT), 29, 45, 83, 89, 91, 92, 93, 154, 168, 182, 244, 301, 302–303, 307, 308; caffeine and, 232; described, 79, 80, 81; eliminating, 303; endurance, 131, 253; goal of, 306; illness following, 214; intensity of, 305; novices and, 303; pace and, 305; quality of, 306; recovery and, 80, 251, 252, 282; scheduling, 80, 303, 305; swimming, 183

Breaststroke, 121

Breathing, 88, 107, 136, 140, 169, 193, 199, 201, 208, 294; bilateral, 96, 98, 99–100, 101, 103; deep, 80; five-stroke, 101; focus on, 207, 249; from hips, 97; offside, 100; onside, 100; relaxed, 190; three-stroke, 36, 101; two-stroke, 101; underwater, 98

Bricks, 131, 162, 260, 303, 309

Build period, 10, 75, 76, 80, 97, 126, 131, 165, 251, 252, 266, 275, 280, 301, 306; described, 60–61; diet for, 223, 307; fatigue from, 302; finishing, 60; muscular endurance and, 145; planning, 89–94; recovery from, 303; strength training during, 188; training load in, 93

Burnout, 13, 59, 62, 266; risk of, 64, 71, 126, 276

Cadence, 43, 152, 162, 166, 175, 180, 308; body alignment and, 170; climbing and, 136; controlling, 242; described, 171–172; drills, 50; dropping, 129, 138, 142; focus on, 145; heart rate and, 172; intervals and, 142; monitoring, 133; stress and, 172
Caffeine, 80, 232
Calcium, 221, 230–232
Calf raise, 192, 195, 195 (fig.)
Calluses, preventing/caring for, 298
Cameron, Julia, 237
Carbo-Pro, 226
Carbohydrate-loading drinks, 227, 285
Carbohydrates, 222, 223, 226, 228, 229; high-GI, 212, 213; intake of, 214; storing, 227; timing of, 213
Cardiac drift, 74
Cardiac response, 151
Catch, 104–105; mastering, 105–106; pull and, 105
Chafing, preventing/caring for, 298–299
Challenged athletes, special considerations for, 299
Change-up intervals, 147
Checklists, 311
Chin-swivel method, 103
Chop to ankle, knee, and waist, 204, 204 (fig.)
Cipollini, Mario, 28
Cleat position, 42–43, 42 (fig.), 43 (fig.)
Climbing, 123, 126, 142, 151, 166; body mass and, 136; cadence and, 136; improving and, 129, 137, 145; intensity and, 165; sitting/standing while, 136
Clothing, 33–35, 50, 51, 52, 166, 297, 298
Cobb, John, 45
Colting, Jonas: quote of, 123
Comfort, 38, 41, 44, 46, 101, 249
Commitment, 20, 21, 64, 238, 251
Comprehensive Metabolic Panel (CMP), 280
CompuTrainer, 49, 127–128
Confidence, 4–5, 15, 100, 138, 250
Consilience (Wilson), 239
Consistency, 14, 20, 78, 88, 125, 183, 191, 274; intensity and, 75; long-term, 13
Cool-downs, 155, 168, 169, 282
Cordain, Loren, 212
Core, 192; focus on, 188; skills, 169; strengthening, 198; support, 206
Core exercises, 45, 198–205, 206; repetition/intensity for, 190
Cornering, braking and, 135–136
Coupling, 155
Cramps, preventing/caring for, 294–295
Crash cycles, 81–82, 83
Creatine, 233, 292
Creatinine, 280
Critical power (CP), 28, 152, 153, 164; aerobic training zones and, 153 (table); power change during, 154
Crosstraining, 59, 165–166
Cryotherapy, 291
Cycling: block, 84; development, 123–138; endurance-based, 124, 125; higher-intensity, 140; indoor, 19; knee trouble and, 194; skills, 131–138; stronger, 18; subthreshold, 145; transition from, 170; zones, 62, 77
Cycling main set ideas, 147–148
Cyclist's palsy, 296

Death weekends, 10
Decoupling, 155, 155 (fig.), 156 (fig.), 157, 158
Dehydration, 158, 223, 228, 229, 285, 293, 294
Depression, 282, 292
Derecruits, 180
Descending, 137
Diet, 78; analyzing, 217; balanced/natural, 219; changing, 220; low-fat, 219; low-fiber, 311; muscle loss and, 221–222; optimal, 211–215, 222; performance and, 215; training and, 215. See also Eating; Feeding; Food; Nutrition
Dips, 192
Distance, 11, 15, 28, 103, 174; dominant leg, 132–133; Ironman, 26, 29, 30, 31, 32, 37, 62, 63, 121; per stroke, 98, 104; time versus, 65–66
Downhill strides, 175
Drafting, 130, 137–138, 306
Drills, 173–178; balance, 99, 101, 110; cadence, 50; explosive, 174; fist, 105; kick, 35, 110; side-kick, 97–98, 101, 104, 117; stroke, 110, 308; swimming, 101–104, 117
Dual leg lift, 202, 202 (fig.)
Duration, 62, 65, 90, 125, 139, 166, 303
Dynamic hip drive, 207, 207 (fig.)

Eating: assessment of, 216–217; goals and, 238; mindless, 217; poor, 215. See also Diet; Feeding; Food; Nutrition
Eccentric exercise, 284–291
Economy, 25–26, 76, 171; cycling, 126–128; flexibility and, 88; improving, 32, 49, 85, 127–128, 131, 133, 162, 172, 174–175, 176, 207, 242; positioning, 42; power and, 96; running, 165, 182
Economy of movement, 58, 85, 103
Effort: cardiac response and, 151; heart rate and, 138; maximum, 141; pace and, 139; short-duration, 151
Elbow drop, 105
Electrolytes, 234, 281, 294
Elite athletes, 159, 305; workouts for, 181
Emotions, 5, 159
Endurance, 13, 21, 26, 57, 59, 61, 64, 66, 92, 104, 191, 198, 244, 253, 267, 275–276, 301, 331; aerobic, 89, 154, 155, 158, 167; anaerobic, 16; building, 14, 15, 18, 19, 20, 29, 31, 32, 71, 83, 89, 91, 96, 124, 125, 126, 128, 131, 163–164, 165, 183, 187, 253, 276; cycling, 124–128, 167; focus on, 15, 19, 27, 29, 30, 187; high-intensity training and, 79; rating, 28–29; running, 32, 167, 179, 182, 260; steady-state, 83, 125, 140; strength training and, 210; stroke, 119; swimming, 32, 95, 110–113, 164
Endurance training, 15, 16, 26, 79, 89, 90, 144, 154, 274, 280, 281; diet for, 211–212; healthy approach to, 279; importance of, 125
Energy, 24, 25, 216, 303
Energy bars, 311
Equipment: controlling, 242; cycling, 36–50; risk/fears with, 246; running, 50–51, 175; swimming, 33–36, 35–36 (table), 101
Excessive trunk lean, 170, 170 (fig.)

Fartlek, 164
Fat, 219, 220, 222, 223
Fat oxidation, 25, 74

Fatigue, 10, 11, 25, 74, 76, 78, 103, 136, 174, 280, 295; deep, 62; eliminating, 302; generating, 16; Ironman-distance, 63; managing, 80; premature, 159; risk of, 276; running and, 182; training and, 165

Fears, 137, 246–248; facing, 240, 245, 248–249, 308

Feeding: as long as workout lasted, 226; before the work-out, 224; during the workout, 224; immediately after workout, 226; until next workout, 226–227. *See also* Diet; Eating; Food; Nutrition

Ferritin, 280

Fingers down, 106

Finish, 14–17, 124

Fins, 102; long/short, 35, 101, 110; pros/cons of, 35–36 (table)

Fist drill, 105

Fitness, 58, 71, 73, 136, 303; aerobic, 63, 64, 72, 124, 155, 156, 157, 169; body composition and, 215; breaks and, 63; cardiovascular, 284; components of, 23–26; improving, 10, 23, 58, 75, 89, 282; level of, 179; lost, 78, 241; maintaining, 75; measuring, 23, 61, 76; race, 80; running, 10; swimming, 104

Flexibility, 286, 299; ankle/fins and, 110; back pain and, 41; benefits of, 87–91; commitment to, 207–208; for hips, 208–210, 208 (fig.), 209 (fig.), 210 (fig.); stretch-ing and, 88

Fly-kick sets, 110

Focus, 5, 15, 19, 27, 29, 35, 80, 97, 125, 129, 131, 145, 187, 188, 207, 215, 266, 309; building, 240, 243, 249; mental, 17, 244; soft, 30; training, 252

Food: acidic, 221, 222; alkaline, 221, 222, 231; as self, 216; as signal, 215; choosing, 215–216, 218, 220; energy-dense, 217, 311; high-quality, 31; natural, 219; nutri-ent-dense, 217, 220; pre-race, 311; processed, 222; recovery, 60, 80, 223; stress and, 215. *See also* Diet; Eating; Feeding; Nutrition

Foot strike, 166

Force, 26, 27, 59, 124; focus on, 30; rating, 28–29

Form, 169; holding, 142, 242; running, 172–173

Forward rotations, 107, 107 (fig.)

Frames, 36, 37, 38

Freestyle, 97

Frequency, 19, 63, 75, 89, 96, 162

Front bench drill, 176, 177, 177 (fig.)

Full pulls, 106, 107, 108, 108 (fig.)

Functional threshold (FT), 126, 140, 141, 162, 164, 343; aerobic capacity and, 24–25; improving, 27, 71, 75, 76, 85

Functional threshold heart rate (FTHR) test, 343

Functional threshold power (FTP), 152, 153, 156, 158, 159

Fundamentals, 21, 58, 85–87, 96

Gastrointestinal (GI) problems, 285, 293

Gatorade, 227

Gearing, 47–49, 48 (table)

Gels, 227, 228–229, 311

Genetics, 24, 162

Geometry, 37–38

Glucose, 226

Glutamine, 233, 234

Glycemic Index (GI), 212, 213–214 (table), 311

Glycogen, 24, 25, 74, 219, 223

Goals, 14, 63, 83, 168, 252, 302, 306, 309; achieving, 10, 237, 240, 243; be your, 238–239; focus on, 129, 243; identifying, 237, 240, 275; inflating, 17; long-term, 237, 238; physiological, 222; reasonable, 244, 250; refining, 29; sharing, 240; ultimate, 274; undermin-ing, 238–239

Group rides, guidelines for, 129–130

Half pulls, 106, 107, 107 (fig.), 108

Hamstring curls, 192, 194, 194 (fig.)

Hamstring tendinopathy, 286, 288 (fig.), 289 (fig.); protocol for, 288–289

Hamstrings, stretching, 296

Handlebars, 38, 42, 44

Hands-on head running, 176

Harmony, 238, 239

Head imbalance, 171, 171 (fig.)

Head position, 98, 105, 117

Health baseline, 279–281

Heart rate, 26, 28, 52, 126, 159; average, 174; cadence and, 172; critical power and, 151, 152; cycling, 335–337 (table); data for, 76; decline of, 154, 168, 260; effort and, 138; heat stress and, 158; intensity and, 140; intervals and, 142; pace and, 74, 305; performance and, 72; power and, 151, 152, 152 (table), 153, 155–156, 155 (fig.), 156 (fig.); profile, 151; resting/exercising, 71; RPE and, 76; spikes, 49, 126; training, 150

Heart rate monitors (HRMs), 33, 52, 71, 76, 150, 151, 159

Heart rate zones, running, 338–340 (table), 341–342 (table)

Heat, applying, 291

Heel strike, 169–170

Hellemans, John: pace scale by, 74

Helmets, 40

Herremans, Marc, 299

Hiking, 163, 165–166

Hills, 41; repeats, 84; running, 164, 165, 166

Hinault, Bernard: on climbing, 137

Hip-drive exercises, 206–207

Hip flexors, 170, 188, 206

Hips: breathing from, 97; stability, 166

Horizontal pedaling, 132

Hydration, 32, 74, 78, 166, 218, 219, 293, 294, 309; appropriate, 16; controlling, 242

Hypertension, 234

Hyponatremia, 285

Hypothermia, 34

Ibuprofen, 284, 285

Ice, treating with, 283, 291

Iliotibial band syndrome, 286, 289 (fig.), 290 (fig.); protocol for, 289–290

Illness, 13, 62, 71, 215, 241; BT workouts and, 214; risk of, 64, 182

Immune function, 211, 280

Improvement, 95; long-term, 63; potential for, 27; training for, 17–18

In and up, 203, 203 (fig.)

Increased cadence, 133

Induráin, Miguel, 45

Injury, 10, 13, 18, 62, 191, 233, 241; avoiding, 50, 125, 192, 282; concerns about, 32, 188, 190; history of, 82, 188;

lower-leg, 50; minor, 266; overuse, 163, 170, 260, 282–284; preventing, 85, 207, 279, 284; responses to, 283 (table); risk of, 64, 176, 182, 183, 276; running, 161, 167; symptoms of, 283 (table); training and, 15, 142, 165; treating, 215, 282–284

Intensity, 59, 61, 62, 63, 65, 78, 83, 89, 91, 99, 182, 190, 191, 244, 303; climbing and, 165; consistency and, 75; controlling, 140; crashing, 84; described, 71–75; dropping, 17; goal-race, 92; heart rate and, 140; interval, 139; maintaining, 306; nutrition and, 159, 160; overtraining and, 292; subthreshold, 25; training, 72, 73, 93, 215; zones, 16, 77

International Triathlon Union, 162, 300

Intervals, 84, 148, 180; cadence and, 142; change-up, 147; cruise, 131; duration of, 131, 139; guidelines for, 138–140; heart rate and, 142; intensity of, 131, 139; maximum-effort, 141; mental strength in, 139–140; muscular endurance and, 138; rest, 141; threshold, 308, 309; warming up for, 142

Iron, 230–232, 280

Isolated Leg Training (ILT), 26, 128, 132, 133

Kemmerling, Todd: quote of, 95

Key Three, 63, 223

Kick drills, 35, 110

Kickboards, 101, 110; pros/cons of, 35–36 (table)

Kicking, 109–110

Knee extension, 192, 194, 194 (fig.)

Knee lift, 177, 177 (fig.)

L-glutamine, 233–234

Lactate, 25, 78, 129, 139, 151, 158

Lat pulldowns, 192, 196, 196 (fig.)

Laughlin, Terry, 101

Leaning tower, 86, 86 (fig.)

Leg presses, 191, 192, 193, 193 (fig.)

Leg turnover, 171

Lewis, Carl, 28

Lifting, 19, 187

Limiters, 5, 28–30, 168, 300; A-priority race, 81; balance as, 101; catch as, 106; choosing, 118; cycling, 123, 124; endurance as, 29, 110, 123, 167, 182, 303; identifying, 18–19, 92; muscular endurance as, 29, 128, 131, 260; personal, 142; physiological, 61; power as, 233; running as, 162, 163, 179; speed as, 29; strength and, 93; swimming as, 29, 117, 253; TT as, 131; working on, 118, 138

Lines, 87, 87 (fig.)

Long-course meters (LCM), swimming, 118, 119

Long, slow distance, 125–126

Loping run, 178, 178 (fig.)

Low-energy shock-wave therapy, 291

Low walking, 178, 178 (fig.)

Lower abdominal/oblique combo, 201, 201 (fig.)

Lung capacity, 46, 100, 171

Lunge, 205, 205 (fig.)

Manz, F.: research by, 221

Marching drill, 173, 173 (fig.)

Massage, 285, 291

Masters athletes, special considerations for, 299

Masters group, swimming with, 121–122, 253

Maximum heart rate tests, note on, 344–345

Maximum strength (MS) phase, 190, 191, 192, 198

McGee, Bobby, 179, 180

Meal-replacement drinks, 227

Medicine Ball core strength exercises, 204–205

Mental skills, 19, 63, 80, 240, 301, 311

Mental strength, 18, 242, 244, 250; importance of, 30, 31–32

Metabolic efficiency, 25, 26, 58, 76

Mind, 237, 243–244

Mirror Drill, 172–173, 173 (fig.)

Molina, Scott: quote of, 23

Movie Screen, 250

Muscle mass, 198, 299; loss of, 214, 221–222

Muscles: rebuilding, 219, 223; swimming, 109

Muscular endurance, 27–28, 32, 39, 79, 83, 91, 93, 145, 152, 233; building, 35, 97, 113, 128, 164–165, 167; cycling, 124, 125, 128, 164, 182; gym-based, 190; gym strength and, 90; in hilly terrain, 129; intervals and, 138; running, 164; speed and, 167; sport-specific, 90; swimming, 114–116, 121; trainer sessions, 143–144 (table); training, 140–142, 167; transition to, 128; workouts, 267, 305, 306

Muscular imbalances, 188, 192

Neck pain, preventing/caring for, 295

Neurological system, 239

Neuromuscular blockade, 291

Neuromuscular system, 163, 239

Nitrogen, loss of, 221

Nonsteroidal anti-inflammatory drugs (NSAIDs), 283, 284, 285

Novices: base training of, 257 (table), 258 (table); BT and, 303; peak training of, 259 (table); race week and, 309; training by, 252–253; training plan/tactics of, 254–256 (table)

Numb feet and hands, preventing/caring for, 296

Nutrition, 21, 32, 63, 78, 166, 279, 331; appropriate, 16, 219; balance in, 211; controlling, 140, 242; focus on, 18, 215; guidelines for, 222; importance of, 30, 31; improving, 182, 234; intensity and, 159, 160; lifestyle and, 216, 217; performance and, 18, 211, 213, 220; planning, 169; race-day, 295; recovery and, 18, 211, 213, 219, 226; risks/fears with, 246; running and, 182; sports, 223, 227–229, 235; strategy for, 211, 218, 235, 238, 307; swimming and, 95; timing, 225 (table). See also Diet; Eating; Feeding; Food

Obliques, 200, 200 (fig.)

Offside arm, 98

Omega-3 fats/oils, 220, 230

Omega-6 fats, 220

Open arm carriage, 171, 171 (fig.)

Over and around, 202, 202 (fig.)

Over the barrel, 106

Overload, 89; described, 79, 81–84; recovery and, 292

Overtraining, 13, 71, 76, 82, 292

Pace, 13, 20, 25, 32, 71, 72, 73, 75, 76, 80, 117, 174, 241; annual, 10; average, 162; changes in, 131; comfortable, 119; conservative, 244; controlling, 242; effort and, 139; electrolyte problems and, 234; heart rate and, 74, 305; initial, 78; interval, 138–139; maintaining, 27; mental/physical, 245; mistakes with, 160; overall, 164; qualitative description of, 152; risks/fears with, 247; scale, 74; SS, 167, 168; superthreshold, 28; threshold, 304, 308

Paddles, 113; pros/cons of, 35–36 (table)

Pains, preventing/caring for, 292–299

Paleo diet, 212, 234

Paleo Diet for Athletes, The (Cordain and Friel), 211–212

Patellofemoral syndrome/patellar and quadriceps tendinopathy, 286, 288 (fig.); protocol for, 288

Patience, 30, 32, 183, 191, 245, 249

Peak period, 75, 89, 94, 126, 251, 280, 301–303, 305–308; bike maintenance during, 311; BT for, 304 (table); consideration for, 306–308; described, 61; workouts during, 302–303, 305–306

Pedal recovery, 133

Pedaling, 132–133, 158; dead spots in, 49; economic, 126, 127; leg-speed variation while, 127

Pedals, buying, 39

Performance, 17, 20, 26, 58, 71, 73, 187, 266; caffeine and, 232; checking, 150; creatine and, 233; diet and, 215; drop in, 5, 78, 280, 292; endurance, 24, 85; heart rate and, 72; improving, 10, 19, 23, 30, 46, 61, 64, 81, 101, 188, 213, 234, 237, 243, 292; nutrition and, 18, 211, 213, 220; optimal, 16, 301, 307, 309; recovery and, 93; risks/fears with, 247; skills and, 84–88; sleep and, 230, 234; supplements and, 232; training and, 307; ultimate, 244; ultraendurance, 26; visualizing, 139

Periodization, 89, 124, 222–223, 251, 274; importance of, 57; strength training, 188, 189 (table)

Physiology, 23, 64, 71, 75, 86, 123, 126, 187

Pike, 200, 200 (fig.)

Piriformis syndrome, 286, 290 (fig.); protocol for, 290

Plans, 152, 160, 251, 274; skills and, 85; sticking to, 240–241; structuring, 188–190

Plyometrics, 176–178

Power, 25, 71, 75; aerodynamics and, 41; anaerobic, 27; bike position and, 41; economy and, 96; effectiveness of, 152; generating, 45, 49, 151, 159; heart rate and, 151, 152, 152 (table), 153, 155–156, 155 (fig.), 156 (fig.), 157; outputs, 76, 151, 155; superthreshold, 28; swimming, 121; testing, 154; training and, 72, 150. *See also* Critical power; Functional threshold power

PowerBar, 228

Power Cranks (PC), 49–50

Power meters, 33, 39, 45, 52–53, 260; cycling with, 150–160

Power-Tap, 52–53, 152

Power zones, 152–153, 153 (table); heart rate and, 152 (table); power testing and, 154

Prep period, 92, 188, 252, 266; baseline exam in, 279–280; crosstraining and, 85; described, 58–59; trail running and, 165

Preparation, 145, 241; controlling, 242; mental, 311; risks/fears with, 248; tips for, 309

Pressing the T, 98

Prilotherapy, 291

Progression, swimming, 101

Progression drill, 117

Propulsive swimming, 104–109; balance swimming and, 106

Protein, 220, 222, 227, 228; muscle rebuilding and, 223; nitrogen and, 221; powder, 226

Pull, 36; catch and, 105; preparation for, 113

Pull-buoys, 35, 36, 101, 110, 113; pros/cons of, 35–36 (table)

Push, learning to, 244–245

Qualifying, training for, 18–20

Quick feet, 177, 177 (fig.)

Race-simulation workouts, 60, 61, 91, 159, 244, 266, 275, 276, 302, 307; described, 148, 149, 150

Race-specific muscular endurance, 147

Race week, 302; body composition for, 307; considerations for, 308–309, 311–312; plans and, 241; recovery and, 308; rest during, 309; workouts during, 308–309, 310 (table), 311

Racing: capacity, 24; considerations for, 180; Ironman-distance, 26, 29, 30, 31, 32, 37, 62; mind and, 243–244; plans and, 241; power-based, 159–160; smart, 20

Rand, Ayn: quote of, 3

Range of motion, 34, 44, 198, 299

Rate of perceived exertion (RPE), 71, 72, 76, 141, 152

Rear bench drill, 177, 177 (fig.)

Rear Superman, 199, 199 (fig.)

Rebuilding phase, 62, 282

Recovery, 20, 58, 61, 64, 76, 78–81, 110, 125, 139, 167, 168, 174, 176, 187, 229, 303, 308; active, 75, 182, 282–291; additional, 302; compromising, 93, 165; creatine and, 233; described, 65, 95; ensuring, 306; exercise and, 224; extended, 14, 15; flexibility and, 88; goals and, 238; importance of, 10; improving, 169, 213, 307; inadequate, 62, 76, 282; long-term, 13; nutrition and, 18, 211, 213, 223–224, 226–227; overload and, 292; pedal, 133; performance and, 93; post-race, 61–62; sleep and, 305; time for, 16, 17, 75, 145, 251; walking, 173, 308; yoga and, 88

Recovery drill, 108–109, 109 (fig.)

Recovery drinks, 227, 228, 311

Recovery week, 59, 76, 82, 93, 189

Recruitment, 126–127, 191

Rehabilitation, 283, 284

Reinertsen, Sarah, 299

Relaxation, 32, 110, 133, 295

Remer, T.: research by, 221

Repetitions, 190, 191, 192, 198

Resistance, 4, 49, 134; increasing, 106, 137, 285

Rest, 14, 20, 25, 81, 139, 305; active, 282, 283–284; complete, 282; focus on, 309; intervals and, 141; musculoskeletal deconditioning and, 282; overtraining and, 292; significance of, 10

Rest, ice, compression, and elevation (RICE), 282

Rhabdomyolysis, 285

Risks, 5, 246–248

Roosevelt, Theodore: quote of, 279

Rotator cuff tendinopathy, 286 (fig.); protocol for, 286

Run emphasis, 65

Run/walk endurance workout, 179

Run/walk protocol, 179, 180, 253

Run/walk volume and pace workout, 180

Runners: base training of, 263 (table); build training of, 264 (table); peak training of, 265 (table); training by, 260; training plan/tactics of, 261–262 (table)

Running: balanced, 169; block, 84; crashing, 82; development, 161–165, 167–169; downhill, 166, 175; drills, 173–178; endurance, 164, 165; fatigue and, 182; form, 169; high-cadence, 162; high-frequency, 75; high-intensity, 167, 182; improving, 162, 169; key training sessions for, 179–181; long/considerations for, 180; long-course, 164; nutrition and, 182; recovery, 64, 182; strength training and, 167; stress of, 161; technical improvements to, 162, 166; technique, 169–172; tempo, 165; trail, 87, 165, 166; transition, 145, 165, 170

Running Research News (Anderson), 232

Russian twist, 203, 203 (fig.)

Saddle height, 43, 44 (fig.)

Saddle position, 43, 44 (fig.)

Saddle sores, preventing/caring for, 297

Saddles, 36, 37, 42, 297

Sampson, Patty H.: quote of, 211

Scott, Dave: quote of, 57

Scott, Steve, 27

Seated row, 192, 195, 195 (fig.)

Self-coaching, 10, 14

Self-image, 239, 240

Setups, traditional, 45

Shilt, Jeff, 300

Shimano Total Integration (STI), 38

Shoes: buying, 39; cycling, 50; running, 33, 50–51, 78; too small, 296, 297

Shoulder roll, 105

Side-kick, 102; drills, 97–98, 101, 104, 117

Side-kick extended, 102, 103

Side stitches, preventing/caring for, 294

Sideways crossovers, 176

Sideways running, 176

Single-leg squat touches, 86, 86 (fig.)

Single-stroke change, 101, 103

Skills, 16, 21, 62, 79, 92, 103, 164, 174; cycling, 124–128; developing, 19, 57, 89, 122, 138; fundamental, 58, 85–87; mental, 19, 63, 80, 240, 301, 311; movement, 84, 85, 87; performance and, 84–88; running, 169; stability, 85

Skills reverse brick, 174, 175

Skip drill, 173, 173 (fig.)

Slalom ride, 134

Sleep: overtraining and, 292; performance and, 230, 234; recovery and, 305; training and, 16; weekend, 16, 20

Sodium, 234, 295, 311

Soft-tissue therapy, 284, 291

Solutions, 246–248

Speed, 13, 50, 59; adding, 106; aerobics and, 87; bike position and, 87; fins and, 110; free, 182; FT, 164; improving, 26–27, 30, 58; muscular endurance and, 167; play, 164; rating, 28–29; running, 168; subthreshold speed, 260; success and, 183; swimming for, 104; threshold, 167–169; training, 306

SpinScan, 127–128

Spin-ups, 26, 50, 133

Spinning, 15, 47, 142, 276, 308

Spinning bikes, riding, 127

Sports bars, 227, 228, 229

Sports drinks, 224, 227–228, 229, 295, 311

Squad training, pros and cons of, 121–122

Squats, 191, 192–193, 193 (fig.)

SRM training system, 53

Stamina, 20, 130

Stance Line, 170, 171, 172, 176, 177

Standing, 147

Standing-hip drive, 206–207, 206 (fig.)

Standing straight arm, 108, 108 (fig.)

Standing straight-arm pulldown, 197, 197 (fig.)

Starches, 219–220

Stationary trainers, 49

Stems, adjustable, 44

Stowe, Harriet Beecher: quote of, 237

Straight-arm pulldowns, 192, 197

Strategies, 160, 250, 309, 311; dietary, 229; plans and, 241

Strauss, Rich, 104

Strength, 13, 57, 92, 244; building, 19, 31, 71, 89, 113, 187; cycling, 128–130; flexibility and, 88; identifying, 18–19; nutrition and, 18; plans, 166, 188, 191; routine, 295, 296; run-specific, 176–178; solid base of, 14; targets, 191 (table); workouts, 305–306

Strength maintenance (SM), 190, 289

Strength training, 29, 81, 231, 260, 299; endurance and, 210; focus on, 187, 188; general tips for, 191–192; high-intensity, 19, 90; periodization, 188, 189 (table); running and, 167; traditional, 188

Stress, 76, 87, 161, 231; adaptation to, 106, 191; aerobic, 99; breathing, 100; cadence and, 172; food and, 215; heat, 72, 74, 158; mental, 78; physical, 279; psychological, 25; removing, 302; training, 166, 276

Stretch-cord exercises, 106–109

Stretching, 80, 110, 127, 142, 169, 192, 206, 208, 245, 252, 296, 311; flexibility and, 88; poor, 295; post-workout, 60; program, 198; static, 284, 285; value of, 88

Strides, 164, 173, 174, 182, 308; downhill, 175; length of, 170; rate, 180; short, 172; tips for, 175; uphill, 176

Stroke, 49, 118, 119, 121; distance per, 98, 104; drills, 110, 308; improving, 100, 101

Stroke mechanics, 36, 82, 101, 104; focus on, 29, 35, 96, 97

Success, 242, 252; achieving, 238; critical factors for, 30–32; hiding, 238–239; Ironman-distance, 11, 28; long-term, 13; speed and, 183; strategies for, 249; traits for, 3–6

Supercompensation, 81

Supermans, 198–199, 199 (fig.)

Supplements, 221, 229–234

Sustained speed (SS), 167, 168, 173

Swim cords, 109

Swim functional threshold pace test, 343

Swim vertigo, preventing/caring for, 293

Swimming, 305–306; balance and, 97–98; bilateral, 99, 100; block, 84; crashing, 82; development of, 96–100; drills, 101–104, 117; effective, 110; equipment for, 33–36, 35–36 (table); for speed/fitness, 104; fundamentals and, 96; glossary for, 347; Ironman-distance, 121; long-distance, 103; nutrition and, 95; offside improvement with, 99; propulsive, 104–109;

side, 104; sock, 109; technique for, 99, 103, 104; three-stroke, 103, 117; videotaping, 97; zones, 62, 333–334 (table)
Swiss Ball bridge, 202, 202 (fig.)
Swiss Ball crunch, 201, 203, 203 (fig.)
Swiss Ball exercises, 201–203
Swiss Ball oblique crunch, 203, 203 (fig.)
Switching off, 180
Swivel breaths, 103

Tapering, 301
Technical skills, 14, 175; improving, 58, 249
Technique, 16, 191, 244, 305; building, 15, 96, 106, 174; controlling, 242; perfect, 190; swimming, 103, 104, 106, 109, 122; swimming workouts, 117–120
Tempo, 84, 165, 307
Tendinitis, 286
Testing, 75–78, 169, 343–345; schedule/sample, 77 (table)
Testosterone, 280, 292
Thermoregulation, 299
Thoughts, controlling, 239–241
Threshold, 304, 308, 309; aerobic, 155, 156, 157, 159. *See also* Functional threshold
Threshold/subthreshold workouts, 181
Tight shoulders, 170–171, 171 (fig.)
Time, distance versus, 65–66
Time trialing (TT), 78, 124, 154, 343; cleat position and, 42; strength workouts, 146; team, 130; training for, 131; workout, 146
Timing, 100, 174, 190
Toe drill, 173, 173 (fig.)
Total Immersion series, 101
Traditional back extension, 202, 202 (fig.)
Training, 11, 25, 31, 159, 187, 224; abilities, 27–28; aerobic, 26, 174; aids, 52–53; balanced, 63–66, 71–79; consistency with, 191, 274; crash course on, 57; cycles, 17, 65; daily hours for, 66–68 (table); focus on, 30, 125; goals and, 238; high-intensity, 26, 74–75, 125, 164, 267; injury and, 15, 142, 165; mental, 238; moderation in, 14, 15; nutrition for, 215, 223–224, 226–227; obstacles to, 300; optimal, 13; patience with, 191; performance and, 307; periodization and, 274; planning, 241, 274; power-based, 150, 151, 152, 154–158, 331; protocol for, 33; safe, 11; satisfaction with, 191; sleep and, 16; small-group, 17; steady-state, 93; stress of, 279; structured, 62, 252; swimming, 35, 95, 110–120; triad, 26–27; understanding, 266, 306; volume and, 252; weekly, 10, 69–70 (table), 274. *See also* Endurance training
Training and Racing with a Power Meter (Allen and Coggan), 152
TrainingPeaks.com, 155
"Training with Power Guide" (Friel), 152
Training zones, 71, 73 (table), 77; adjusting, 76; defining/
by sport, 333–342; heart rate, 73
Transition, 58, 62–63, 103, 162, 175; bike-to-run, 60; goal of, 63
Triathlons, 164; challenge of, 3, 332
Triceps dip, 196, 196 (fig.)
Triceps extension, 108, 192, 197, 197 (fig.)
Triple 3s, 147
Twisting sit-ups, 198
Twisting "throw," 205, 205 (fig.)
Two-legged jumps, 178, 178 (fig.)

Ultraendurance, 25, 27, 183
Ultrasound, 285, 291
Underperformance, 20, 156, 292

Veterans: base training of, 271 (table); build training of, 272 (table); peak training of, 273 (table); training by, 266–267; training plan/tactics of, 268–270 (table)
Video analysis, 98
Video Camera, 250
Visualization, 139, 245, 248, 249, 250
Vitamins, 223, 226, 227, 230, 231–232
VO$_2$max, 23, 78–79, 85, 126, 162, 167, 168; estimating, 24; improving, 27; pace, 74; testing, 76, 169; training, 79
Volume, 16, 63–65, 78, 89; building, 161; crashing, 82, 84; cycling, 125; dropping, 17, 301; endurance and, 32; overtraining and, 292; running, 64, 168; total, 65

Waiting, pushing and, 245
Warm-ups, 155, 168, 169, 294, 308; cycling, 129; deeper race, 344; interval, 142; protocols, 343–345; shorter race, 344; swim test, 343–344; thorough, 78
Water, 222, 223, 311
Weather, 78, 246
Weekend warriors, stresses by, 231
Weight lifting, 19, 45, 58, 62, 187, 221; aerobic training and, 90; considerations with, 166; quality, 192
Weight training, 190–197, 198
Wheels, 33, 36, 38, 40
Wide elbows, 171, 171 (fig.)
Wilson, Edward: on mind, 239
WKO+ software, 154, 156
Working athletes, training by, 274–275, 275 (table)
Workouts, 10, 14; anaerobic, 64, 78; back-to-back, 83–84; challenge, 83; distance freestyle, 36; distances/ durations of, 15; duathlon-type, 19; endurance, 16, 30; feeding during, 224; frequency of, 17, 161, 252; group training, 17; high-intensity, 16, 24, 75, 79; intensity/ length of, 14; key, 65, 267; muscular endurance, 27, 114–116; power, 28; scheduling, 65, 251; structure of, 276; subthreshold, 169; swim technique, 117–120

Yoga, 87–91, 207, 208, 276

ABOUT THE AUTHORS

JOE FRIEL has trained endurance athletes since 1980. His clients have achieved top performances in U.S. and foreign national championships, world championships, and the Olympic Games. While Friel is among triathlon's preeminent coaches, he has also worked extensively with amateur and professional road cyclists, mountain bikers, triathletes, duathletes, swimmers, and runners from all corners of the globe.

Friel is the best-selling author of *The Triathlete's Training Bible, Your First Triathlon, The Cyclist's Training Bible, Cycling Past 50, Precision Heart Rate Training* (coauthor), and *The Mountain Biker's Training Bible.* He holds a master's degree in exercise science and is a USA Triathlon and USA Cycling certified coach. He is a featured columnist for *Inside Triathlon* and *VeloNews* magazines, and writes feature stories for other international publications and Web sites.

Joe Friel speaks at seminars and camps around the world on training and racing for endurance athletes and provides consulting services for corporations in the fitness industry. Every year he selects a group of the brightest coaches with the greatest potential and closely oversees their progress as they advance into the ranks of elite-level coaches.

For more information on personal coaching, seminars, developmental coach mentoring, certification of coaches in the Training Bible methodology, coaching symposia, and consulting, visit www.TrainingBible.com. Register to receive Training Bible's monthly newsletter, receive regular updates on Joe Friel's training blog, or find a coach.

GORDON (GORDO) BYRN has been active in triathlon since 1998. He has posted numerous strong Ironman results, including an 8:29 at Ironman Canada and several podium finishes at international events. In 2002, he raced, and won, Ultraman Hawaii, a three-day ultra-endurance triathlon that covers over 500 kilometers.

In recent years, Byrn was active in the European and Asian private equity industries. While he remains involved in the financial world through his advisory business, Byrn now focuses his time on coaching endurance athletes and speaking on his experiences in both corporate and athletic arenas. For more information on training, coaching, and applying the lessons of athletic success in your life, visit www.EnduranceCorner.com.